Public Health at the Crossroads
Achievements and Prospects
Second Edition

This book is an introduction to public health as a discipline and a critique of its recent development. Identifying poverty as the greatest continuing threat to health worldwide, the authors, both of them prominent public health academics, researchers and advocates, review epidemiological, demographic and public health trends internationally, and argue that the prospects for public health will improve only if health in a broad sense becomes a central concern of the policy-making process.

This extensively revised edition of *Public Health at the Crossroads* provides an overview of major health trends, summarises the current state of the world's health, and presents updated estimates of the global burden of disease. It examines the pattern of modern epidemics, the impact of disability, and the causes of premature death in rich and poor countries alike.

In a challenge to clinicians and public health practitioners and students at all levels, and with examples drawn from diverse geographical and medical areas, Beaglehole and Bonita argue for an inclusive vision of public health based on the application in public policy of improved epidemiological understanding of the causes of disease. Of interest to all health professionals, it will be essential reading for those in public health and related fields.

DR RUTH BONITA, B.A., Dip. Ed., M.P.H., Ph.D., M.D. (*Hons.*)

Dr Bonita's prime research interest for the past two decades has been the epidemiology, prevention and management of cardiovascular disease, in particular, stroke. Most of this work has been undertaken at the University of Auckland in New Zealand where, until recently, she was Professor of Public Health and Epidemiology. In 1999 she was appointed as Director of Surveillance in the Non-Communicable Disease Cluster at the World Health Organization in Geneva. Her interests have now shifted from an academic research base to international health concerns and, in particular, mapping the advancing epidemics of NCDs and the major risk factor that predict them. She has co-authored a successful textbook *Basic Epidemiology* published by WHO (1993) and now translated into 35 languages. *Public Health at the Crossroads: Achievements and Prospects* (Cambridge University Press, 1997) is the second book also co-authored with Robert Beaglehole, her colleague and partner of 35 years.

DR ROBERT BEAGLEHOLE, M.B., Ch.B., M.Sc., M.D., D.Sc., F.R.A.C.P., M.R.C.P.(UK), F.A.F.P.H.M., F.R.S.(NZ)

Dr Robert Beaglehole, a New Zealand Public Health Physician, trained in medicine in New Zealand and then in epidemiology and public health at the London School of Hygiene and Tropical Medicine and the University of North Carolina at Chapel Hill. Formerly Professor of Community Health at the University of Auckland, New Zealand, he is currently working as a Director in the Evidence and Information for Policy Cluster at the World Health Organization in Geneva. He has published over 200 scientific papers and several books on epidemiology and public health, including *Global Public Health: A New Era* and *Global Public Goods for Health*, both published by Oxford Univsersity Press.

Reviews of the first edition of *Public Health at the Crossroads*

Public health really is at a crossroads. Drs Robert Beaglehole and Ruth Bonita trace the origins of the field (the tortuous route we have travelled), the many contemporary challenges (that health really is a global issue), and some future promising directions (how a broader approach to public health grounded in an appropriate epidemiology can inform future social policy). The book is refreshing, truly multidisciplinary, based on relevant data and international in its application. Although given separate attention, the authors highlight the striking structural similarities in the public health problems of the poor and the wealthy countries. *Public Health at the Crossroads* is essential reading for those who wish to look beyond traditional public health and the mechanics of everyday epidemiology to new possibilities and more appropriate strategies and methods.

John B. McKinlay, Ph.D.
Sonja M. McKinlay, Ph.D.
New England Research Institutes
Watertown, MA, USA

This sweeping, panoramic view of the state of health in the world provides a marvellous perspective on the problems of health and disease old and new, among poor and rich nations alike. Again and again the authors zoom in for close-up examinations of the causes of infant and child deaths, the yawning gaps between poor and rich, the historical background and evolutionary development of modern public health movements, capsule summaries of health and the services that provide it, in nations around the world, and much more. Beginning students of public health and epidemiology, those who are midway in their training, and established scholars in the field will learn much from this up-to-the-minute, user-friendly discourse. I recommend it without reservation.

John Last, M.D.
Emeritus Professor of Epidemiology and
Community Medicine, University of Ottawa, Canada

After a century 'on the road', public health faces important choices. This book examines, in broad social context, the historical journey of public health and its prospects for revitalisation as we enter a new century. Epidemiologists and public health practitioners face a widening challenge: population health problems that range from local to global levels; entrenched social-economic disparities as sources of poor health; and the emerging hazards of a rapidly changing, interdependent world. The book has a fine sense of public health as both a scientific and a social enterprise.

A. J. McMichael
Professor of Epidemiology
London School of Hygiene and Tropical Medicine, UK

Public Health at the Crossroads

Achievements and Prospects

Second Edition

ROBERT BEAGLEHOLE
and
RUTH BONITA

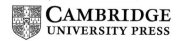

CAMBRIDGE UNIVERSITY PRESS
Cambridge, New York, Melbourne, Madrid, Cape Town, Singapore, São Paulo, Delhi

Cambridge University Press
The Edinburgh Building, Cambridge CB2 8RU, UK

Published in the United States of America by Cambridge University Press, New York

www.cambridge.org
Information on this title: www.cambridge.org/9780521832915

First published 1997
Reprinted 1999, 2001
Second edition 2004
Third printing 2008

Printed in the United Kingdom at the University Press, Cambridge

A catalogue record for this publication is available from the British Library

Library of Congress Cataloguing in Publication data

Beaglehole, R.
Public health at the crossroads: achievements and prospects/Robert Beaglehole
and Ruth Bonita, – 2nd ed.
p.   cm.
Includes bibliographical references and index.
ISBN 0 521 83291 8 – ISBN 0 521 54047 X (pb.)
1. World health. I. Bonita, R. II. Title.
RA441.B43 2004
362.1 – dc22   2003065260

ISBN 978-0-521-83291-5 hardback
ISBN 978-0-521-54047-6 paperback

Contents

Preface

This revised edition assesses the achievements and the current state of epidemiology and public health with a focus on the last 50 years. The main challenges facing epidemiology and public health are identified and strategies for the future discussed. The prime audience for this book is students of epidemiology and public health, who will continue to shape the future of these disciplines.

Public health is the collective action taken by society to protect and promote the health of entire populations; in contrast, clinical medicine deals only with the health problems of individuals. Public health is broad and inclusive, although it is often considered from only a narrow medical perspective. Epidemiology, with its focus on the causes of disease at the population level and the methods for their control, is the most important science contributing to public health. Many other disciplines also contribute, for example, biostatistics, medical sociology, health economics, and various qualitative approaches. Epidemiology is central to public health because of its population focus and quantitative methods.

Epidemiology and public health remain at a crossroads. The choice is between a narrow focus on health service issues and the health problems of individuals on the one hand, or a refocus on the major underlying causes of population health on the other. The main argument of this book is that both epidemiology and public health are still failing to fulfil their potential to improve the public's health. The problem lies both with the public health professions – which have narrowed their professional concerns – and because there is a disjunction between the ideas and ideals of public health and the way society organises itself in relation to health.

Despite promising beginnings with the work of Snow and many others on cholera and other major causes of mortality in the middle of the last century, and path-breaking work a century later on the tobacco-caused lung cancer epidemic, epidemiology is still peripheral to the health endeavour. Internationally, public health has been marginalised, as collective responsibility for social welfare in general has been replaced by an emphasis on market forces and individualism. At the national level, the ongoing debates about health care reforms have been narrowly focused on cost containment and medical care services and have not embraced the need for a re-emphasis on public health services and the health of entire populations. Given the growing threats to public health, the prospects for epidemiology and public health will improve only if population health becomes a more central concern of the entire policy-making process.

As the purpose of public health is to improve health, this revised edition, which has three main sections, begins with an extensively updated overview of major health trends and a summary of the current state of the world's health. It also reviews recent estimates of the global burden of disease and identifies the major unresolved health problems. This is followed by a discussion of the causes of modern epidemics. The framework for Part I is the health transition and the forces which propel it. Part II describes the development of epidemiology and considers epidemiology's contribution to the improvement in health status. Criticisms of epidemiology are discussed and the major challenges facing epidemiology outlined.

Part III describes the global state of the organisation and delivery of public health services. Case studies of several wealthy countries are used to illustrate different approaches to the organisation of public health activities. In most countries public health remains marginalised and the emphasis is still on medical care services. These services know no limit and, with the ageing of the world's population especially in poor countries, could easily claim even the small proportion of health budgets spent on public health services. The impact of recent reviews of public health in the United Kingdom, United States of America, Sweden and New Zealand is described. The situation in Japan is outlined because of the major recent health improvements in Japan. In a few poor countries, public health has at various times assumed a more central role in public policy. Two such countries, China and Cuba, have made impressive gains in health status over the last few decades although recent trends in both countries are a cause for concern. The third poor country to be considered is India, and here the focus is on the state of Kerala which, despite enduring and widespread poverty, has achieved a remarkably high standard of health, although this too is now threatened by factors outside the health sector.

The book concludes by drawing together the achievements, the present dilemmas and the future prospects for public health; alternative pathways for epidemiology and public health are outlined. Recent worldwide political, economic and environmental changes present the most important challenges to public health in the twenty-first century; public health practitioners must adopt a truly global perspective. For epidemiology and public health to move centre stage, it will be necessary to recognise and confront these challenges. A major shift in emphasis is required if public health is to develop with a focus on environmental sustainability, equity and community partnerships. This process will be easier if public health practitioners rediscover the reforming values of their nineteenth-century predecessors and reconnect with the aspirations and energy of the people and communities they serve. In the short term the initiative must come from public health practitioners. A tremendous responsibility falls on all of us. We need to rediscover our passion for public health so that it moves forward and fulfils its potential to improve the health of populations globally.

Acknowledgements

This book has benefited from invaluable feedback from many friends and colleagues to whom we are indebted: in particular, Tim Armstrong, Bruce Aylward, Toni Ashton, Andrew Ball, Peter Davis, Anna Howe, Marilyn Fingerhut, Rod Jackson, Tord Kjellström, Colin Mathers, Tony McMichael, Alan Norrish, Neil Pearce, George Salmond, David Skegg, Alistair Woodward and Alan Wylie.

Country profiles and their updates benefited from input from Kjell Asplund, Warwick Armstrong, Don Bandaranayake, Pedro Brito, Gilliam Durham, Bobbie Jacobson, Kazunori Kodama, Walter Holland, Vivian Lin, Martin McKee, John Powles, Roger Rosenblatt, KR Thankappan, Stig Wall, Hirotsugu Ueshima and Hiroshi Yanagawa.

The mechanics of assembling the material and preparing the manuscript for the first edition could not have taken place without considerable effort from Joanna Broad, Dale Cormack-Pearson, Raewynne Menzies, Wendy Smidt and Rachael Taylor. April Lindsay assisted in the revisions for the second edition.

We would like to acknowledge the support and encouragement of our children, Rob and Anna Beaglehole.

PART I

Global health

The first part of this book

- considers the health transition and the forces that propel it (Chapter 1);
- outlines the current state of global health (Chapter 2); and
- describes the major causes of premature death and disease (Chapter 3).

1

Health, disease and the health transition

1.1 Introduction

This chapter sets the global health scene by introducing definitions central to an understanding of health and disease, and describes the populations and country groupings that will be used in our comparisons. It also introduces the health transition which provides a framework for explaining and describing major trends in health and disease.

1.2 Health status or disease status?

Health has a wide variety of meanings ranging from an ideal state to the absence of a medically defined and certified disease. Health as an ideal state has been encapsulated in the original and inspirational World Health Organization (WHO) definition: 'health is a state of complete mental, physical and social well-being and not merely the absence of disease or infirmity'[1]. The definition reflects the optimism at the end of the Second World War. Unfortunately, health, in this vision, is unattainable. While individuals may very occasionally be in this state, populations as a whole will never be free of premature death, disease or disability because of their close interaction with a changing environment. The adaptive fit between human biology and the human-made environment is inevitably imperfect[2].

In the 1980s WHO promoted a more realistic definition of health which emphasises the ability to function 'normally' in one's own social setting. 'Health' here is a means to an end but again requires the absence of disability, disease or handicap, despite the fact that many people consider themselves to be in 'good health' even in the presence of a disabling disease. By contrast, and in the opinion of many modern market orientated 'health reformers', health is more like a commodity which can be provided or even 'bought' in discrete packages.

A simple subjective categorisation by individuals into one of three current states of health, for example, 'good; fair; poor', has been shown to predict future health outcomes with a surprising degree of accuracy; expectations for health clearly differ between young and old people, and by culture and gender[3]. With further research, this type of subjective information may provide additional dimensions to death statistics; however, it is not yet useful either for international comparisons or for assessing trends over time because of the differences in survey instruments and cultural differences in reporting health. To address these problems, WHO has recently undertaken a multicountry survey using a standardised health survey status instrument together with new statistical methods for adjusting biases in self-reported health[4].

Of more use, both theoretically and practically, is a definition which states that health is created by removing obstacles and by providing the basic means by which individual goals can be achieved[5]. The foundations of health are common to all and include basic requirements such as adequate food, safe water, shelter, safety and hope. In addition, information, education and a sense of community are essential if people are to develop their potential. These foundations have a more profound long-term effect on health status than the activities of the health system[6]. The chosen definition of health has important implications for health policy. It determines whether the emphasis is on a multi-sectoral approach to improving health or whether the focus is on selected diseases and technological solutions[7].

The main source of 'health' data remains death statistics. Epidemiologists are often criticised for concentrating on this narrow aspect of health. Death statistics, however, provide an important starting point because of the gross disparities they reveal and for historical purposes, there is no alternative. In addition, death has a deep significance in all societies.

The most useful source of death information is the data supplied to the WHO by member countries. These data depend upon two essential components: an estimate of the population at risk and the identification of deaths. Only a minority of countries conduct regular censuses to determine the age distribution of their populations. Even in wealthy countries such as the United States of America, population counts are not always accurate, especially for minority groups[8].

Counting deaths is even more difficult. Only about 66 of the 192 member states are in a position to provide national death statistics to the WHO[9]; a further

50 provide incomplete data, but which can be adjusted for incompleteness. In the absence of national death registration systems for two-third's of the world's population, estimates – often based on data from sentinel surveillance sites as in India and China – are used to assess the burden of death[10]. A great failure of epidemiology and public health is that insufficient attention has been given to ensuring that adequate vital health data are collected. WHO and other groups have recently given considerable attention to the development and use of summary measures of population health status and these will be described and discussed in Chapter 2.

As very few countries can provide useful data on deaths going back more than a few decades, trends over time must be interpreted with great caution. Even the available data are limited by the lack of attention to quality. The problems with death data include:

- changes in diagnostic and death certification fashions;
- periodic revisions of the WHO disease classification system;
- the contribution of multiple causes to death, especially in ageing populations; and
- the generally low and declining use of post-mortems.

Fortunately, many of the known limitations of mortality data tend to cancel out each other and, from a population perspective, the available data are extremely useful in studying overall trends, even if flawed at the individual level. In addition, modern modelling techniques can take account of unmeasured errors in the basic mortality data[11]. The great attraction of death as a key indicator of health status is that it can be measured more easily than morbidity (sickness). It is often assumed that morbidity changes in parallel with mortality, although this is by no means always true, especially in older people.

Death data are used for a number of purposes. They

- allow comparisons among and within countries;
- demonstrate trends in longevity or life expectancy and various related measures;
- show trends in death rates for different age groups; and
- provide information about the leading causes of death.

Even a cursory inspection of the available mortality data reveals a tremendous burden of premature death in all countries, especially in poor countries, as described in Chapter 2.

1.3 Categorising countries

A striking feature of the global health picture is the great diversity between and, to a lesser extent, within countries. Various classifications are used to group the more than 200 countries in the world, but no system is satisfactory. The World Bank categorises countries according to their gross national product and by eight demographic regions[12]. The regional categories are further simplified into two groups, the former socialist economies of Europe and the established market economies where relatively uniform age distributions are leading to older populations, and the other six regions where the age distributions are younger. These latter countries correspond to the low and middle income countries and contain 85% of the world's population. WHO in its most recent assessment of global health status, has divided its six regions into 14 subgroups based on five mortality strata; these five groupings are further broken down into three epidemiological groups: Developed countries; High Mortality Developing countries; and Low Mortality Developing countries. This classification has no official status but is useful for analytical purposes[13].

The United Nations uses the terms 'developed' and 'less developed' or 'developing' to categorise countries into two broad groups which are similar to the two main World Bank groups. This nomenclature, however, assumes a continuum; the 'developing' countries will not necessarily follow the pattern of wealth generation of the small number of 'developed' countries. Other labels include 'North' and 'South', 'First World' and 'Third World' countries, 'industrialised', 'non-industrialised', and 'newly industrialising'; 'countries in transition' is often used to label countries undergoing economic and social transitions, especially as a result of the dissolution of the former Soviet Union. All of these terms are unsatisfactory and simplistic because, within broad groups of countries, there is enormous diversity in social, economic and health characteristics.

The terms 'rich' (or 'wealthy') and 'poor' are perhaps the most helpful because this simple dichotomy emphasises an important basic distinction between countries. Furthermore, it helps to remind us that rich countries have largely achieved and maintained their position at the expense of the poor countries. For these reasons, we prefer these terms.

1.4 The health transition: a critique

1.4.1 What is the 'health transition'?

The health transition is a framework for describing and explaining the spectacular shifts in the patterns and causes of death that have taken place in most countries[14]. Demographers originally used the term 'demographic transition' or 'mortality transition' to describe the change from high fertility and high mortality rates in 'traditional' societies to low fertility and low mortality rates in 'modern' societies. A broader term, the 'epidemiological transition', was introduced to describe, in addition to mortality, the long-term changes in patterns of sickness and disability that occurred as societies changed their demographic, economic and social structure[15]. 'Health transition' is a more appropriate term because it includes the social and behavioural changes which parallel, and propel, the epidemiological transition[16].

1.4.2 Health transition: periods, pathways and models

The health transition, as originally described by Omran, consists of three periods:

- the era of pestilence and famine;
- the era of receding pandemics; and
- the era of non-communicable diseases (originally called 'man-made' or 'degenerative' diseases, and now often called 'chronic' diseases)[15].

The main distinguishing feature has been described as the transition from a pattern dominated by infectious diseases with very high mortality, especially at younger ages, to a pattern dominated by non-communicable diseases and injury with lower overall mortality, which peaks at older ages. The main determinant of this mortality transition was the control of infectious disease with the consequent mortality decline precipitating the fertility decline. The basic premise of Omran's theory was that, in progressing from high to low mortality levels, all populations experience a shift in the major causes of death and disease[17].

In the era of pestilence life expectancy was low, less than 30 years, and probably higher in men than in women. The major causes of death were due to malnutrition, epidemic infectious diseases, and complications of pregnancy and childbirth. In many western countries the second stage of the transition was established early in the eighteenth century[18] and was dominated by infectious diseases and malnutrition; people lived, on average, up to 50 years. In Western Europe this period lasted until the early twentieth century with the influenza pandemic of 1918–20 being the last major pandemic. The era of non-communicable diseases is characterised by low fertility rates, growth of the population, and an increase in the importance of cardiovascular disease and cancer. In this era, life expectancy is greater in women than men, exceeding

55 years, and ultimately reaches over 80 years. These three periods overlap, and progress is not necessarily linear, progressive or uniform within countries; nor are mortality declines necessarily associated with improvements in morbidity and disability[19].

Recently, a fourth phase of the health transition has been proposed in an attempt to account for the resurgence of 'old' infectious diseases and the emergence of new infectious diseases in association with non-communicable diseases[20,21]. Patterns of mortality and morbidity in this fourth stage have been explained largely on the basis of individual lifestyle[21]. This interpretation is limited because it exaggerates the role of determinants of disease at the level of the individual, underplays the power of social and economic determinants of epidemics, and has often led to victim blaming.

The pathway from high infectious disease mortality rates is highly variable and not all countries have experienced high rates of non-communicable diseases. In North and Western Europe and North America the benefits of the decline in infectious diseases were, in part, offset by rises in cardiovascular disease and cancer death rates. The increase in non-communicable diseases has been less in Japan, China, and Southern European countries – especially for coronary heart disease, but greater in countries of Eastern and Central Europe. Non-communicable age-specific disease death rates will probably increase in poor countries as economic and social changes occur, although data to substantiate this suggestion are still sparse[22].

It is unlikely that the evolution of the health transition in poor countries will simply be a replication of the pattern of the wealthy countries. In some countries, population growth, poverty, environmental degradation, and the 'demographic' trap, may prevent the transition from high mortality and fertility to low mortality and fertility[23]. This outcome is especially likely in sub-Saharan Africa. Even so, it is important to note that most poor people today have lower death rates than wealthy people a century ago[24].

Three models of the transition, depending on the time and rate of change, have been proposed[15]:

- classical or western;
- accelerated (such as occurred in Japan); and
- the delayed or contemporary model, which describes the incomplete transition in poor countries.

Other variations on these models have been proposed to account for the rapidity of the decline in mortality rates this century in middle income countries such as Singapore and South Korea[25]. It has been suggested that there are as many models as there are societies[17]. Different transition models can occur in different populations within a single country. For example, in New Zealand the European (Pakeha) population followed the classical model; more recently the Maori population made an incomplete health transition and has, in turn, been followed by Pacific populations resident in New Zealand, although unacceptably high rates of infectious diseases are still a feature of both these populations in New Zealand[25]. Some middle income countries, such as Mexico, are following the 'prolonged and polarised model' characterised by overlapping stages (for example, the reappearance of infectious diseases such as malaria that had previously been controlled and high rates of other infectious diseases such as HIV/AIDS), and by polarisation, that is, an exacerbation of social class inequalities in mortality rates. The most disadvantaged populations experience high rates of both infectious and non-communicable diseases with the excess mortality of the poorest population mostly due to communicable diseases[26,27].

1.4.3 What propels the health transition?

There are three major forces underlying the health transition:

- the health determinants;
- the demographic; and
- the therapeutic.

The main driving force includes the underlying social, economic, political and cultural factors which determine health and are responsible for, and propel, the health transition by reducing infectious disease mortality rates[28]. The importance of these factors is apparent from a comparison of the health effects of rapid economic and social changes in the so-called Tiger Economies of East Asia beginning in the 1960s, with the rapidly contracting economies of Central and Eastern Europe in the early 1990s[29]. Of major importance has been the attainment of modest levels of per capita income and widespread literacy, especially for women[30]. Also included in this category are the important public health interventions, which reduce the population's exposure to health hazards, for example, improvements in personal hygiene as a result of public information campaigns in the early nineteenth century[17].

Some changes, such as urbanisation and the associated changes in behaviour, occur with industrialisation; other more recent changes are superimposed by global marketing and promotion forces, for example nutritional changes and the increase in cigarette smoking[22]. An increasing frequency of these risk factors in the population leads to increases in age-specific death rates. A specific component of the health transition is the nutrition transition, which is the shift over many centuries in the customary diet from that typical of hunter–gatherers to one high in total fat and refined carbohydrates. These dietary changes, together with changing patterns of physical activity, have resulted in the emergence of non-communicable disease epidemics including obesity. This nutrition transition is as variable as the mortality transitions[31].

The demographic component refers to the ageing of populations as a result of declining fertility and declining death rates, particularly in children. The ageing of the population is the prime driving force for the emergence of the non-communicable diseases of adulthood, which have a long latent period and become much more frequent with increasing age. As populations age, the absolute number of these diseases will inevitably increase, even if the age- and cause-specific death rates decline.

The third driving force, the therapeutic component, includes factors that tend to reduce the risk of dying once disease has become established. Effective health services are essential for the achievement of good population health and interact with the independence of women and higher educational levels. The most effective health services are not necessarily those which are technologically advanced, but rather those which are either free or inexpensive, effective and readily accessible. From a historical perspective, this contribution to the health transition has been small because of the ineffectiveness of most medical interventions. The therapeutic component has been of much more importance recently in poor countries and has contributed to the major decline in child mortality that has taken place in these countries over the last few decades[30]. In addition, over the last two decades effective and cheap interventions have become available for the most important non-communicable diseases[32].

1.4.4 The health transition: a critique

The health transition remains a useful framework for describing the changing patterns of mortality. An analysis of extensive cause of death data for the period 1950–1995 confirmed that as all-cause mortality declines, the composition of mortality by cause changes systematically in many age groups with different patterns occurring by age and sex[11]. Nevertheless, the theory has limitations. Firstly, it fails to explain differences in death rates between countries and has limited ability to predict changing patterns of disease with 'modernisation'. The recent deterioration in life expectancy at middle age in some Central and Eastern European countries and the devastating impact of HIV/AIDS in Africa – both counter-transitions – and the increasing inequalities in health in all countries, were not predicted by the health transition theory. In addition, the original formulation viewed the transition in linear and progressive terms when the reality is now recognised to be much more complex, even within a country.

By focusing on the important social and economic causes of changing death rates, the health transition offers potential for understanding health trends and thus improving health in all countries. However, as originally formulated, the transition theory downplayed the importance of early and late nineteenth century public health interventions[17].

Secondly, as originally formulated, the epidemiological transition theory with its dichotomy of diseases – infectious or non-communicable – ignores the interaction between disease types; nor were violent deaths, either intentional or unintentional, originally considered. The theory does not easily account for the marked declines that have occurred in mortality rates for some major non-communicable diseases, for example, heart disease and stroke. Furthermore, there is a tendency to view the health transition in isolation from the momentous social and economic changes that propelled the transition, especially the nineteenth-century European version[33].

Further elaboration of the health transition theory is required. Careful reconstruction of national time series, cause-specific, mortality patterns is a necessary first step; regional and within country patterns also require exploration[18]. The variability of change according to particular historical, regional and cultural contexts would aid detailed explanation and prediction. Unusual countries and regions might shed useful insights, for example, the island of Nauru, which attained great wealth through the exploitation of its phosphate deposits, which led to high non-communicable disease rates, and the oil rich states of the Middle East with their high mortality rates. The central and influential role of social and community endeavour in propelling the transition and its close interaction with underlying structural changes in the nature and organisation of societies, also require investigation[33]. Health transition research has focused largely on mortality differentials in a single society; more explanatory power would result from cross-country comparisons[34]. With further elaboration, testable hypotheses based on the health transition may be developed.

In summary, although the health transition theory is a useful descriptive tool, it remains a blunt instrument with only limited predictive powers. Epidemiologists, among others, face a major challenge in developing the theory so that it becomes a useful and powerful framework for the study of disease and mortality in populations, both from historical and contemporary perspectives and for prediction.

1.5 Summary

This introductory chapter has set the scene for the rest of the book by introducing various concepts of health and disease and describing the country and population groupings, which we concentrate on in the next chapters. The health transition is still a useful model for describing broad changes in patterns of fertility and mortality and morbidity. Unfortunately, it requires more elaboration before it will be of much predictive value. The next chapter describes the major historical trends in mortality and summarises the current state of the world's health.

Chapter 1   Key points

- Operational definitions of health suitable for summarising trends in the status of populations are evolving rapidly.
- Reliable cause-specific death data are available for only a minority of countries.
- All categorisations of countries are simplistic and mask great variation within groups and countries; estimation is used to fill the gaps.
- The health transition theory provides the best framework for describing changing patterns of death, but its predictive power is weak.

References

1. *World Health Organization Constitution.* Geneva: WHO, 1946.
2. Dubos, R. *Mirage of Health.* New York: Harper, 1959.
3. Mossey, J.M. & Shapiro, E. Self-rated health: a predictor of mortality among the elderly. *Am. J. Pub. Hlth* 1982; **72**: 800–8.
4. Murray, C.J.L., Tandon, A., Salomon, J.A. & Mathers, C.D. New approaches to enhance cross-population comparability of survey results. In: Murray, C.J.L., Salomon, J.A., Mathers, C.D., Lopez, A.D., eds. *Summary Measures of Population Health: Concepts, Ethics, Measurement and Applications.* Geneva: World Health Organization, 2002.
5. Seedhouse, D. The way around health economics' dead end. *Hlth Care Anal.* 1995; **3**: 205–20.
6. Murray, C.J.L. & Chen, L.C. In search of a contemporary theory for understanding mortality change. *Soc. Sci. Med.* 1993; **36**: 143–55.
7. Rifkin, S.B. & Walt, G. Why health improves: defining the issues concerning 'comprehensive primary health care' and 'selective primary health care'. *Soc. Sci. Med.* 1986; **6**: 559–66.
8. Hahn, R.A. & Eberhardt, S. Life expectancy in four U.S. racial/ethnic populations: 1990. *Epidemiology* 1995; **6**: 350–5.
9. World Health Organization. *World Health Statistics Annual.* Geneva: WHO, 1993.
10. Lopez, A.D. Counting the dead in China: measuring tobacco's impact in the developing world. *Br. Med. J.* 1998; **317**: 1399–400.
11. Salomon, J.A. & Murray, C.J.L. The epidemiologic transition revisited: compositional models for causes of death by age and sex. *Pop. Dev. Rev.* 2002; **28**: 205–28.

12. World, Development Report. *Investing in Health: World Development Indicators.* New York: Oxford University Press, 1993.

13. World Health Organization. *World Health Report, 2002. Reducing Risks, Promoting Healthy Life.* Geneva: World Health Organization, 2002.

14. Feachem, R.G.A., Kjellstrom, T., Murray, C.J.L., Over, M. & Phillips, M.A. *The Health of Adults in the Developing World.* New York: Oxford University Press, 1991.

15. Omran, A.R. The epidemiologic transition: a theory of the epidemiology of population change. *Milbank Mem. Fund Q.* 1971; **49**: 509–38. Reprinted in *Bull. WHO* 2001; **79**: 161–70.

16. Caldwell, J.C. Introductory thoughts on health transition. In: Caldwell, J., Findley S., Caldwell, P., Santow, G., Cosford, W., Braid, J. & Broers-Freeman, D. (eds.). *What We Know about Health Transition: The Cultural, Social and Behavioural Determinants of Health.* Australian National University, Canberra: 1990; **1**: xi–xiii.

17. Caldwell, J.C. Population health in transition. *Bull. WHO* 2001; **79**: 159–60.

18. Mackenbach, J.P. The epidemiologic transition theory. *J. Epidemiol. Commun. Hlth* 1994; **48**: 329–32.

19. Riley, J.C. Why sickness and death rates do not move parallel to one another over time. *Soc. Hist. Med.* 1999; **12**: 101–24.

20. Olshansky, S.J. & Ault, A.B. The fourth stage of the epidemiologic transition: the age of delayed degenerative diseases. *Milbank Mem. Fund Q.* 1986; **64**: 355–91.

21. Rogers, R.G. & Hackenberg, R. Extending epidemiologic transition theory: a new stage. *Soc. Biol.* 1987; **34**: 234–43.

22. Yusuf, S., Reddy, S., Ounpuu, S. & Anand, S. Global burden of cardiovascular diseases. Part 1: general considerations, the epidemiologic transition, risk factors, and impact of urbanisation. *Circulation* 2001; **104**: 2746–53.

23. King, M. & Elliott, C. Legitimate double-think. *Lancet* 1993; **341**: 669–72.

24. Kunitz, S.J. Explanations and ideologies of mortality patterns. *Pop. Dev. Rev.* 1987; **13**: 379–408.

25. Pool, I. Cross-comparative perspectives on New Zealand's health. In: Spicer, J., Trlin, A. & Walton, J.A. (eds.). *Social Dimensions of Health and Disease: New Zealand Perspectives.* Palmerston North: Dunmore Press, 1994.

26. Frenk, J., Bobadilla, J.L., Sepulveda, J. & Cervantes, M.L. Health transition in middle-income countries: new challenges for health care. *Hlth Pol. Plan* 1989; **4**: 29–39.

27. Heuveline, P., Guillot, M. & Gwatkin, D.R. The uneven tides of the health transition. *Soc. Sci. Med.* 2002; **55**: 313–22.

28. Wilkinson, R. & Marmot, M. (eds.). *The Solid Facts.* Copenhagen: WHO Regional Office for Europe, 1998.

29. Hertzman, C. & Siddiqi, A. Health and rapid economic change in the late twentieth century. *Soc. Sci. Med.* 2000; **51**: 809–19.

30. Caldwell, J.C. Routes to low mortality in poor countries. *Pop. Dev. Rev.* 1986; **12**: 171–220.

31. Popkin, B.M. Special Issue Editor. The Bellagio Conference on the Nutrition Transition and its Implications for Health in the Developing World. August 20–24, 2001 Bellagio, Italy. *Pub. Hlth Nutr.* 2002; **5**: 93–280.

32. Yusuf, S. Two decades of progress in preventing vascular disease. *Lancet* 2002; **360**: 2–3.
33. Davis, P. A sociocultural critique of transition theory. In: Spicer, J., Trlin, A. & Walton, J.A. (eds.). *Social Dimensions of Health and Disease: New Zealand Perspectives*. Palmerston North: Dunmore Press, 1994.
34. Caldwell, J.C. Health transition: the cultural, social and behavioural determinants of health in the Third World. *Soc. Sci. Med.* 1993; **36**: 125–35.

2

Global health: past trends and present challenges

2.1 The global picture: measures of progress

Tremendous improvements have occurred in the health of people in the 200 years since the health transition began. One measure of these changes is that most poor people now live longer, on average, than the wealthiest people a century ago. Despite these gains, there remains a tremendous preventable burden of premature death and disease worldwide[1].

In this chapter we review the major global trends in mortality and summarise the current state of health of the world's population. The health status of four main population groups will be described: children, women of child-bearing age, adults, and older people. Children are considered because the vast majority of child deaths are still due to preventable infectious diseases, superimposed on a background of poverty and malnutrition. Furthermore, the main focus of international public health, stimulated by UNICEF (United Nations Children's Fund), continues to be on children. The separate consideration of deaths in association with pregnancy and birth (maternal mortality) is justified because of the tremendous global variation in maternal mortality and because the vast majority of these deaths are preventable. Even so, maternal deaths make up only a very small proportion of the total number of deaths worldwide each year, despite the great deal of attention that they receive from international aid organisations.

Deaths in adults are important for five reasons. Firstly, adults make up one-half of the population of the world and about 80% (or 45 million) of all deaths occur in adults; about one-third of these adult deaths (16 million) are undoubtedly premature, that is, before the age of 60 years[1]. Secondly, adult death rates show considerable regional variation, emphasising the preventive potential. Thirdly, the nature of adult health problems is quite different from those that continue to preoccupy policy-makers in poor countries. The major causes of death in adults in all countries are non-communicable diseases and injuries, and these conditions do not respond to the same strategies that have been used in reducing infectious disease death rates. Adult diseases have received attention in wealthy countries, but the problems of adult non-communicable disease and injuries in poor countries have been neglected[2]. A fourth reason is that adults represent the most economically productive segment of society, and maximising their well-being is the one way of ensuring a reduction in the deaths among small children. A final justification for a focus on adults is the ageing of the population in all countries. This trend is reflected in the changing pattern of diseases worldwide and, in turn, has major implications for health services and societies, in general.

2.1.1 Life expectancy

The dramatic reduction in death rates over the last 200 years can be explained by a number of factors. The most important relate to changes in the cultural, social, economic and behavioural determinants of health and, to a lesser extent, to public health interventions; medical interventions explain only a small amount, although they have had more impact over the last few decades, especially in poor countries. The decline in death rates has led to a major improvement in life expectancy. Life expectancy, the simplest measure of the health of a population, is the average number of years of remaining life, and is always an estimate because it is based on the risk of dying at successive ages within the current population; it assumes no change in death rates in the future.

Our hunter–gathering forebears were lucky to live, on average, 25–30 years; over ensuing centuries, the situation improved very slowly[3]. In the first half of the seventeenth century, for example, life expectancy in western Europe was still not much more than about 25 years, regardless of sex and social class. In nineteenth-century England and Wales, life expectancy increased by only 7 years, from 41 years in 1841 to 48 in 1901 for the total population[4], in contrast to the rapidity of changes in most countries over the last half century.

Life expectancy at birth has increased by 20 years from a global average of 46 years in 1950[5]. Even in the past two decades life expectancy has increased 3 years for men (reaching 63 years in 2000) and 2 years for women (reaching 67 years in 2000). Life expectancy ranges from 81.4 years for women in wealthy countries such as Western Europe, North America, Japan, Australia and New Zealand down to 48.1 years for men in sub-Saharan Africa (Fig. 2.1).

The exceptions to the worldwide increases in life expectancy at birth during the 1990s were in Africa – largely due to HIV/AIDS – and in the former Soviet countries of Eastern Europe. In the latter case, male and female life expectancies at birth declined by 3.2 years and 2.7 years, respectively, over the

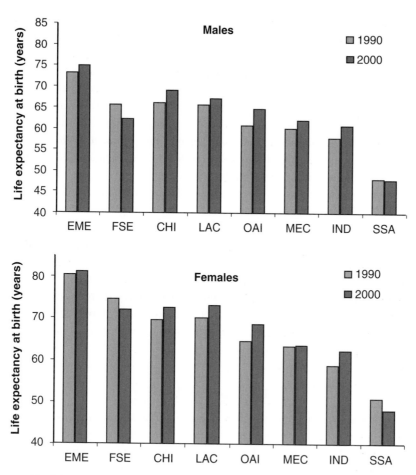

Fig. 2.1. Gains in life expectancy at birth from 1990 to 2000, by sex and region. *Note*: Regional groupings are those used in the Global Burden of Disease Study[9]. EME includes Western Europe, North America, Japan, Australia and New Zealand; FSE includes the former socialist countries of Eastern Europe and Central Asia; OAI includes Asian and Pacific countries apart from India (IND), China (CHI), Japan, Australia and New Zealand; MEC includes Middle Eastern countries and North African countries; LAC, Latin America and Caribbean; SSA, sub-Saharan Africa.

10-year period between 1990 and 2000. The life expectancy at birth of Russian men was only 58 years in 2001, possibly related to an increase in death rates from heart disease, trauma and injury associated with alcohol consumption, and an increase in infant mortality[6]. Continuing economic and industrial disruption in Russia suggests that there is little hope for major improvements in Russian vital statistics, although there has been some recovery over recent years[7]. In almost all countries, women have longer life expectancy than men, except for some countries in the Eastern Mediterranean region, North Africa, and Asia[8].

Life expectancy at birth may disguise smaller inter-country differences in the duration of later life. Even for people in poor countries, once they survive to reach middle age, life expectancy begins to approach that of people in developed countries. As with increases in life expectancy at birth, there has been an increase in the average length of remaining life once a person reaches 65 years of age. At this older age, the most rapid improvements have occurred in the last few decades, largely because of the decline in death rates from heart disease and stroke, two of the major causes of death in adults.

Substantial variations in life expectancy also occur within countries by ethnicity, geographical location and social class. The health gains of the past decade have mainly benefited the better off[10, 11]. In the United States of America, a white male at birth now has a life expectancy, after adjusting for census undercount and misclassification on death certificates, almost 7 years greater than that of a male African–American[12]. Data from two Dutch villages in the eighteenth century showed that the upper class group had more than a 10-year advantage in life expectancy compared with the lower class group[13]. Relative class inequalities in some wealthy countries are still similar to those observed 200 years ago in the Dutch villages[14].

2.1.2 Counting the dead

The best known measure of health status is the cause of death based on the death certificate. This provides an invaluable source of information on patterns of death and trends over time. Unfortunately, complete cause-specific death registration data are available routinely for only a minority of the world's countries. Less than one-third of the world's population is covered adequately by national vital registration systems and there is a wide regional variation ranging from 80% population coverage in the European region to less than 5% population coverage in the Eastern Mediterranean and African regions of the World Health Organization. However, the use of sample registration systems has extended the coverage to the equivalent of three-quarters of global mortality. Survey data and indirect demographic techniques provide information on levels of child and adult mortality for the remaining 25% of estimated global mortality[8].

For most poor countries, indirect methods are required to estimate trends for specific causes of death. The two most populous countries in the world, China and India, systematically collect sample mortality data. In China, a nationally representative sample of the population from 145 disease surveillance centres (DPS) covers about 1% of the total Chinese population[15]. Data on the age, sex and cause of 725 000 deaths are also collected annually from the vital registration system operated by the Ministry of Health, covering a population of 121 million (66 million in urban areas, 55 million in rural areas). A third source of data on mortality in China is an annual 1 per 1000 household survey which asks about deaths in the past 12 months[16]. From these three low-cost information sources in China, it has been possible to extrapolate to the national level and contribute to estimates of global patterns and causes of death.

In India, the Sample Registration System has collected data successfully on rural mortality and fertility since the mid-1960s through continuous recording by resident enumerators as well as through retrospective half-yearly population surveys[17]. Data are collected on vital events in rural and urban sampling units, which cover a population of about 6 million people. Comparison of these data with other survey and demographic estimates suggests that under-reporting of child deaths is minimal and is around 15% of adult deaths. The Medical Certificate of Cause of Death (MCCD) also provides information for deaths in urban India. A high coverage of all deaths (estimated at 95%) has been achieved using these multiple approaches.

An alternative to the medically certified death certificate, the verbal autopsy, has also been shown to be economical and useful in improving the quality of cause of death information where health workers have minimal training[18-20]. Verbal autopsy information is, however, still far from ideal, and of relatively limited use for certain groups of causes of death with similar symptom patterns. WHO is exploring the use of verbal autopsy in population surveys to identify injury deaths, particularly deaths related to war and civil conflict[21].

These multiple sources have been used by WHO, together with information derived from specific epidemiological studies, to estimate life tables and cause of death patterns for all regions of the world[1, 22, 23]. In countries with a substantial HIV epidemic, separate estimates are made of the numbers and distributions of deaths due to HIV/AIDS and these deaths are incorporated into the life table estimates[24]. The major gap in mortality data is the sub-Saharan African region where, apart from South Africa, no country has the necessary empirical data required for estimating mortality rates for specific causes of death.

2.1.3 Fifty-six million deaths worldwide

The distribution of the 56 million deaths estimated to have occurred in 2001 by broad cause of death is shown in Table 2.1. Approximately three-quarters occur in developing countries, reinforcing the fundamental importance of improving mortality statistics as a measure of health status in developing countries. Overall, almost one-fifth (18.3 million) of all deaths are Group I conditions: 11 million

Table 2.1. *Estimated deaths (millions), by level of development and broad cause of death, 2001*[1]

	Group I	Group II	Group III	All causes	(%)
Developing countries	17.48	21.39	4.08	42.95	(75.9)
High mortality	*14.65*	*10.02*	*2.28*	*26.95*	
Low mortality	*2.83*	*11.37*	*1.80*	*16.00*	
Developed countries	0.90	11.69	1.02	13.61	(24.1)
Total	18.38	33.08	5.10	56.56	(100)

Group I: Communicable, maternal, perinatal, nutritional conditions.
Group II: Non-communicable diseases.
Group III: Injuries.

deaths are from infectious and parasitic diseases, with the remainder due to a combination of respiratory infections (4 million), perinatal conditions (2.5 million), maternal conditions and nutritional deficiencies (each approximately 500 000). Almost 60% of deaths are due to Group II: non-communicable diseases (33 million). Injuries (group III) are responsible for 9% of deaths globally (approximately 5 million).

Communicable diseases are responsible for over half (54%) of the deaths in high mortality developing countries, 18% in low mortality developing countries, but for only 6% in developed countries. Conversely, even in the high mortality countries non-communicable diseases account for about one third of all deaths (10 million); twice as many deaths from non-communicable diseases occur in developing countries as in developed countries. The remainder are due to intentional and unintentional injuries, the majority of which occur in high mortality developing countries.

Table 2.2 shows the distribution of these deaths by broad cause of death in four age bands. Almost 1 in 5 of all deaths occur in children under 5 years of age; 99% of these deaths are in poor countries. More than 1 in 4 of all deaths (28%) occur in young adults (15–59 years). Similar numbers of deaths occur in men and women for group I and group II conditions, but twice as many Group III (Injury) conditions occur in men compared to women.

Figure 2.2 shows the percentage distribution of death by selected causes globally. Cardiovascular disease (heart disease and stroke) explains 30% of all deaths and cancer 13%; a further 16% are due to other non-communicable diseases (e.g. respiratory disease). Respiratory infections, mostly in children, explain 7% of deaths and perinatal and neonatal causes a further 4.5%. More than 1 in 10 deaths (11%) are due to other infectious and parasitic diseases, excluding AIDS, malaria and TB, which together explain 8.4% of all deaths.

Table 2.2. *Estimated deaths (in millions), by age, gender and broad cause of death, 2001*[1]

Age	Group I		Group II		Group III		All causes	
	Male	Female	Male	Female	Male	Female	Total	(%)
0–4	4.89	4.51	0.45	0.45	0.18	0.18	10.66	(18.8)
5–14	0.36	0.43	0.11	0.12	0.28	0.15	1.45	(2.4)
15–59	2.82	2.61	4.30	2.94	2.31	0.95	15.93	(28.1)
60–69	0.56	0.35	3.92	2.86	0.29	0.15	8.13	(14.4)
70+	0.90	0.95	7.95	9.98	0.32	0.30	20.3	(35.8)
Total	9.53	8.85	16.73	16.35	3.38	1.73	56.57	(100)

Group I: Communicable, maternal, perinatal, nutritional conditions.
Group II: Non-communicable diseases.
Group III: Injuries.

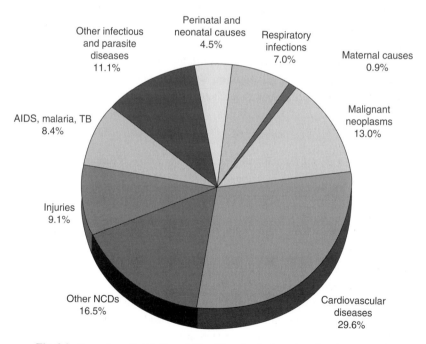

Fig. 2.2. Percentage distribution of 56 million deaths by selected main causes of death, 2001.

2.2 Infant and child deaths

2.2.1 Past trends

Improvement in infant and child death rates has led to the universal increase in life expectancy at birth. These gains have been impressive. In poor agrarian societies last century only one out of two babies survived to the age of 15 years[3]. Infant death in the first year of life (infant mortality) is now a rare event in many countries, occurring only about 3 times in every 1000 births in countries with the lowest rates. In contrast, in countries with the highest rates, as many as one in eight babies still die in the first year of life.

Infant mortality rates are falling in most countries and regions (Table 2.3), but the degree of variation between countries has increased over the last 40 years, reflecting general global inequities in health.

Infant mortality rates declined in the least developed countries by 40% between 1960 and 2001 compared with a 56% decline in developing countries, and 84% decline in industrialised countries for the same time period[28].

Death rates in children in the first 5 years of life (child death rates), are more reliable for regional comparisons because population surveys are used for estimating child death rates. Progress has been made in all regions in reducing death rates (Table 2.3). As with infant mortality rates, however, there has been a worsening of the relative gap between rich and poor countries. Between 1960 and 2001, under 5 mortality rates declined by 44% in least developed countries (from 278 to 157 per 1000 live births), by 60% in developing countries (from

Table 2.3. *Regional summaries of Under 5 and Infant Mortality rate, 1960 and 2001*[28]

	Under-5 mortality rate		Infant mortality rate (under 1)	
	1960	2001	1960	2001
Sub-Saharan Africa	253	173	152	107
Middle East and North Africa	250	61	157	47
South Asia	244	98	148	70
East Asia and Pacific	212	43	140	33
Latin America and Caribbean	153	34	102	28
CEE/CIS and Baltic States	103	37	78	30
Industrialised countries	37	7	31	5
Developing countries	223	89	141	62
Least developed countries	278	157	170	100
World	197	82	126	57

223 to 89 per 1000 live births), and by 81% (from 37 to 7 per live births) in industrialised countries[28]. While there was a sixfold variation in child mortality rates between wealthy industrialised countries and sub-Saharan Africa – the region with the highest child mortality rates in 1960 – by 2001 there was a 24-fold variation. Improvements occurred in sub-Saharan Africa during the 1950s and 1960s, but the rate of progress has slowed since 1970. In countries that have recently experienced civil wars, such as Iraq, Somalia, Rwanda, Zaire and the former republics of Yugoslavia, child mortality rates have deteriorated. These wars have claimed the lives of millions of children and left four to five million others crippled, either physically or mentally, for life[23,25].

2.2.2 The present

The wide variation in infant mortality rates for different regions of the world are shown in Fig. 2.3.

More than 10 million children under 5 years of age die each year, mostly from preventable causes and almost all are in poor countries[1,26]. This is 3 million fewer child deaths (14% reduction) since 1990. Even so, if these children had

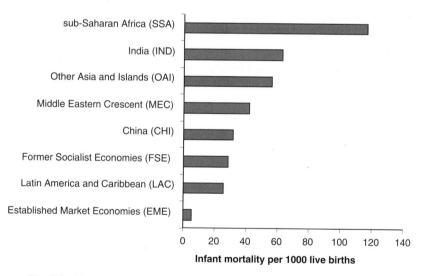

Fig. 2.3. Global variation in infant mortality rates, 2000.
Note: Regional groupings are those used in the Global Burden of Disease Study[10]
EME includes Western Europe, North America, Japan, Australia and New Zealand;
FSE includes the former socialist countries of Eastern Europe and Central Asia,
OAI includes Asian and Pacific countries apart from India, China, Japan, Australia and New Zealand; *MEC* includes Middle Eastern countries and North African countries.

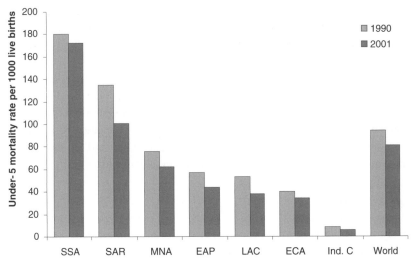

Fig. 2.4. Trends in under-5 mortality rate by region, 1990–2002.
Note: Regional groupings: AFR: sub-Saharan Africa; SAR: South Asian Region; MNA: Middle East and North Africa; EAP: East Asia and Pacific; LCR: Latin America and Caribbean; ECA: East and Central Asia; Ind. C: Industrialised countries.

the same death rate as children in Japan or in the United States of America, there would have been only one million child deaths. Just six countries (India, Nigeria, China, Pakistan, DR Congo, Ethiopia) account for 50% of worldwide deaths in children under 5 years, and 42 countries for 90%[26]. In poor countries children still die of the infectious diseases that have plagued populations since the beginning of large settlements centuries ago[27]. Seven out of ten deaths in children under the age of 5 years still occur in low income countries and can be attributed to just five preventable conditions: pneumonia, diarrhoeal diseases, malaria, measles and undernutrition. The infectious disease deaths are the direct result of poverty, low birthweight and the absence of comprehensive health services. The vast majority of these deaths can be prevented, often at very low cost, by a combination of social and health policy measures and public health and medical interventions[1]. Trends in under 5 mortality since 1990 are shown in Fig. 2.4.

At the Millennium Summit in 2000, representatives from 189 countries committed themselves to sustaining development and eliminating poverty. The Millennium Development Goals (MDGs) summarise these commitments and provide a framework for measuring progress (see Chapter 10). There are eight overarching development goals with 18 health-related targets and outcomes or indicators established for 2015[29]. A number of indicators relate to child health including the prevalence of underweight children under 5 years of age, infant mortality rate (0–1 year) per 1000 live births, and percentage of 1-year-old children immunised for measles. The child health goal is a reduction of under-5 mortality by two-thirds between 1990 and 2015[30].

Substantial progress has been made in many countries with immunisation coverage, measles reduction, polio eradication, elimination of iodine deficiency, breast feeding, the control of guinea worm, and the provision of safe water and sanitation. However, unless strategies for delivery of known and effective interventions are greatly improved, it is unlikely that the MDG for reduced child mortality will be achieved[31].

Measles provides an example of progress that has been made in reducing infectious disease death rates in children in poor countries. Measles, a relatively mild disease for a healthy child, can be devastating in poor communities. Unfortunately, an earlier goal of controlling measles by the year 2000, specifically a 90% reduction in cases and a 95% reduction in deaths compared with pre-immunisation levels, was not met in many poor countries[1]. Almost three-quarters of the estimated 745 000 deaths from measles occur in children under 5 years of age, the majority of whom live in poor countries[1]. The cornerstone of WHO/UNICEF strategic plan on measles mortality reduction and regional elimination for the years 2001–2005 is to provide two opportunities for measles vaccination (either through a second dose or through mass campaign). It is expected that this will achieve high levels of population immunity, enhancement of measles surveillance, and improved case management of measles. The overall goal is to reduce global measles mortality by half in 2005, relative to 1999[32].

The successes in controlling polio are due to improvements in both childhood nutrition and immunisation campaigns, with half the poor countries reaching the internationally agreed target of 80% coverage for the major vaccine preventable diseases of childhood[33]. In 1988 when a global programme to eradicate polio was announced by WHO, 125 countries on five continents were known to have indigenous transmission of wild polio virus with 350 000 cases of polio. By 2002, polio was on the brink of eradication with only seven countries (India, Nigeria, Pakistan, Egypt, Afghanistan, Niger and Somalia) still endemic and only 483 virologically confirmed cases that year[34]. The greatest threats to polio eradication are problems in strategy implementation in just seven countries[35]; virtually all of the world's polio cases (99%) are concentrated in just three countries – India, Nigeria and Pakistan. A further $89 million has recently been provided by Rotary International to address the problems in these countries; this brings the contribution by Rotary International in a public-private partnership with WHO and UNICEF to a total of $500 million[36].

Although infectious disease deaths still occur in wealthy countries, particularly in marginalised populations, they have largely been prevented in wealthy countries because poverty and malnutrition are much less common and less severe, and preventive child health services are effective. In contrast to poor countries, child mortality in wealthy countries is dominated by sudden infant death syndrome, congenital disorders and injuries (mostly unintentional). Even these are increasingly preventable; for example, sudden infant death rates have declined dramatically in several countries over a short period as a result of epidemiological research and public health campaigns[37]. Congenital defects show marked social class gradients, indicating the importance of environmental factors and the potential for preventive strategies.

2.3 Maternal deaths

2.3.1 Past trends

Maternal mortality rates have improved dramatically over the last two centuries, as determined by the data from few countries, which have kept long-term population records. In Sweden, for example, the rate declined continuously from 1750, with a tremendous improvement occurring in the first 100 years when maternal mortality rates halved from about 1000 per 100 000 births to about 500 in the 1850s[38].

In the 1880s maternal mortality rates in Western European countries were at least 500 per 100 000 births. Rates fell markedly between 1880 and 1910 in Scandanavian countries, but in most other countries they remained high until the 1930s. Since then, reform of obstetric practice, in particular concern about puerperal sepsis, led to a rapid decline in mortality rates. Marked country differences still remain, however (Fig. 2.5)[39]. Only 65 countries have maternal mortality ratios less than 50 per 100 000 live births; 42 of these countries are in the European region (not shown).

2.3.2 The present

Although maternal deaths make up less than 1% of all deaths (Fig. 2.2), exact estimation is difficult. Maternal mortality includes causes of death directly attributable to pregnancy, deaths caused by pre-existing conditions, and deaths due to causes unrelated to the pregnancy. The official definition excludes incidental causes but in practice this does not always occur. Several methods exist to estimate the likely number of maternal deaths but, as with all global health estimates, considerable uncertainty remains. In most of the world, maternal mortality is underestimated because of the absence of an adequate vital

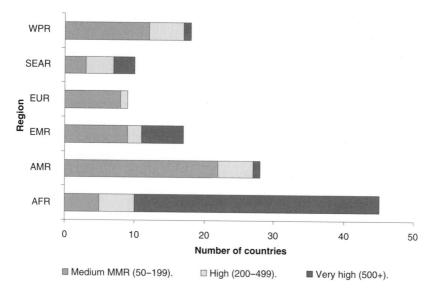

Fig. 2.5. Maternal mortality ratios for WHO regions, 2000. Number of countries by level of MMR (per 100 000 births). AFR, African region; AMR, Americas region; EMR, Eastern Mediterranean region; EUR, European region; SEAR, South-east Asia region; WPR, Western Pacific region.

registration system. There have been few population-based studies of the causes of maternal mortality in poor countries and this hampers an understanding of the real situation[40].

The vast majority of the estimated half million maternal deaths, occur in poor countries. The main cause of maternal mortality worldwide is unsafe abortion[41]. A recent decision by the US Government to freeze funds for the United Nations Fund for Population Activities (UNFPA) will have major consequences for maternal health. The loss of the US contribution will cut UNFPA's budget by around 10% leading, by some estimations, to approximately 2 million unwanted pregnancies which, in turn, will lead to 800 000 abortions that otherwise could have been avoided[42].

The global variation in maternal death rates is greater than for any other population subgroup. The highest maternal mortality rates are in sub-Saharan Africa, where the lifetime risk in women in east Africa is 1 in 12 compared with 1 in 4000 women in northern Europe[43,44]. Young adolescents in Africa and Asia receiving no prenatal care have up to a 5% chance of dying during pregnancy[45].

The Millennium Development Goal for improving maternal health is a reduction by three-quarters by 2015, of the maternal mortality ratio[46]. There are two associated indicators: the maternal mortality ratio and the proportion of births attended by skilled health personnel. This goal is unlikely to be met in most of sub-Saharan Africa without major action for the provision of expanded family planning services and screening, referral, and improved services for antenatal and obstetric care, although it has been estimated that cost-effective interventions are available (\$3 per woman and \$230 per death averted)[47,48]. Other important effects of childbirth, apart from maternal mortality, include morbidity and long-term disability that can result from childbirth in less than ideal circumstances. For example, it has been estimated that there are over 100 acute morbidity episodes for every maternal death[49]. Sustaining affordable improvements in safe motherhood depends on improving the functioning of health systems, as a whole, at the same time as making maternity care a priority[43].

2.4 Adult deaths

2.4.1 Past trends

There are marked regional and country variations in adult mortality. As with child and infant mortality, adult mortality has improved, although differences between countries remain great. Most countries have experienced a fall in total mortality in both men and women over the last 40 years although death rates increased, especially in men, in Central and Eastern Europe. The greatest improvements have occurred in Japan with the lowest total mortality rates in both men and women. The situation in at least some poor countries is also improving, although reliable data are available for only a few countries, for example, Sri Lanka, Chile, Costa Rica and Cuba, where the chances of dying have fallen consistently since the 1950s, except for men in Sri Lanka[50].

2.4.2 The present

The top ten disease and injury causes of death in 2001 for developed countries and developing countries are shown in Table 2.4. In developed countries, ischaemic heart disease and cerebrovascular disease (stroke) are together responsible for 36% of mortality, and death rates are higher for men than women. This proportion has decreased only slightly from 38% in 1990[8]. The increase in cardiovascular mortality in Eastern European countries has been offset by continuing declines in many other developed countries. Lung cancer is the third leading cause of death, again with a nearly three-fold male excess. Another largely tobacco-related cause, chronic obstructive lung disease, is the fifth leading cause of death, accounting for 3% of deaths in developed countries. Suicide accounts for nearly 2% of deaths in developed countries, a proportion

Table 2.4. *Ten leading causes of death, developed and developing countries, 2001*[8]

Developed countries[a]	% of total deaths	Developing countries	% of total deaths
1 Ischaemic heart disease	22.2	1 Ischaemic heart disease	16.9
2 Cerebrovascular disease	13.8	2 Lower respiratory infections	14.8
3 Trachea, bronchus, lung cancers	4.5	3 Cerebrovascular disease	14.1
4 Lower respiratory infections	3.7	4 HIV/AIDS	13.2
5 COPD [b]	3.0	5 Perinatal conditions	10.4
6 Colon and rectum cancers	2.6	6 Diarrhoeal diseases	9.4
7 Stomach cancer	2.0	7 COPD [b]	9.3
8 Self-inflicted injuries	1.9	8 Tuberculosis	6.8
9 Diabetes mellitus	1.8	9 Malaria	4.9
10 Cirrhosis of the liver	1.7	10 Road traffic crashes	4.7

[a] Developed countries includes European countries, former Soviet countries, Canada, USA, Japan, Australia, New Zealand.
[b] Chronic obstructive pulmonary disease.

that has remained unchanged since 1990. Road traffic crashes are no longer in the top ten causes of mortality, as there has been a decline in death rates due to road traffic crashes of nearly 30% since 1990.

The leading causes of mortality are very different in developing countries. While the three leading causes of death include ischaemic heart disease and cerebrovascular disease, together claiming one-third of all deaths in developing countries, six of the top ten causes of death in developing countries are infectious and perinatal causes. Acute lower respiratory infections (primarily pneumonia) are the second leading cause of death (60% of these among children aged under 5). HIV/AIDS is the fourth leading cause of death for developing countries, accounting for over 10% of all deaths or 2.9 million deaths in total. More than 80% of these deaths occurred in Africa, making HIV the leading cause of death in this region, claiming almost one in four deaths. About 1 in ten of all adult AIDS deaths are caused by tuberculosis[51]. Tuberculosis, responsible for a total of 1.6 million deaths in 2001 and road traffic crashes (responsible for 1.2 million deaths) are ranked in the top 10 in developing countries. One in 8 of all deaths from tuberculosis are attributable to HIV[51]. Chronic obstructive lung disease kills more people (1.5 million) in the Western Pacific Region (primarily

China) than anywhere else in the world, with 60% of global mortality from the disease occurring there[8].

Other leading causes of death in developing countries include two major causes of childhood mortality, perinatal conditions and diarrhoeal diseases, which claim a total of 2.5 and 2.0 million lives each year respectively, and malaria (1.1 million deaths, mostly in children under 5 years of age). While death rates due to perinatal conditions have declined slightly compared with 1990, death rates due to diarrhoeal diseases have declined substantially, from an estimated 2.9 million deaths in 1990[1].

There were an estimated 1.2 million lung cancer deaths in 2001, an increase of nearly 30% in the 10 years from 1990. This represents one in six (17%) of all cancer deaths; three-quarters occurred among men. This was an increase of nearly 30% in the decade since 1990. Stomach cancer, which until recently was the leading site of cancer mortality worldwide, has been declining in all parts of the world where trends can be reliably assessed and now causes 850 000 deaths each year, or about two-thirds as many as lung cancer. Liver cancer is the third leading site, with 616 000 deaths a year, more than half (60%) of which are estimated to occur in the Western Pacific Region.

The chance of an adult dying prematurely (arbitrarily defined as between the age of 15 and 59 years) varies markedly between countries and by broad cause (Fig. 2.6). Almost one-third (31%) of all deaths in developing countries

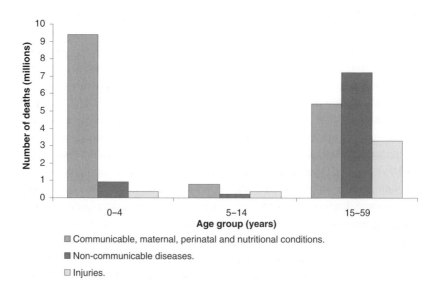

Communicable, maternal, perinatal and nutritional conditions.

Non-communicable diseases.

Injuries.

Fig. 2.6. Premature deaths by broad cause and age group, men and women combined, 2001.

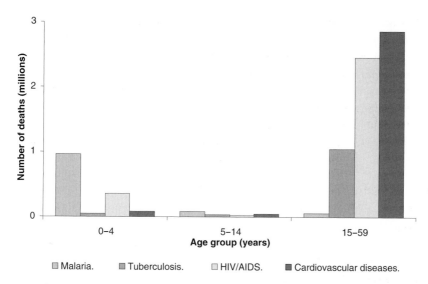

Fig. 2.7. Premature deaths by selected cause and age group, men and women combined, 2001.

occur at young adult ages (15–59 years), compared with 15% in richer regions. Differences in the risk of premature death are largely explained by variations in non-communicable disease death rates, although communicable disease deaths remain important, largely in sub-Saharan Africa, and to a lesser extent, in India.

It is perhaps surprising that the risk of premature death in men and women from non-communicable diseases is higher in poor countries than in the wealthy countries, apart from Central and Eastern European countries. Non-communicable diseases, largely cardiovascular disease (CVD), are the major cause of premature death in this age group, responsible for half of all deaths. Injuries are an important cause of death in men in all regions (one-quarter of all deaths in men aged 15–59 years) and the risk of dying from injury is especially high in Central and Eastern European countries (one-third of all deaths in this age group). A cause of concern is the relatively early age of CVD deaths in the developing countries compared with the developed countries[2]. It is noteworthy that there are almost as many premature deaths from cardiovascular diseases as AIDS, malaria and TB combined (Fig. 2.7).

Even within wealthy countries there are striking variations between ethnic and cultural groups. For example, in the United States of America premature mortality in African–American men and women is 90% and 80% higher than in white men and women, respectively. The death experience of African–American men in the United States is comparable to that among men in some of the poorest nations in the world, such as The Gambia and India.

In poor countries, the leading causes of deaths for adult women are cardiovascular diseases, cancer, tuberculosis, digestive diseases and respiratory infections. For men, the ranking is cardiovascular diseases, digestive diseases, unintentional injuries, tuberculosis, cancer and respiratory infections.

2.4.3 Recent trends in causes of adult deaths in wealthy countries

In the early years of last century, infectious diseases such as tuberculosis were still the leading causes of adult mortality. However, from about the 1920s, heart disease and stroke became increasingly important, especially in men, along with several kinds of cancer, notably lung cancer. A feature of the trends in the United States of America and many other wealthy countries, is the decline in cardiovascular death rates since the mid-1970s. The greatest decline in cause-specific death rates has occurred in Japan where stroke death rates have declined by over 70% in the last few decades. This illustrates the point that non-communicable disease death rates do not always increase as the health transition occurs; stomach cancer rates have also fallen and coronary heart disease death rates are low in Japan. It remains to be seen whether heart disease rates will stay low in Japan because the diet is slowly changing in an adverse direction, and cigarette smoking is common, especially in men.

There have been several major exceptions to the recent favourable trends in adult mortality patterns, for example, AIDS and deaths due to injury. The most notable and long-standing exception, and numerically the most important, however, has been the emergence over the last 50 years of the tobacco-caused epidemics, particularly lung cancer. In some countries, such as the United Kingdom, the United States of America and Australia, the lung cancer epidemic has peaked in men, but is still increasing in women. When the substantial effects of tobacco are discounted, there is little evidence that the overall incidence of cancer is rising[52]. Some cancers, for example, stomach cancer, are declining rapidly, perhaps as a result of dietary changes[53]. It appears that, in the United Kingdom, the United States of America and Sweden, rates of some non-smoking-caused cancers may be increasing, for example, testicular cancer, melanoma and oesophageal cancer[54]. These trends are important. Although tobacco smoking is the most important preventable cause of cancer and several other diseases, about 70% of cancer cases are not directly linked to smoking;

other important environmental causes of cancer remain to be discovered. In many countries, particularly the poorer countries, the tobacco related epidemic is only just beginning, as it takes approximately 20 years of heavy smoking before lung cancer appears.

2.4.4 Recent trends in causes of adult deaths in poor countries

The adult health situation in poor countries is much less clear[50]. The major reason for this uncertainty is the lack of routine cause specific mortality statistics; very few poor countries have 100% medical certification of death[55]. Where data are available, trends in cause specific death rates of adults in poor countries are variable. Some countries such as Chile and Costa Rica have experienced recent increases in life expectancy, and there has been an apparent decline in death rates for the major causes of death[50]. These declines in non-communicable disease death rates are surprising and would not have been predicted on the basis of the health transition as two forces underlying the transition, the demographic and health determinants components, have been acting to increase the age-specific rates of non-communicable diseases. It is extremely unlikely that the health care component is sufficiently powerful to control the increase in the mortality rates. In Cuba there has been an increase in non-communicable disease death rates, especially in men. In most poor countries, death rates from injury have increased in men. Even if the age-specific rates are declining in some poor countries, the total burden of non-communicable disease in these countries will increase with the ageing of the population. Interpretation of adult mortality trends in poor countries must be cautious until more reliable data are available.

2.4.5 Deaths in older people

The rapidity of ageing is without precedent; for example, it took over 100 years for Belgium to double the proportion of its 60+ population from 9% to 18%. China will take 34 years and Singapore only 20 years to achieve the same population ageing[56]. It is essential that ageing worldwide be taken seriously in terms of both research and the development of appropriate health and social policies; it is unlikely that poor countries will be able to implement adequate support systems, given their economic status and the lack of political will. As longevity increases in all countries, the health experience of elderly people assumes greater importance, both socially and economically.

In 2000, 6.9% of the world's population was over the age of 65 years and projections suggest that, by 2015, the world's elderly population will be 8.3% of

Table 2.5. *Proportion of total population aged 65 years and over in 2000, by level of development and projections to 2015*[5]

	Total population (millions)		Population aged 65 and above (as % of total)	
	2000	2015	2000	2015
High income countries	878	929	14.7	18.3
Middle income countries	2675	3037	6.6	8.5
Low income countries	2397	3096	4.5	5.2
World	5950	7062	6.9	8.3

the total, with the bulk of this increase occurring in poor countries (Table 2.5)[57]. The proportion of people 65 years and over in 2000 in high income countries was 14.7% compared with 4.5% in low income countries. More older people live in low and middle income countries, about 285 million people, in contrast to the 130 million people in this age group in high income countries. Yet the percentage increase of the older population in developing countries is much higher than in developed countries.

Projections to 2015 suggest that two-thirds of the 500 million people 65 years and over will be living in poor and middle income countries. In this older age group the majority of deaths are from non-communicable diseases.

2.4.6 Avoidable deaths

Several estimates have been made of the proportion of deaths that are either avoidable (preventable) or amenable to the effects of health services. One method uses current knowledge to determine the proportion of deaths from each disease which is considered preventable. Another uses, as a reference population, a country or population subgroup with low mortality and takes this experience as an ultimately achievable goal for all countries. In this latter method, potentially preventable deaths are those which would not have occurred if the death rates were the same as in the reference population. This method is based on actual death rates and therefore most appropriately reflects what is achievable. Using Japan as the reference population, over 90% of deaths in children less than 5 years and over 70% of adult deaths in the age group 15–59 years in poor countries are avoidable[2]. Even among older people, there is much room for improvement. For example, in wealthy countries it has been estimated that about one in five of all deaths in men and one in 12 of all deaths in women in the age group 70 years and over are directly related to cigarette smoking[52].

Achieving such major reductions in death rates will not be easy. Indeed, some might consider it an impossible goal. In view of the tremendous reductions in death rates that have occurred in Japan in the last half century, however, cautious optimism is appropriate. Reducing death rates globally to the Japanese level will require a range of policy measures; there is no simple 'magic bullet' intervention. Unfortunately, the improvements in mortality in Japan are not readily explainable, although it does appear that the Japanese commitment to relative income equality has been one factor in their success[58]. Above all, political will is now required to make reducing death rates a global and national priority.

2.5 Disease and disability

2.5.1 Measuring the impact of disease and disability

Premature deaths, because of the great potential for prevention they represent, are a major challenge for public health. Death alone as an indicator of health status, however, fails to account for the full burden of disease and disability. Various attempts have been made to develop more comprehensive health indicators. The global burden of disease (GBD) project developed a new summary measure that combines the impact of premature mortality with that of disability and captures the impact on populations of important non-fatal disabling conditions[59]. Disability adjusted life years (DALYs) combines time lost through premature death and time lived with disability. One DALY can be thought of as one lost year of 'healthy' life and the measured disease burden is the gap between a population's health status and that of a normative reference population (with life expectancy at birth of 82.5 years for females and 80.0 years for males). The DALY provides a way to link information at the population level on disease causes and occurrence to information on both short-term and long-term health outcomes, including impairments, disability and death. In this measure causes of death that occur early in life are weighted more heavily than those that occur later in life and do not take into account competing risks[60], but rather measure years lost against a normative standard[61].

The WHO undertook a new assessment of the GBD in 2000 based on an extensive analysis of mortality data for all regions of the world, together with systematic reviews of epidemiological studies and population health surveys. These revisions drew on a wide range of data sources, and various methods were developed to reconcile often fragmented and partial estimates of epidemiological parameters that are available from different studies. In some regions, however, and for many diseases, the necessary data on disease incidence and duration are simply not available. This gap is especially apparent for the adult diseases, which, as we have seen, make up the bulk of the deaths worldwide. For more precise estimates, data are required for subgroups of disease. Furthermore, the method summarises the disease experience on a regional basis, often without any assurance that the data are applicable to the entire region. The data on disability are particularly poor, apart from a few diseases, for example, stroke, which have been extensively studied in wealthy countries. Even for stroke, there is a real problem in differentiating stroke related disability from generalised disability[62]. This is an important limitation of the DALYs measure because disability contributes as much as half of all DALYs.

The GBD project in general, and the DALY measure in particular, have stimulated considerable debate, in part due to the limitations of the basic data, the extrapolations from these data to entire regions, the assumptions that are needed for these estimates, and even the justification for the project[63, 64]. The greatest degree of uncertainty relates to the sub-Saharan estimates because of the scarcity of epidemiological, data[65]. The GBD project includes an assessment of all causes of disease and injury burden. Where the evidence is uncertain, incomplete or even non-existent, the best possible inferences based on the knowledge base that is available, are used to assess the uncertainty in the resulting estimates[66]. This has generated controversy among epidemiologists, who are more used to reporting only assessments with narrow uncertainty intervals primarily based on sampling error[63].

The social values and disability weights incorporated into the DALYs have also attracted criticism. Some critics have argued against the use of age weights that give lower value to years of life lived in early childhood and older ages[64, 66] and some recent national burden of disease studies have used time discounting but not age weights[67].

However, perhaps the most persistent criticisms have been that burden of disease analysis may result in incorrect policy decisions with an end result penalising the poor and elderly people by according priority to young and middle ages[68] or by fuelling competition for resources between advocates for communicable disease and noncommunicable disease prevention strategies[69] when many of the global forces underlying these disease categories are similar[67, 70]. These criticisms stem from a concern that priorities for health action might be set solely on the basis of the magnitude of burden of disease. However, the different diseases, injuries and risk factors contributing to loss of health are important factors, as are cost-effectiveness of interventions and other information relating to equity and social values in informing health policy in relation to the potentials for improvement of population health[1].

2.5.2 The global disease burden

The leading causes of DALYs worldwide for the year 2000 are shown in Table 2.6. Lower respiratory infections, perinatal conditions, HIV/AIDS and unipolar depressive disorders are the three leading causes of DALYs for men and women combined. The global burden of diarrhoeal diseases, conditions arising in the perinatal period, and congenital anomalies have all declined, from a combined total of 16.3% of total DALYs in 1990 to 12.6% in 2000. Reflecting the huge increase in HIV incidence between 1990 and 2000, HIV/AIDS has leapt from the 28th leading cause of DALYs (0.8%) in 1990 to third leading cause (6.7%) in 2001.

The total DALYs are similar in magnitude for men and women. A main sex difference is for depression, which is the fourth leading cause of disease burden in women but ranks seventh for men. Road traffic injuries are a leading cause of overall disease and injury burden in men (3.4%) but not in women (1.6%). When DALYs rather than deaths are considered, the public health importance of injuries becomes more apparent. In parts of South Asia, Eastern Europe and the Western Pacific, 20% or more of the entire disease and injury burden is due to injuries alone.

Table 2.6 also highlights the marked contrast in epidemiological patterns between different regions of the world, even more so than comparisons based on deaths. Thus in the more developed countries, the share of disease burden due to communicable, maternal, perinatal and nutritional conditions is typically around 5%, compared with 70–75% in Africa (not shown). Specifically, the leading causes of disease burden in Africa in 2001 were HIV/AIDS (20.6%), malaria (10.1%) and acute lower respiratory infections (8.6%), compared with ischaemic heart disease, depression, alcohol dependence and stroke in the developed countries. Table 2.6 also highlights the differences between high mortality and low mortality developing countries; the latter epidemiological subgroup has disease burdens similar to that of developed countries.

Given that, in the calculation of the disease burden, deaths that occur early in life are weighted more heavily than those that occur later in life, it is noteworthy that in young adults (15–59 years) injuries and non-communicable diseases account for 2.5 times as many DALYs as communicable disease. Conversely, the bulk of disease burden in children under 5 years is for communicable disease (Fig. 2.8).

Table 2.6. *Ten leading causes of disease burden (DALYs) globally and in developed and developing countries, 2001*

			Low mortality		High mortality	
Developed countries[a]		% total DALYs	Developing countries	% total DALYs	Developing countries	% total DALYs
1	Ischaemic heart disease	9.4%	1 Unipolar depressive disorders	5.9%	1 HIV/AIDS	9.0%
2	Unipolar depressive disorders	7.2%	2 Cerebrovascular disease	4.9%	2 Lower respiratory infections	8.2%
3	Cerebrovascular disease	6.0%	3 Lower respiratory conditions	4.1%	3 Diarrhoeal diseases	6.3%
4	Alcohol use disorders	3.5%	4 Road traffic injuries	4.19%	4 Childhood cluster diseases	5.5%
5	Dementias	3.0%	5 COPD[b]	3.8%	5 Low birth weight	5.0%
6	Hearing loss, adult onset	2.8%	6 Ischaemic heart disease	3.2%	6 Malaria	4.9%
7	Road traffic injuries	2.5%	7 Birth trauma	2.6%	7 Unipolar depressive disorders	3.1%
8	COPD[b]	2.6%	8 Tuberculosis	2.4%	8 Ischaemic heart disease	3.0%
9	Osteoarthritis	2.5%	9 Alcohol use disorder	2.3%	9 Tuberculosis	2.9%
10	Lung cancer	2.4%	10 Hearing loss	2.2%	10 Road traffic injuries	2.0%

[a] Developed countries include Established Market Economies (EME) and Former Socialist Economies (FSE).
[b] Chronic Obstructive Pulmonary Disease

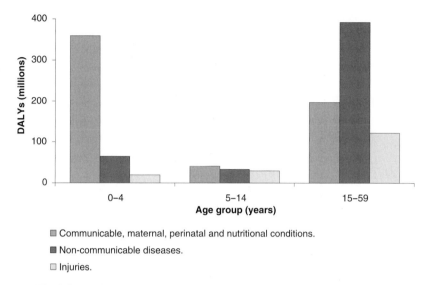

Communicable, maternal, perinatal and nutritional conditions.
Non-communicable diseases.
Injuries.

Fig. 2.8. Burden of disease (in million DALYs), by broad cause, age group, men and women combined, 2001[8].

2.5.3 Health expectancy measures

Another form of summary measure of population health, health expectancy, has been used since the 1970s to report on average levels of population health. Disability-free life expectancy (DFLE) was calculated and reported for many countries in the 1980s and 1990s[71,72]. Unfortunately, DFLE estimates based on self-reported health status information are not comparable across countries due to differences in survey instruments and cultural differences in reporting of health[61].

In the World Health Report 2000, WHO reported for the first time on the average levels of population health for its 191 member countries using disability-adjusted life expectancy (DALE). DALE measures the equivalent number of years of life expected to be lived in full health[22]. Updated estimates of healthy life expectancy for the year 2000 were published in the World Health Report 2001 using improved methods and incorporating cross-population comparable survey data from 63 surveys in 55 countries[23]. To reflect the inclusion of all states of health better in the calculation of healthy life expectancy, the name of the indicator used to measure healthy life expectancy was changed from DALE to HALE (healthy life expectancy). Some commentators have argued that the data demands and complexity of the calculations make healthy life expectancy an impractical measure for use as a summary measure of population health[73]. Although the concept of healthy life expectancy is relatively simple

Table 2.7. *Life expectancy (LE), healthy life expectancy (HALE), and lost healthy years as per cent of total LE (LHE%), at birth and at age 60, by sex and total, WHO regions and world, 2001*[1]

WHO Region	Persons			Males			Females		
	HALE (years)	LE (years)	LHE% (%)	HALE (years)	LE (years)	LHE% (%)	HALE (years)	LE (years)	LHE% (%)
At birth									
AFRO	39.2	48.0	18.4	37.3	46.7	20.1	41.1	49.3	16.7
AMRO	63.2	73.7	14.3	60.4	70.4	14.1	65.9	77.0	14.4
EMRO	51.8	62.4	17.1	50.6	61.1	17.2	52.9	63.7	16.9
EURO	63.2	72.2	12.4	60.3	68.1	11.4	66.1	76.3	13.3
SEARO	52.3	61.8	15.3	52.0	60.7	14.2	52.6	62.8	16.3
WPRO	63.6	72.0	11.6	61.9	69.9	11.4	65.4	74.1	11.8
World	56.0	65.0	13.8	54.3	62.7	13.4	57.7	67.2	14.2
At age 60									
AFRO	8.8	15.1	42.2	7.4	14.1	47.3	10.1	16.2	37.6
AMRO	15.0	21.3	29.4	13.6	19.4	30.2	16.5	23.1	28.7
EMRO	9.9	16.4	39.7	9.1	15.6	41.5	10.7	17.2	38.1
EURO	13.9	19.3	28.2	12.5	17. 2	27.2	15.2	21.4	28.9
SEARO	10.4	16.3	36.2	10.0	15.5	35.4	10.8	17.2	36.9
WPRO	14.4	19.6	26.2	13.3	18.1	26.5	15.6	21.1	25.9
World	12.9	18.4	30.0	11.6	16.7	30.3	14.2	20.2	29.7

AFR, African region; AMR, Americas region; EMR, Eastern Mediterranean region; EUR, European region; SEAR, South-east Asia region; WPR, Western Pacific region.

to understand, health encompasses multiple domains and mortality risks, and with the additional requirement to ensure comparability of estimates across countries, any acceptable methods used to compute healthy life expectancy inevitably will be complex.

The first estimates of HALE show that overall, global HALE at birth is 56.0 years in 2001, 9.0 years lower than total life expectancy at birth of 65.0 years (Table 2.7). Japan had the highest average healthy life expectancy of 74.5 years at birth in 2001. The bottom ten countries are all in sub-Saharan Africa where the HIV/AIDS epidemic is most prevalent, resulting in HALE at birth of less than 40 years. The male to female gap overall is lower for HALE than for total life expectancy; the global HALE for females at birth is just over 3 years greater than that for men. Thus, although women live on average 4.5 years longer than men, they spend a greater amount of time with disability.

A similar pattern can be seen for regional healthy life expectancies at age 60; HALE ranged from a low of 7.4 years for men in the African region to a high of around 16.5 years for women in the Americas. The equivalent 'lost' healthy years at age 60 are a higher percentage of remaining life expectancy, owing to the higher prevalence of disability at older ages. These range from around 40–50% in Africa to around 25–30% in developed countries.

2.6 Inequalities in health

The focus so far in this chapter has been on inequalities in health at the regional level, particularly for conditions that are preventable. Even within countries, major inequalities are apparent and occur irrespective of whether the population is categorised by social class, income, occupation, education or ethnicity. Inequalities in health status have always existed, but it is only over the last few decades, and primarily in the United Kingdom, that social class inequalities have received systematic research attention; epidemiologists usually consider social class as a 'nuisance' variable, rather than as a powerful explanatory variable. The findings from the United Kingdom have now been replicated in most other western countries, although the vital statistics of the United States of America only report basic data about the health of the nation in terms of race, sex, and age[74]. Evidence is also emerging on the existence of health inequalities in Central and Eastern European countries[75,76].

Entrenched health inequalities reflect the failure of social policy to address social and economic deprivation. Inequalities have also been seen either as a biological phenomenon associated with random variation in the population distribution of health[77] or as the unintended consequences of success in expanding the advantages of the upper social classes[78]. Random variation is an unlikely explanation given that the extent, and even the direction, of health inequalities can change surprisingly quickly. From a human rights perspective, the health of one group of people should not be valued more highly than that of other groups.

Social class patterns have changed over the last 40 years. For example, from the 1930s to the 1950s coronary heart disease rates were highest in the upper social classes in the United Kingdom, but by the 1970s the pattern had reversed[79]. Despite the continuing decline in mortality rates, social class gradients have either remained constant or increased; Japan is an exception in that social class differences in mortality have apparently narrowed since the 1950s[80]. Even within occupational groups that are far from deprived, such as British civil servants, there is a sharp social class effect[81]. This indicates the importance to health of relative deprivation, in addition to the more widely recognised effects of absolute deprivation.

It is more difficult to assess the links between social class and mortality for women than it is for men because of the way social class is usually measured. In most national vital registration systems, a woman's position is based on her husband's occupational status, ignoring the independence of a woman's life separate from her spouse. In an attempt to overcome this problem, a variety of additional data derived from a British longitudinal study linking census and mortality data have been examined[82]. High mortality rates among women were associated with working in a manual occupation, being a single woman in a manual occupation, living in a rented house, and having no access to a car. When these indicators are combined, mortality rates were found to be two to three times higher than for women with none of these disadvantages[81]. These data indicate that it is necessary to use multiple measures to reflect accurately the relationship between a woman's life circumstances and mortality.

Several possible explanations for the health inequalities have been advanced: misclassification of social class, particularly in women and retired people; a downward drift because of ill health; inequalities in the distribution of major risk factors for disease; generalised susceptibility to ill health in lower social classes; inequalities in the distribution of income; and internalised racism. Epidemiological research allows several of these explanations to be rejected. Misclassification and downward drift can be ruled out on the evidence from long-term epidemiological studies. Inequalities in the distribution of known risk factors for cardiovascular disease or cancer explain only a part of the inequalities in death and disease. An important reason for inequalities in health appears to be the distribution of wealth within a country[83]. In countries where income distribution is relatively equal, health inequalities are less than in countries where there are gross disparities in wealth. This explanation will be explored in more depth in the next chapter. At a more general level, health inequalities reflect social policies which neglect the needs of poor people. A case has been made for routine reporting of total health inequality estimates alongside average levels of health in populations and groups. This would allow meaningful comparisons of inequality across countries and an understanding of the determinants of inequality[84].

2.7 Explaining trends in mortality

The historical improvements in mortality rates have been obvious and dramatic. We cannot assume, however, that life expectancy will continue to increase into the next century, especially given the experience in many African countries and some Central and Eastern European countries where life expectancy fell in the 1990s.

 * The explanations for these trends are difficult to disentangle, and the health transition theory provides only limited guidance. In part, our difficulty stems

from the multi-factorial nature of the causes of death. Another problem is our limited ability to relate changes in possible causes and mortality trends at a population level in any meaningful quantitative manner. A further complication stems from the focus on mortality trends in Western Europe, justified on the basis of the availability of better long-term data from this region. The population of Western Europe, however, is only a small (and diminishing) proportion of the world's population. Furthermore, most countries of the world, including the most populous (China and India), have experienced major mortality declines only in the last few decades. The causes of the mortality decline in Western Europe in the nineteenth century will be different from the causes operating in China and India in the twenty-first century.

Various explanations have been advanced for the decline in mortality rates, which gathered speed in nineteenth-century Europe. McKeown proposed that steady improvements in nutrition beginning in the eighteenth century, together with improvements in water supply and sanitation services, an increase in the general standard of living following the Industrial Revolution, and a reduction in birth rates propelled the health transition[71]. The development of effective medical measures was too late to make a major contribution to the mortality decline in Europe and other western countries. For example, it has been estimated that, at most, only 3.5% of the total decline in mortality in the United States of America between 1900 and 1973 could be ascribed to medical measures introduced for the major infectious diseases[72]. On the other hand, targeted public health interventions including vaccination, personal hygiene campaigns, and improved child health care services, were of major importance[3,85].

McKeown's thesis generated controversy, which was fuelled by critics of medicine, such as Illich[86], who were concerned at the medicalisation of modern society and the power of the health professionals. Ironically, McKeown's ideas also encouraged many economists indirectly in the belief that improvements in health for the entire population would come from unrestrained economic development and that a reduction in social and health inequalities should not be necessarily a priority of social policy. One unfortunate effect of this policy has been a widening of income inequality. For example, the lowest 10% of the population in the United Kingdom, in terms of income in the early 1990s, were about 17% worse off than they were in the late 1970s.[87]

The more recent decline in mortality in poorer countries has some parallels with nineteenth-century Europe. For example, the dramatic gains in China in the last four decades were associated with major improvements in food supply (despite occasional devastating famines) as well as public health campaigns directed at the control of infectious diseases; literacy, especially for females, has also been of major importance[88]. The most recent declines in mortality, however, have been influenced greatly by public health and medical care advances[89]. For example, smallpox, a major scourge of humankind for centuries, has been eradicated, and for a period, malaria was controlled in many parts of the world, and children have benefited from global efforts to increase immunisation coverage, oral rehydration therapy for diarrhoea, and appropriate care for acute respiratory infections.

The modern decline in mortality from non-communicable diseases in rich countries also shows the influence of both public health campaigns and medical care[90]. The major influence in the early stages of the decline in coronary heart disease mortality beginning in the late 1960s and early 1970s, appears to have been changes in diet and smoking habits, although the evidence is incomplete. More recent trends have occurred as a result of major reductions in community risk factor levels, accounting, for example, for much of the decline in coronary heart disease death rates in Finland since1970[91,92]. Risk factor levels have improved as a result of public health campaigns directed primarily at the population as a whole. Medical care of established cardiovascular disease has been shown to be effective in reducing case fatality, especially in hospitalised patients, but from a population perspective, is making smaller contributions to the mortality declines than improvements in population levels of risk factors[93]. In contrast, lung cancer rates are declining in men in some countries purely as a result of the dissemination of research findings and public health campaigns; medical and surgical therapy has little impact on lung cancer death rates.

Evidence from population groups, which have undergone the health transition in the last few decades, for example, New Zealand Maori, indicate the importance of health policies nested in the context of positive social policies. The New Zealand governments of the early decades of the last century, and in particular the Labour Government of 1933–38, implemented a wide range of policies to strengthen the welfare state; collectively these policies had a dramatic and beneficial impact on Maori mortality rates[94].

There are important lessons to be learnt from the health transition in both rich and poor countries. Historically, social and economic developments, which improved nutritional status and sanitary systems and increased the literacy of women, together with public health interventions, have been of major importance. General developments have interacted with more specific public health measures directed towards the control of infectious diseases and, more recently, non-communicable disease. Medical care services do have an impact on population mortality trends, especially on child mortality in poor countries; for adults this impact is smaller, although these services are of tremendous importance in relieving suffering. The major gains in health status in the future will come most effectively and efficiently from public health measures.

2.8 Emerging issues

A feature of the current global health status picture is the 'double burden' of disease. Countries that are still struggling with old and new infectious disease epidemics must now also deal with the emerging epidemics of chronic non-communicable disease such as heart disease, stroke, diabetes and cancer. In both developing and developed regions, alcohol, tobacco, high blood pressure and high cholesterol are major causes of disease burden and are covered in greater detail in Chapter 3. Just five risk factors – unsafe sexual practices, alcohol and tobacco use, indoor air pollution, occupational exposures – account for at least 20% of the world's disease burden[1].

The non-communicable disease burden becomes especially evident as populations age and as population risk factor profiles change, partly in response to globalisation (see Chapter 10). In the developed countries the ageing of the population is occurring in a relatively slow and predictable manner, and in some, such as Japan and Sweden, the rate of ageing is already slowing down. Already more than half (57%) of the world's population over the age of 65 years live in developing countries. The proportion of the world's population over 65 years, currently 7%, will more than double (to 16%) in the next 50 years. The most explosive ageing will occur in some of the poorer regions of the world, particularly in India, Indonesia, and China; within the next half century, the number of people aged 65 years or more will increase six-fold in the South East Asian region of the WHO.

In the absence of preventive action, these rapid demographic changes, particularly in poorer regions of the world, will lead to an increase in the burden of non-communicable diseases. The non-communicable disease epidemics are essentially preventable according to existing knowledge. Over the last 50 years an extensive body of research has accumulated in different settings using a variety of methods including laboratory, clinical methods, and quantitative and qualitative population sciences. It is well known, for example, that the major established risk factors common to many non-communicable diseases (smoking, high blood pressure, inadequate diet, lack of physical activity), are responsible for most of the occurrence of premature cardiovascular disease in developed countries[93, 95]. This research has identified appropriate strategies for the prevention and control of noncommunicable disease and some of these lessons have been applied with good effect in wealthy countries. Efforts to reduce population cardiovascular disease risk factor levels, for example, have contributed to an important decline in cardiovascular disease death rates in many developed countries[92, 96], and tobacco-attributable mortality is now declining among men in several of these countries. Much more can be achieved on the basis of existing knowledge.

The causes of the non-communicable disease epidemics in developing countries appear to be largely the same as in wealthy countries[97]. The challenge will be to translate this knowledge into effective action in developing countries in order to avoid the predictable, but largely preventable, burden of non-communicable diseases, in particular, cardiovascular diseases. It has been estimated, for example, that the combination of personal and non-personal health interventions could lower the incidence of cardiovascular disease events by as much as 75%[98].

It is difficult for poorer countries to focus on medium-term preventive strategies in the face of more immediate health problems, even though over 40% of all deaths in the poorest 20% of the world's population are already due to non-communicable diseases. The 'double burden' of disease is being superceded by the 'triple burden'. To the unfinished agendas of infectious and non-communicable disease prevention and control is being added new health threats consequent on the new phase of globalisation (see Chapter 1). These new challenges potentially will worsen regional and national health inequalities[99].

2.9 Summary

The lack of routine collection of vital events severely hampers efforts to describe worldwide health trends. From the data that are available, however, death rates are declining and life expectancy is continuing to increase, except in countries in sub-Saharan Africa and Central and Eastern Europe. Despite these improvements, major inequalities in mortality between regions, and within regions, have remained almost unchanged over the last few decades. Indeed, improvements in global health status, as measured by gains in life expectancy and other measures and the reductions in preventable deaths, have been accompanied by a widening health and poverty gap between and within countries. Investment in health research and development remains focused largely on the health problems of the 10% of the world's richest populations and only 10% of funds available for health research is directed at improving the health of 90% of the world's population. This disparity, referred to as the 10/90 disequilibrium[100], requires urgent attention.

People living in poor countries not only face lower life expectancies than those in richer countries but also live a higher proportion of their lives in poor health[99]. Richer countries should be much more active in seeking ways to improve the health of the world's poor. WHO has been a strong advocate for efforts to increase the resources available for this purpose. The recent WHO Commission on Macroeconomics and Health took an optimistic view of the relationship between health expenditure/interventions and health outcomes[101]. It concluded that the bulk of the global disease burden is the result of a relatively small set of conditions, each with an existing set of effective interventions. The main problems are the funding of these interventions and access of poor populations to them. The Commission estimated that the essential interventions to target these problems could be provided for a per capita cost of around \$34 per person per year or a total annual increase in health expenditures of around \$17 billion by 2007 and \$29 billion by 2015, above the level of 2002.

Routine health status measures of health trends and inequalities are required to heighten awareness of their significance among policy makers, donors and international agencies. Better and more comprehensive data is a first step in the development of a stronger strategy to improve overall health and reduce inequalities in health status throughout the world. There is insufficient emphasis given to disease surveillance in most national health systems, a serious impediment to setting disease prevention and control priorities and for measuring progress. Additionally, there is as yet insufficient emphasis in national health data collection on the need for cross-population comparability. Despite the growing pressures of shrinking public sector resources, there is an urgent need for centralised organisations to collect data. There is a danger of this process becoming increasingly fragmented as a result of growing reliance upon private and voluntary sector organisations to collect such data.

The global health scene has been characterised by major steps forward but with some disturbing features. The measurement of health status is multi-faceted and must take account of differences between and within nations that inevitably impinge on the comparability of data. As a first and essential step, there is need for better national and regional heath surveillance systems. Without such data, particularly in poorer regions of the world, it will be difficult to know if, and how much, progress is being made in improving global health status and reducing growing health inequalities.

The health transition continues unevenly. In wealthy countries, child and maternal mortality rates are low, and the major causes of adult deaths are cardiovascular diseases, which are declining in most countries, and cancer. In poor countries the trends are variable, although statistics are scarce; however, most poor people today have lower mortality rates than wealthy people a century ago, indicating the important influence of the social, political, and economic environment on health status. Childhood infectious disease death rates have declined, but much preventable infectious disease remains.

The trend data that are available indicate that major improvements in death rates can occur over a relatively short time. The major feature of the current patterns of health worldwide is the enormous variation in the mortality and disease burden, especially between regions and countries, but also within countries. Most of the differences in the burden of disease between regions is due to differences in premature death; disability rates are more equal across regions. Furthermore, most of the regional mortality variations are due to the infectious diseases which are readily preventable. Yet, poor countries also experience the greatest burden from non-communicable diseases. While these too are largely preventable, they require more complex strategies than the prevention of infectious diseases.

Chapter 2   Key points

- Major global improvements have occurred in health status over the last five decades as measured by declining death rates and increasing life expectancy.
- The global inequalities in relative death rates have not changed substantially, and death rates have increased recently in some Sub Saharan African and Central and Eastern European countries.
- Detailed cause of death information is available for only one-third of the world's population; sample registration systems provide information on a further 40%.
- Of the 56 million deaths each year, half occur before the age of 60 years and 80% occur in poor countries. One-third of deaths are due to communicable diseases and almost half to non-communicable diseases and injuries; the epidemics of non-communicable diseases will inevitably increase as the world's population ages.
- Premature deaths are responsible for about 60% of the Disability Adjusted Life Years lost; disability is responsible for the remaining 40%.
- Entrenched inequalities in health status exist in all countries.

References

1. World Health Organization. *World Health Report 2002. Reducing Risks, Promoting Healthy Life*. Geneva: World Health Organization, 2002.
2. Yusuf, S., Reddy, S., Ounpuu, S. & Anand, S. Global burden of cardiovascular diseases. Part 1: general considerations, the epidemiologic transition, risk factors, and impact of urbanisation. *Circulation* 2001; **104**: 2746–53.
3. Powles, J. Changes in disease patterns and related social trends. *Soc. Sci. Med.* 1992; **35**: 377–87.

3M SelfCheck™ System

Customer name: LIN, TING-TING

Title: Public health at the crossroads :
achievements and prospects / Robert
Beaglehole and Ruth Bonita.

ID: 30114014348521

Due: 05-10-15

Total items: 1
28/09/2015 17:40
Overdue: 0

Thank you for using the
3M SelfCheck™ System.

4. Woods, R. The role of public health initiatives in the nineteenth-century mortality decline. In: Caldwell, J., Findley, S., Caldwell, P., Santow, G., Cosford, W., Braid, J. & Boers-Freeman, D. (eds.). *What We Know About Health Transition: The Cultural, Social and Behavioural Determinants of Health.* Canberra: Australian National University Printing Service, 1990; **1**: 110–15.

5. United Nations Development Programme. *Human Development Report 2002: Deepening Democracy in a Fragmented World.* New York: Oxford University Press, 2002.

6. Plavinsky, S.L., Plavinskaya, S.I. & Klimov, A.N. Social factors and increase in mortality in Russia in the 1990s: prospective cohort study. *Br. Med. J.* 2003; **326**: 1240–2.

7. Hertzman, C. & Siddiqi, A. Health and rapid economic change in the late twentieth century. *Soc. Sci. Med.* 2000; **51**: 809–19.

8. Bonita, R. & Mathers, C. Global health status at the beginning of the 21st century. In: Beaglehole, R. (ed.). *Global Public Health: A New Era.* Oxford: Oxford University Press, 2003.

9. Murray, C.J.L. & Lopez, A.D (eds.). The global burden of disease: a comprehensive assessment of mortality and disability from diseases, injuries and risk factors in 1990 and projected to 2020. *Global Burden of Disease and Injury Series*, Vol. 1. Cambridge: Harvard University Press, 1996.

10. Tüchsen, F. & Endahl, L.A. Increasing inequality in ischaemic heart disease among employed men in Denmark 1981–1993: the need for a new preventive policy. *Int. J. Epidemiol.* 1999; **28**: 640–4.

11. Drever, F. & Whitehead, M. *Health Inequalities: Decennial Supplement.* London: The Stationery Office, 1997.

12. Hahn, R.A. & Eberhardt, S. Life expectancy in four U.S. racial/ethnic populations: 1990. *Epidemiology* 1995; **6**: 350–5.

13. Schellekens, J. Mortality and socioeconomic status in two eighteenth century Dutch villages. *Population Studies* 1989; **43**: 391–404.

14. Najman, J.M. Health and poverty: past, present and prospects for the future. *Soc. Sci. Med.* 1993; **36**: 157–66.

15. Lopez, A.D. Counting the dead in China: measuring tobacco's impact in the developing world. *Br. Med. J.* 1998; **317**: 1399–400.

16. World Development Report. *Investing in Health: World Development Indicators.* New York: Oxford University Press, 1993.

17. TATA Institute of Fundamental Research. The Third International Workshop on Medical Certification of Causes of Death for India. *Proceedings of the International Meeting on Verbal Autopsy and on the Epidemiological Aspects of the Sample Registration System.* New Dehli, 2001.

18. Chandramohan, D., Maude, G., Rodrigues, L.C. & Hayes, R.J. Verbal autopsies for adult deaths: issues in their development and validation. *Int. J. Epidemiol.* 1994: **23**: 313–22.

19. Hoj, C., Stensballe, J. & Aabz, P. Maternal mortality in Guinea Bisseau: the use of verbal autopsies in a multi ethnic population. *Int. J. Epidemiol.* 1999; **28**: 70–6.

20. Morris, L., Danel, I., Stupp, P. & Sarbanescu, F. Household surveys to evaluate reproductive health programmes. In: Khlat, M. (ed.). *Demographic Evaluation of Health Programmes.* UNFPA, French Ministry of Cooperation. 1996; 75–87.

21. Murray, C.J.M., King, G., Lopez, A. *et al.* Armed conflict as a public health problem. *Br. Med. J.* 2002; **324**: 346–9.
22. World Health Organization. *World Health Report 2000. Health Systems: Improving Performance.* Geneva: WHO, 2000.
23. World Health Organization. *World Health Report 2001. Mental Health: New Understanding, New Hope.* Geneva: WHO, 2001.
24. Salomon, J.A. & Murray, C.J.L. Modelling HIV/AIDS epidemics in sub-Saharan Africa using seroprevalence data from antenatal clinics. *Bull. WHO* 2001; **79**: 596–607.
25. UNICEF. *The State of the World's Children.* New York: Oxford University Press, 1996.
26. Black, R., Morris, S. & Bryce, J. Where and why are 10 million children dying every year? *Lancet* 2003; **361**: 2226–34.
27. Horton, R. The infected metropolis. *Lancet* 1996; **347**: 134–5.
28. UNICEF. *The State of the World's Children 2003.* New York: Oxford University Press, 2003.
29. World Health Organization. *Millennium Development Goals: WHO's Contribution to Tracking Progress and Measuring Achievements.* Geneva: WHO, 2003.
30. http://www.developmentgoals.org/.
31. Bryce, J., el Arifeen, S., Pariyo, G. *et al.* Reducing child mortality: can public health deliver? *Lancet* 2003; **361**: in press.
32. World Health Organization and UNICEF. Measles mortality reduction and regional elimination; Strategic Plan 2001–2005. WHO/V and B/01.03; also at http://www.who.int/vaccines-documents/DocsPDF01/.
33. UNICEF. *The State of the World's Children.* New York: Oxford University Press, 1994.
34. Expanded Programme on Immunization. Progress towards the global eradication of poliomyelitis, 2001. *Wkly Epidemiol. Rec.* 2002; **77**: 97–108.
35. Aylward, R.B., Acharya, A., England, S., Agocs, M. & Linkins, J. Global health goals: lessons from the worldwide effort to eradicate poliomyelitis. *Lancet* 2003; **362**: 909–14.
36. World Health Organization. Changing epidemiology of Polio prompts tactical shift in world's largest public health initiative. WHO Press Release, 13 May 2003.
37. Dwyer, T. & Ponsonby, A.L. The decline of SIDS – a success story for epidemiology. *Epidemiology* 1996; **7**: 323–5.
38. Högberg, U. & Wall, S. Secular trends in maternal mortality rates in Sweden, 1750–1980. *Bull. WHO* 1986; **64**: 79–84.
39. WHO/UNICEF/UNFPA. *Maternal Mortality in 2000: Estimates Developed by WHO, UNICEF and UNFPA.* Geneva: WHO, 2003.
40. Malcoe, L.H. National policy, social conditions, and the aetiology of maternal mortality. *Epidemiology* 1994; **5**: 481–3.
41. Tonks, A. Pregnancy's toll in the developing world. *Br. Med. J.* 1994; **108**: 353–4.
42. Editorial. Undermining international family planning. *Lancet* 2002; **359**: 539.
43. Goodburn, E. & Campbell, O. Reducing maternal mortality in the developing world: sector-wide approaches may be the key. *Br. Med. J.* 2001; **322**: 917–20.
44. Department for International Development. *Better Health for Poor People: Strategies for Achieving International Development Targets.* London: DFID, 2000.
45. UNICEF. *Children and Development in the 1990s.* New York: UNICEF, 1990.

46. Sahn, D.E. & Stifel, D.C. Progress toward the millennium development goals in Africa. *World Development Report* 2003; **31**: 23–52.

47. Jowett, M. Safe motherhood interventions in low-income countries: an economic justification and evidence of cost effectiveness. *Hlth Pol.* 2000; **53**: 201–28.

48. World Health Organization and United Nation's Children Fund. *Revised 1990 Estimates of Maternal Mortality. A New Approach by WHO and UNICEF.* Geneva: World Health Organization, 1996.

49. Koblinsky, M.A., Campbell, O.M.R. & Harlow, S. Mother and more: a broader perspective in women's health. In: Koblinsky, M.A., Timyan, J. & Gay, J. (eds.). *The Health of Women: A Global Perspective.* Boulder: Westview Press, 1992.

50. Feachem, R.G.A., Kjellstrom, T., Murray, C.J.L., Over, M. & Phillips, M.A. (eds.). *The Health of Adults in the Developing World.* New York: Oxford University Press, 1991.

51. Corbet, E.L., Watt, C.J., Walker, N. *et al. The Growing Burden of Tuberculosis: Global Trends and Interactions with the HIV Epidemic. J. Am. Med. Assoc.* 2003; **163**: 1009–21.

52. Peto, R., Lopez, A.D., Boreham, J., Thun, M. & Heath, C. *Mortality from Smoking in Developed Countries 1950–2000: Indirect Estimates from National Vital Statistics.* Oxford: Oxford University Press, 1994.

53. Coggon, D. & Inskip, H. Is there an epidemic of cancer? *Br. Med. J.* 1994; **308**: 705–8.

54. Davis, D.L., Dinse, G.E. & Hoel, D.G. Decreasing cardiovascular disease and increasing cancer among whites in the United States from 1973 through 1987: good news and bad news. *J. Am. Med. Assoc.* 1994; **271**: 431–7.

55. Lopez, A.D. Assessing the burden of mortality from cardiovascular disease. *WHO. Stats. Quart.* 1993, **46**: 91–6.

56. Ebrahim, S. Ageing, health and society. *Int. J. Epidemiol.* 2002; **31**: 715-18.

57. See Ref. 5.

58. Marmot, M.G. & Davey-Smith, G. Why are the Japanese living longer? *Br. Med. J.* 1989; **299**: 1547–51.

59. Murray, C.J.L. & Lopez, A.D (eds.). The global burden of disease: a comprehensive assessment of mortality and disability from diseases, injuries and risk factors in 1990 and projected to 2020. *Global Burden of Disease and Injury Series,* Vol. 1. Cambridge: Harvard University Press, 1996.

60. Lai, D. & Hardy, R.J. Potential gains in life expectancy or years of potential life lost: impact of competing risks of death. *Int. J. Epidemiol.* 1999; **28**: 894–8.

61. Mathers, C.D., Vos, T., Lopez, A.D. & Ezzati, M. *National Burden of Disease Studies: A Practical Guide.* Edition 2.0. Geneva: WHO, 2001.

62. Bonita, R., Solomon, N. & Broad, J.B. The prevalence of stroke and stroke related disability: estimates from the Auckland Stroke studies. *Stroke* 1997; **28**: 1898–902.

63. Sayers, B. McA., Bailey, N.T.J. *et al.* The disability adjusted life year concept: a comment. *Europ. J. Pub. Hlth* 1997; **7**: 113.

64. Williams A. Calculating the global burden of disease: time for a strategic reappraisal? *Hlth Econ.* 1998; **8**: 1–8.

65. Cooper, R.S., Osotimehin, B., Kaufman, J.S. & Forrester, T. Disease burden in sub-Saharan Africa: what should we conclude in the absence of data? *Lancet* 1998: **351**: 208–10.

66. Murray, C.J.L. & Lopez, A.D. Progress and directions in refining the global burden of disease approach: response to Williams. *Hlth Econ.* 2000; **9**: 69–82.
67. Mathers, C., Vos, T. & Stevenson, C. *The Burden of Disease and Injury in Australia.* Canberra: Australian Institute of Health and Welfare, 1999.
68. Barendregt, J.J., Bonneux, L. & Vander Maas, P.J. DALYs: the age-weight on balance. *Bull. WHO* 1996; **74**: 439–43.
69. Gwatkin, D.R., Guillot, M. & Heuveline, P. The burden of disease among the global poor. *Lancet* 1999; **354**: 586–9.
70. Barker, C. & Green, A. Opening the debate on DALYs. *Hlth Pol. Planning* 1996; **11**: 179–83.
71. McKeown, T. *The Role of Medicine – Dream, Mirage or Nemesis.* London: Nuffield Provincial Hospitals Trust, 1976.
72. McKinlay, J.B. & McKinlay, S.M. The questionable effect of medical measures on the decline of mortality in the United States in the twentieth century. *Milbank Mem. Fund Q.* 1977; **55**: 405–28.
73. Almeida, C., Braveman, P., Gold, M.R. *et al.* Methodological concerns and recommendations on policy consequences of the World Health Report 2000. *Lancet* 2001; **357**: 1692–7.
74. Moss, N. & Krieger, N. Report on the Conference of the National Institutes of Health. *Pub. Hlth Rep.* 1995; **110**: 302–5.
75. Shkolnikov, V., McKee, M. & Leon, D. Changes in life expectancy in Russia in the mid-1990s. *Lancet* 2001; **357**: 917–21.
76. Gavrilova, N.S., Semyonova V.G., Evdokushkina, G.N. & Gavrilov, L.A. The response of violent mortality to economic crisis in Russia. *Population Res. Pol. Rev.* 2000; **19**: 397–419.
77. St.Leger, A.S. Inequalities and health. *Lancet* 1994; **343**: 538.
78. Charlton, B.G. Is inequality bad for the national health? *Lancet* 1994; **343**: 221–2.
79. Marmot, M.G. & McDowall, M.E. Mortality decline and widening social inequalities. *Lancet* 1986; **ii**: 274–6.
80. See Ref. 58.
81. Marmot, M. Social differences in mortality: the Whitehall Studies. In: Lopez, A.D., Caselli, G. & Valkonen, T. (eds.). *Adult Mortality in Developed Countries: From Description to Explanation.* Oxford: Oxford University Press, 1995.
82. Moser, K.A., Fox, A.J. & Jones, D.R. Unemployment and mortality in the OPCS longitudinal study. *Lancet* 1984; **ii**: 1324–9.
83. Wilkinson, R.G. Income distribution and life expectancy. *Br. Med. J.* 1992; **304**: 165–8.
84. Gakidou, E. & King, G. Measuring total health inequality: adding individual variation to group-level differences. *Int. J. Equity Hlth* 2002, **1**: 3.
85. Szreter, S. The importance of social intervention in Britain's mortality decline *c.* 1850–1914: a re-interpretation of the role of public health. *Soc. History Med.* 1988; **1**: 1–37.
86. Illich I. *Limits of Medicine. Medical Nemesis: The Expropriation of Health.* Harmondsworth: Penguin, 1981.
87. Dean, M. Absolute effects of relative poverty. *Lancet* 1994; **344**: 463.
88. Caldwell, J.C. Routes to low mortality in poor countries. *Pop. Dev. Rev.* 1986; **12**: 171–220.

89. Warren, K.S. McKeown's mistake. *Hlth Transition Rev.* 1991; **1**: 229–33.
90. Critchley, J.A. & Capewell, S. Substantial potential for reduction in coronary heart disease, mortality in the UK through changes in risk factor leads. *J. Epidemiol. Commun. Hlth* 2003, **57**: 243–7.
91. Jousilahti, P., Vartiainen, E., Tuomilehto, J., Pekkanen, J. & Puska, P. Effect of risk factors and changes in risk factors on coronary mortality in three cohorts of middle-aged people in Eastern Finland. *Am. J. Epidemiol.* 1995; **141**: 50–60.
92. Vartiainen, E., Jousilahti, P., Alftahan, G. *et al.* Cardiovascular risk factor changes in Finland, 1972–1997. *Int. J. Epidemiol.* 2000; **29**: 9–56.
93. Magnus, P. & Beaglehole, R. The real contribution of the major risk factors to the coronary epidemics. Time to end the 'only 50% myth'. *Arch. Intern. Med.* 2001; **161**: 2657–60.
94. Pool, I. Cross-comparative perspectives on New Zealand's health. In: Spicer, J., Trlin, A. & Walton, J.A. (eds.). *Social Dimensions of Health and Disease: New Zealand Perspectives.* Palmerston North: Dunmore Press, 1994.
95. Stamler, J., Stamler, R., Neaton, J.D. *et al.* Low risk-factor profile and long-term cardiovascular and non-cardiovascular mortality and life expectancy. Findings for 5 large cohorts of young adult and middle-aged men and women. *J. Am. Med. Assoc.* 1999; **282**: 2012–18.
96. Kuulasmaa, K., Tunstall-Pedoe, H., Dobson, A. *et al.* For the WHO MONICA Project. Estimation of contribution of changes in classic risk factors to trends in coronary-event rates across the WHO MONICA Project populations. *Lancet* 2000; **355**: 675–87.
97. Eastern Stroke and Coronary Heart Disease Collaborative Research Group. Blood pressure, cholesterol, and stroke in eastern Asia. *Lancet* 1998; **352**: 1801–7.
98. Murray, C.J.L., Lauer, J.A., Hutubessy, R.C.W. *et al.* Effectiveness and costs of interventions to lower systolic blood pressure and cholesterol: a global and regional analysis on reduction of cardiovascular-disease risk. *Lancet* 2003; **361**: 717–25.
99. McMichael, A.J. & Beaglehole, R. The changing global context of public health. *Lancet* 2000; **356**: 495–9.
100. Global Forum for Health Research. *The 10/90 Report on Health Research 2000.* Geneva: Global Forum for Health Research, 2001.
101. Commission on Macroeconomics and Health. *Macroeconomics and Health: Investing in Health for Economic Development.* Geneva: WHO, 2001.

3

Contemporary global health issues

3.1 Introduction

The worldwide burden of premature death represents a great challenge to those concerned with public health and the state of humanity in general. The most important underlying causes of ill health are the social and economic characteristics of a society, which are the driving forces for the health transition. Unfortunately, these major determinants are often poorly defined and, from a health policy perspective, difficult to act upon and often neglected.

The broad definition of the term 'cause' used in this book refers to any factor that influences health directly or indirectly in either direction. But the mere existence of a cause does not imply necessarily that it will lead to a state of health or disease. For example, motor vehicles are not associated inevitably with death and destruction. Countries with the same number of cars per head of population can have quite different death rates from car crashes because of different approaches to prevention – often associated with different cultural values. In reality it is simplistic to think in terms of a single 'cause' of disease. Complex pathways, mechanisms and multiple systems are involved. For example, the evidence on social class gradients suggests that the underlying causal process associated with social integration may be expressed through different diseases[1].

The health status of a population reflects the interaction between its genetic endowment and environmental conditions. Very often in policy discussions, health is reduced to its personal and family dimensions and the relationship between the health of populations, and the wider social and natural environmental conditions is ignored[2]. There is abundant evidence that the major differences in health and disease between populations are caused by environmental rather

54

than by genetic factors[3]. For example, the striking international differences in death rates from cardiovascular disease, the rapid changes in these rates over time, and the impact of migration on disease rates, all testify to the importance of the environment in determining the health status of a population. The modification of environmental factors is the most logical approach to improving health, but genetic factors are also responsible for some of the differences in disease experience within populations. For example, not all smokers get lung cancer, suggesting that genetic factors may contribute to this important cause of death and disease, although diet and other environmental factors may also be involved[4].

Within populations, it is the interaction of the individual's genetic predisposition with environmental determinants of health that is critically important. Until recently, genetic factors have been thought to be fixed and unchangeable. However, now specific gene–environment interactions responsible for some relatively uncommon diseases (such as cystic fibrosis) have been identified. An increasing number of genes will be found to be associated with specific diseases as a result of the human genome project. Despite the huge cost of this research, it is unlikely, from a global perspective, that major positive health impacts will result from genetic manipulation. Unfortunately, this insight is not appreciated generally and funding for genetic research is much greater than funding for public health research, which has the potential to make a greater impact.

WHO has recently quantified the contribution of selected major risks to health and has assessed the global and regional distribution of disease attributable to 20 leading risk factors ranging from underweight to childhood sexual abuse[5]. This ambitious undertaking is constrained by the limited availability of high quality data on many of these risks, especially in the poorest regions. However, this exercise illustrates that risks are widespread and that all have a global impact, although the burden of many is concentrated almost exclusively in high mortality developing countries; the striking regional variations in the leading risks to health are largely related to the underlying social and economic conditions.

The global distribution of the burden of disease attributable to 20 leading selected risks by level of country development is shown in Fig. 3.1. It has been estimated that the leading five risk factors account for more than one-third of mortality and one-third of disability as measured by DALYs. The leading ten risk factors account for 42% of all deaths and 33% of DALYs. The inclusion of the additional risk factors makes only a marginal difference.

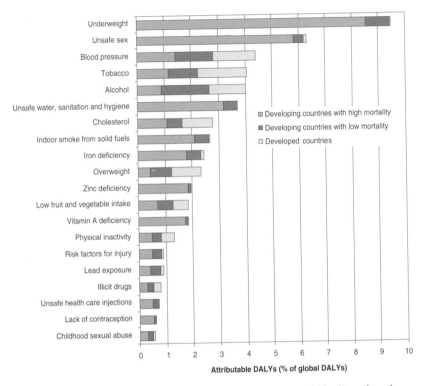

Fig. 3.1. Global distribution of burden of disease attributable to 20 leading selected risk factors.

3.2 Underlying socio-economic causes of population health status

3.2.1 Health, wealth and poverty

A basic level of wealth sufficient to supply essential needs such as food, shelter, clothing and warmth is important for health. In traditional societies, wealth was measured in many ways. In most societies, wealth is now measured in terms of personal and family income. Inequalities in wealth – both absolute and relative – and power, lead to inequalities in health by determining the social circumstances in which people work and live and their psychosocial responses to these conditions.

Industrialisation and the wealth it created, has had major and variable impacts on the health of nations. The countries of Europe and North America which industrialised early, ultimately experienced many health benefits, although striking inequalities in health status are still entrenched in these countries. The early experience of industrialisation and the associated massive urbanisation led to appalling living and working conditions for much of the workforce with an overall worsening in health status. Much of the long-term benefit reaped by the wealthy countries has been supported by their former colonies, which continue to provide cheap labour, resources and relatively open markets. Instead of being part of a linear process, wealthy and poor countries act as complementary, but grossly unequal, participants in the overall global process of industrialisation[6].

The relationships between economic development and health are complex. Once a minimum level of per capita income is achieved, social and political priorities have a greater impact on the health status of the population than overall national wealth. Investments in education, health and other social services are especially important. This finding is critical and contrasts with the generally accepted view that the health of a population will improve in a linear fashion as a nation 'develops' and becomes increasingly wealthy. This assumption ignores the evidence that uncontrolled economic growth, which encourages production and consumption, is responsible for much of the global environmental destruction. The main favourable effects of economic growth on health depend on the sound use of the increased capital and the increased amounts spent on improving nutrition, both in quality and quantity, effective public health measures, medical care, effective birth control, improvements in physical environment, and widespread literacy[7].

The WHO Commission on Macroeconomics and Health emphasised the costs to the economy of preventable epidemics, especially from infectious diseases[8]. For example, it is estimated roughly that a high prevalence of malaria can be associated with a reduction of economic growth of 1% or more per year. The Commission argues strongly for massive additional funds for health improvement to promote economic growth. Although this is a strong argument for attracting extra resources into health development, there is a danger that this justification ignores the overwhelming humanitarian reasons for encouraging and assisting countries to respond to their health priorities.

Poverty is perhaps the dominant feature of the world today. The criteria for poverty vary. The World Bank's description of poverty is 'a condition of life so limited by malnutrition, literacy, disease, squalid surroundings, high infant mortality, and low life expectancy as to be beneath any reasonable definition of human decency'[9]. Absolute poverty is defined as a per capita annual income of about US$450[9]. Approximately one-fifth of the world's population, about 1.2 billion people, are estimated to live in absolute poverty – barely surviving on less than 1$ per day; over 70% are women. Nearly half of the world's population, approximately three billion people, live on less than US$2 per day[10]. Clearly, these three billion people have incomes insufficient to meet even their most basic needs (See Box 3.1).

Box 3.1   Women in poverty[11]

Poverty is the condition of the vast majority of the world's women. Almost two-thirds live in countries classified by the United Nations as having 'very low GDP' (<$1000 to <$3000 per capita annually).

In every country, at every socio-economic level, women control fewer productive assets than do men; they also work longer hours but earn less income. Lacking alternatives, women are more often compelled to resort to jobs that are seasonal, labour intensive and carry considerable occupational risks. Thus poverty for women is more intractable than for men, and their health is even more vulnerable to adverse changes in social and environmental conditions.

Women's work is grossly unpaid, unrecognised, and undervalued to the order of US$11 trillion a year. Yet it has been estimated that the total bill to provide basic services to women in every developing country is around $20 billion a year, or only 5% of the total size of public sector budgets in poor countries.

Poverty and powerlessness, two problems which women suffer disproportionately, are serious health hazards. In no country in the world are women offered the same socio-economic and political opportunities as men; women lag behind men on virtually every indicator of social and economic status.

Although there have been slight reductions in world poverty in percentage terms – largely driven by the recent and impressive increases in wealth in China – the absolute number of poor people barely changed in the 1990s (Table 3.1)[10].

At the end of the 1990s, the situation had deteriorated so much in several sub-Saharan countries that more than half, and maybe even three-quarters, of the population in Malawi, Mozambique, Zambia and Zimbabwe, were living below the poverty line[12]. The continuing failure to reduce poverty in sub-Saharan Africa, the world's poorest region, is a major challenge to all countries. The level of income inequality worldwide is 'grotesque'[10]. However, trends over recent decades are ambiguous because of the range of economic

Table 3.1. *Poverty in poor regions of the world, 1985–2000*[10]

Region	% of the population below the poverty line		Number of poor (millions)	
	1990	1999	1990	1999
Sub-Saharan Africa	47.7	46.7	242	300
East Asia and the Pacific	27.6	14.2	452	260
Excluding China	18.5	7.9	92	46
South Asia	44.0	36.9	495	490
Latin America and the Caribbean	16.8	15.1	74	77
Eastern Europe and Central Asia	1.6	3.6	7	17
Middle East and North Africa	2.4	2.3	6	7
Total	29.0	22.7	1,276	1,151
Excluding China	28.1	24.5	916	936

performances across countries and regions, with impressive growth in many East Asian countries and reversals in sub-Saharan Africa. The poorest sub-Saharan African countries now have incomes approximately one-fortieth of the richest countries. The world's richest 1% of people receive as much income as the poorest 57%; the income of the richest 25 million Americans is equal to that of almost two billion people[10]. The distribution of wealth within countries is also very uneven. The greatest inequality in income distribution occurs in the poorest countries. For example, there is a 20- to 30-fold difference between the richest and poorest fifths of the population in Mexico and Brazil[13].

Most wealthy countries that have increased their incomes over the past two decades have also seen rising income inequality, especially in the United Kingdom and the United States. In the United States during the 1980s, the richest 1% increased their share of the nation's wealth from around 31% to 37%, yet in 1991 it was estimated that almost one-fifth of total mortality in people aged 25–74 years of age was attributed to poverty[14]. In the United Kingdom there was a threefold increase in the proportion of children living below the European Union's poverty line in the 1990s and about one in three children are now below this line[15]. In relatively wealthy countries, the vast majority of those in poverty belong to one of five groups: single parents and their children, the elderly, the unemployed, racial and ethnic minorities, and the disabled. Three of these groups (single mothers, the elderly and the disabled) are likely to increase in numbers[16].

Global health

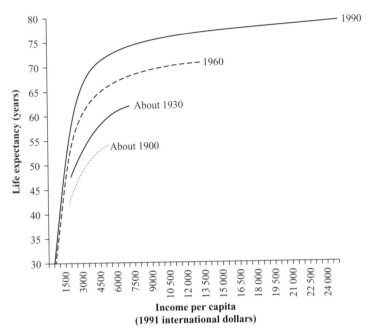

Fig. 3.2. The relation between life expectancy and income per capita.
Source: World Development Report, 1993[9].

Health is not a straightforward function of wealth. The complex relationship between life expectancy and per capita income for selected countries and four periods is shown in Fig. 3.2[9]. As measured by life expectancy at birth, health improves rapidly as average per capita income increases to $5000 (1991 International dollars) per person. It was estimated that a doubling of income from $1000 in 1990 corresponded to a gain in life expectancy of about 11 years, whereas a doubling from an income of $4000 would be associated with a gain of only about 4 years[17]. Above a mean of about $5000, per capita income itself is no longer the critical determinant of health status.

The rich Middle Eastern oil-producing countries (which are mainly Muslim) illustrate the complexity of this relationship. Life expectancy in these countries is relatively low and reflects the relatively low state of development in the region as measured by the Arabic Human Development Index[18]. On the other hand, several countries such as Sri Lanka and China, have much higher levels of life expectancy than would be expected from their per capita incomes[10]. Another indication of the importance of factors other than income is that, over time, a given level of income has become associated with a longer life expectancy. For example, in 1900 an income of $5000 per capita was associated with a life expectancy of about 55 years; in 2000 this income level was associated with a life expectancy of at least 70 years. Much of the improvement in life expectancy at the same level of income is attributed to the benefits of new knowledge stemming from health research and more generally from human development programmes that enable the knowledge to be used.

In general, once countries reach a per capita income of more than $5000, health standards become dependent on the distribution of income and the effect-iveness of government policies[19]. Expenditures on health personnel and health facilities do not cause the variation in life expectancy as much as social factors such as literacy, nutrition, transportation and communications[20]. Poor countries such as Cuba and China have achieved exceptionally high standards of health and demonstrate the importance of female autonomy, literacy and political will to make health a priority, especially for women and children. However, it is noteworthy how rapidly this commitment to health improvement as a national priority can change. China, as we shall see in Chapter 8, has undergone rapid social and economic changes over the last decade, which have had some adverse health effects, especially for rural populations.

As income distribution within a country narrows, life expectancy tends to increase[21,22]. The widening income gap between the rich and poor in the United Kingdom over recent decades is reflected in a slowdown in the decline in mor-tality in young people in Britain[14,15]. Sometimes, policy decisions that seem remote have an unexpected health impact. For example, the value-added tax on fuel in the United Kingdom increased the overall tax burden unevenly and added to the redistribution of wealth from the poor to the rich[23].

Economic inequality may affect health, both directly and indirectly, through psychological and social processes, by effects on self-esteem, and on social relations in general[24]. The advantage of the Japanese workers over British workers is not due to a greater spending on health care in Japan but may be explained by the fact that material rewards for work are more evenly distributed in Japan[25]. In recent decades, income distribution in Japan has become the narrowest of any country. Very low military expenditure has allowed greater investment in other sectors[26]. The relative increase in Japan's economic position compared to other countries may in turn have a positive impact on Japanese self-esteem and thus on health. It would be interesting to explore the general health consequences of the recent and prolonged downturn in the Japanese economy. It is likely that the health effects of increased unemployment in Japan will be evident soon.

The data supporting the association between the distribution of wealth and health has increased over the last decade[27] especially in the USA. However, the international evidence is rather weak[28] and it remains true that there are many ways in which countries differ, apart from the distribution of wealth. Even within countries, the rich differ from the poor in many ways other than income. The health implications of relative deprivation, as opposed to absolute poverty, are very important[29,30]. The profound policy implications of the association of wealth and health make this an essential area for further research. Despite the increasing evidence at this point, it would be hard to convince politicians of the need to narrow income gaps in the interests of health improvement for the general population. However, as the adverse health effects of unrestrained economic growth become more apparent because of the adverse environmental effects, policy choices involving income redistribution, rather than simply economic growth, will become more attractive and perhaps even essential.

The immediate cause of individual or family poverty is either unemployment or underpaid employment. Unemployment has an effect on health directly through poverty but also through other mechanisms involving psychosocial pathways[31]. Poverty is associated with a whole range of adverse health effects. Poor people have less income to spend on nutritious food, clean water, adequate clothing and shelter, all of which are essential to a minimum level of health and well-being. They also have less access to education and political power, which is needed to improve and safeguard health. Even limited economic progress in poor countries would have a major beneficial impact on health, so long as the wealth gained is distributed equitably, and so long as the economic progress is sustainable and not at the expense of the environment. The important contribution of ill health to creating poverty has received increased attention. Most of the world's population is directly responsible for the costs of sickness, since they are not covered by welfare or insurance schemes. These 'out-of-pocket' expenses can have a major impact on household incomes, especially when the illness is chronic or severe and causes households to go into debt and poverty[8].

WHO has identified poverty as 'the greatest single killer'[32]. WHO has recently mapped the distribution of the major risks to health by poverty as defined by high mortality (high child, high adult) developing countries[5]. Although the data are scarce, especially for the poorer high mortality countries, it is clear that several of the major risks to health such as child underweight, unsafe water and sanitation, and indoor air pollution are associated strongly with absolute poverty. The associations of poverty with tobacco and alcohol consumption, lack of breast feeding, and unsafe sex are weaker and more variable between regions and epidemiological groupings.

Poverty alleviation is the most pressing issue facing public health practitioners and society in general[33]. Not only is this the major immediate global health challenge, it is also necessary for developing a sustainable global economy, as stressed by the Commission on Macroeconomics and Health[8]. If public health practitioners are to contribute to the response to this challenge, they will require skills far beyond those required for designing and implementing traditional public health programmes. As a modest start, this and other topics in this chapter will need to be incorporated into public health training programmes. An important first step for all practitioners is the recognition of the need, in the interests of health, for income redistribution policies, both within and between countries. Economic growth alone is insufficient to overcome absolute poverty and will have little impact on relative poverty[24] and will contribute to the long-term deterioration of the global environment.

3.2.2 Other socio-economic causes

Inadequate shelter is a major cause of ill health in all countries. Rapid urbanisation is causing a housing crisis and future prospects look bleak. The world's urban population – people living in cities with more than 750 000 inhabitants – is estimated to have reached 2.9 billion in 2000 and is expected to rise to 4.9 billion by 2030. Virtually all the population growth expected during 2000–2030 will be concentrated in the urban areas of the world, almost all of this in the less-developed regions[34]. Most of the new urban residents will live in slums with poor or non-existent health services[35]. Homelessness is also an increasing feature of cities in rich countries[36]. Policies which have reduced subsidised housing along with changes in the institutional care of people with mental health problems have contributed to this increase.

Approximately 3% of deaths (1.7 million) and 3.7% of DALYs worldwide are attributable to unsafe water, sanitation and hygiene, and about one-third of this burden occurs in Africa[5]. The decade of the 1980s was the International Drinking Water Supply and Sanitation Decade, and 2002 saw a major international conference on water – the Third World Water Forum. About half the population in urban areas in poor countries, and an even greater proportion in rural areas, still lack safe water and adequate sanitation. The relevant Millennium Development Goal is to halve the proportion of the population with no access to safe drinking water. At the World Summit for Sustainable Development in 2002, a sanitation target was added to mirror the water target. The water target probably is achievable, but not the sanitation target[37].

Although the proportion of the world's population provided with safe water and sanitation services increased over the last two decades, during the same period the growth of the population was even greater. The regional situation is less encouraging, especially for sub-Saharan Africa where the number of people not provided with safe water and sanitation is expected to increase between now and 2015. Even if the targets for both water and sanitation are met, there will still be 700 million people without access to improved drinking water in 2015 and approximately 1.7 billion without access to improved sanitation. Lack of adequate drinking water affects women in particular. The gender-based division of labour places women in more frequent contact with polluted water and the risk of infection from water-borne diseases. Improving access to water reduces the disproportionate cost – both financial and labour – borne by the poor for procuring water.

Water and food pollution in developing countries are caused by poor sanitation, poor hygiene, inadequate waste disposal and water treatment. These conditions create major epidemics of diarrhoeal disease, especially among children. The outbreaks of cholera in South America in 1991 and in South Africa in the late 1990s were the result of poor sanitary conditions. Global warming may also have contributed to this outbreak in South America by encouraging the growth of surface water algae which protect the cholera bacteria[38]. This cholera outbreak cost Peru about $1 billion, three times the total amount invested in the country's water supply during the previous decade[39]. WHO estimates that unsafe water, and poor sanitation and hygiene are responsible for almost 4% of the global burden of disease[5].

The World Bank estimates that 80 countries now have water shortages that threaten both health status and national economies. As industrial, agricultural and individual demands escalate, the situation is deteriorating: worldwide the demand for water is doubling every 21 years[40]. The shortage of water is becoming a source of tension between neighbouring states in the Middle East and parts of Africa and threatens to add to the destabilisation in these areas. The World Bank proposes huge investments in sanitation and water schemes and suggests that water be valued as an economic good, rather than a human right, and water services be privatised. It is unlikely that these suggestions will solve the problems of water supply for the poor. Long-term community development projects may be of more benefit. The World Bank has made several loans for water reform conditional on private sector participation but strong government regulation will be required for this to help the poor. The role of private enterprises – mostly European in origin – in the supply of drinking water is controversial. The experience from several Latin American cities has been mixed and has led to increases in the cost of water, which poor people can ill afford. It would be helpful for international lenders to explore new ways of raising money and involving communities in their water and sanitation provision, including greater use of low-cost technologies that are more affordable to maintain.

Malnutrition and deficiency diseases are major problems in poor countries and in some population groups within wealthy countries[5]. The major hazards for both children and adults are protein-energy malnutrition caused by poverty, and vitamin A, iodine and iron deficiencies[40]. Approximately 780 million people (15% of the total world population) are energy deficient. The worst situation is in Africa, which regularly experiences devastating famines with children and women being most at risk. The goal set at the World Summit for Children was to halve the 1990 rate of child malnutrition by the year 2000. In 50 countries with almost 40% of the world's poor, more than one in five children under the age of five are underweight[10,41]. The target date for this goal has now been set back until 2015 and this goal has been incorporated into the Millennium Development Goals. It seems extremely unlikely that this target will be met, especially in sub-Saharan Africa where many countries are experiencing a worsening of the overall nutrition situation. Unfortunately, the UN World Food Summit in 2002 was a failure with little progress being made towards addressing even the acute and severe malnutrition in southern Africa[42].

Inadequate diet, together with infectious diseases, accounts for a large share of the world's disease burden, including as much as a quarter of the burden among children. There is also increasing evidence that inadequate nutrition in pregnancy may be an important factor in the development of a range of adult non-communicable disease[43]. This possible mechanism should not, however, deflect attention from the immediate health gains that could be made from a serious attempt to reduce the burden of non-communicable disease in adult life[44].

The prospect for adequate food supplies to meet the growing world population is not reassuring, especially in the poorest regions that cannot afford grain imports[45]. The distribution of the available food is also a chronic problem. The so-called 'green revolution' of the 1970s and 1980s produced optimism as the technological solution to food production had many successes[46]. However, this revolution also had adverse environmental effects and did little to increase food availability in sub-Saharan Africa. Furthermore, production is now levelling off. For example, the growth in rice yields virtually ceased in the Philippines in the latter half of the 1980s[38] and, globally, per capita grain production has fallen[47]. The available land for crop production is limited, the supply of fresh water is dwindling, and the seas have been over-fished. The centralisation of large-scale agricultural production, often under the control of multi-national companies, has had an adverse impact on local communities and reduced the viability of small-scale farming. Widespread malnutrition will likely increase, especially in sub-Saharan Africa. A new more ecologically sound approach to food production utilising appropriate genetic technology is now required to improve food supply in the poorest parts of the world[48].

Vitamin A (retinol) deficiency is prevalent widely and causes a range of childhood health problems, including ulceration of the cornea in the eye and permanent blindness. According to WHO, 13.8 million children have some eye damage because of vitamin A deficiency. Of these, up to half a million go blind each year and two-thirds of the blinded children die[42]. Including Vitamin A supplementation with routine immunisation has been an important development and has significantly reduced child mortality from all causes.

Iron and iodine deficiencies are also widespread with about 460 million and one billion people, respectively, affected. Together, these two deficiencies are estimated to be responsible for approximately 4% of the global burden of disease and this proportion is higher in the poorest countries[5]. The amount of iron in the diet in poor countries is decreasing rather than increasing. Girls and women are particularly vulnerable. For example, up to 85% of pregnant Indian women are anaemic. Even in richer countries, 15% of pregnant women suffer from anaemia. In many societies, women face a lifetime of nutritional inequity with severe consequences for the next generation. Severe iodine deficiency causes endemic cretinism, a condition characterised by irreversible mental deficiency. Cretinism affects 5.7 million people and over 20 million suffer lesser degrees of mental retardation caused by iodine deficiency. Iodine deficiency also remains a problem in 13 European countries which have been designated as deficient[49].

A non-governmental organisation was established in 1985 with the aim of reducing iodine deficiency disorders substantially by 2000[50]. The successes of the global partnership created by this initiative indicate the power of selective disease prevention programmes, which translate scientific research into international public health action (see Box 3.2). This project demonstrates the application of science to health and development in poor countries. The key factor was that the International Council for the Control of Iodine Deficiency Diseases, a non-governmental organisation, was able to successfully work with the major international agencies and national governments. It provides one model for translating scientific research to international public health[51].

3.2.3 Literacy and education

Education is one of the most important and most readily modifiable social determinants of health. Literacy interacts with the availability of free or inexpensive and effective health services to produce major positive health improvements. Policies to expand schooling are therefore crucial for promoting health, although in the short-term integrated primary health care programmes have the greatest potential. Improving the education of girls is recognised increasingly as a central factor in improving maternal and child health.

Box 3.2   Eradicating iodine deficiency disorders: a global partnership[51]

Iodine deficiency is the most common preventable cause of mental deficiency in the world today. WHO estimates that more than one billion are at risk with at least 20 million suffering from mental deficiency which is totally preventable by the correction of iodine deficiency before pregnancy.

Three steps have been identified as crucial for the success of the eradication programme:

1. The establishment of a scientific base and reconceptualisation of the problem as a population concern.
2. Bridging the gap to a public health programme with the creation of a non-governmental organisation made up of the scientific community and public health professionals from a range of disciplines.
3. Development of a global partnership through the United Nations system.

Unfortunately, levels of literacy and education, especially among women, are still very low in many poor countries as well as in many relatively affluent Arab countries[18]. Progress was made in the 1960s and 1970s in increasing the proportion of children completing primary school in most poor countries. Between 1970 and 1990, the gender gap in education more than halved in poor countries. However, one of the effects of structural adjustment programmes in the 1980s was that governments reduced educational spending to meet debt repayments[52].

Worldwide, primary enrolments have been improving, rising from 80% in 1990 to 84% in 1998. However, more than 100 million of the 700 million school-age children are not in school – 97% of them in developing countries[10]. Improving literacy is one of the most important Millennium Development Goals (MDGs) with the aim of achieving universal primary education by 2015. Unfortunately, not many developing countries have data on which to judge progress towards this goal, and the situation is especially bad in sub-Saharan

Africa where six countries are on track, five are far behind or slipping back and the other 33 countries without data are likely to be performing poorly[10].

Renewed lending by the World Bank for education, following the 1993 World Development Report, has not led to great progress. The mere provision of loans for education does not result inevitably in increased schooling, especially for girls. A change in attitude is also required by those in power as well as a full understanding of the many reasons why parents keep children from school, including the need to supplement the household income. If women's position in society cannot be changed easily by modifying religious or cultural practices, it may be changed more readily by encouraging female education and employment[53].

3.3 Global environmental changes

The major new public health hazard is the threat to our long-term existence posed by global damage to the biophysical and ecological environment[48]. This is the most important new challenge to epidemiology and public health because it transcends national and regional boundaries. The state of the environment ultimately is a much more powerful determinant of health status than either genes or personal behaviour. The value of the world's ecosystem is not considered in commercial markets and this neglect may compromise sustainable development. The real value of this system is huge, although it is not easy to quantify[54].

The evidence that humans are having a deleterious effect on the environment is increasing[55] and only the most sceptical now question this evidence[56], driven it seems by a selective interpretation of the abundant, but complex data[57]. The underlying cause of global environmental change is our inability to live within the constraints imposed by the closed system of our world and the 'ecological footprint' of wealthy countries, which consume far more than their share of the world's resources[58]. The growing inequality between rich and poor countries exacerbates the problem since the poorer regions naturally want to emulate the living standards of the rich. Even if this goal is ever achieved, it will be unsustainable. The ultimate solution is for the rich regions to reduce their exploitation of the globe's resources. Without significant wealth redistribution and lower total energy and material consumption, the ecologically sustainable, human-carrying capacity of the planet probably is much less than the present world population[59]. A truly global perspective will be required if public health practitioners are to play a role in achieving ecologically and socially sustainable development for all the world's population.

Environmental epidemiology has focused on the health impact of air pollution, pesticides and toxic chemicals. It has yet to confront the scientific difficulties adequately posed by 'planetary overload'[38], which includes global environmental hazards such as ozone depletion and global warming. The health impact of global environmental change is indirect and not immediately obvious[60].

In poor countries the immediate health impact of a deteriorating environment is all too apparent: lack of access to safe water, food and sanitation. In wealthy countries the impact usually is more subtle, but ultimately just as important. In many poor urban areas of wealthy countries, the immediate environmental concerns are the same as those facing much of the poor world.

Air pollution is an important major health hazard in most major cities of the world and much of it is caused by road vehicles[61]. About 1.5 billion people are living in a polluted air environment detrimental to health and this exposure is responsible for about 800 000 million deaths each year. This burden occurs predominantly in developing countries[5]. Air pollution is severe in some areas of Central and Eastern Europe, although only limited data are available to estimate its health impact. It is possible that, in the Czech Republic, one of the most heavily polluted countries, air pollution may be responsible for up to 3% of all deaths[62]. Large cities in poor countries are usually the worst affected, with pollution levels similar to those of the severely polluted cities of the wealthy countries about 40 years ago. Air pollution is increasing in many urban areas and there is likely to be an increase in mortality and morbidity, especially from chronic respiratory diseases. Indoor air pollution is a particularly important cause of the disease burden in poor countries and it is estimated to be responsible for about 3% of the global burden of disease[5].

The health hazards of industrial and agricultural chemicals and the toxic waste created by their production and use, also pose increasing problems. Episodes of poisoning because of industrial errors have been catastrophic. For example, in Bhopal, India, at least 3500 people died and 200 000 were injured in 1984 when isocyonate was released from a pesticide factory into the surrounding slums. The impact of this disaster continues to be felt, although there is no accurate record of the number of people whose health has been permanently impaired[63,64]. Attempts to compensate the victims of this disaster adequately have not yet been made[65,66]. It is likely that, as poor countries continue to industrialise and embrace consumerism and Western notions of development, there will be more Bhopal-like disasters[6]. A particularly worrying concern is the increasing number of nuclear reactors that have the potential to expose large numbers of people to ionising radiation (see Box 3.3).

Box 3.3   Health consequences of the Chernobyl accident[67]

- The largest ever radiation accident involving a nuclear reactor occurred on 26 April 1986 at the Chernobyl nuclear power plant in the Ukraine; five million people in the Ukraine, Belarus and the Russian Federation were exposed to ionising radiation.
- At the time of the accident, 300 of the 444 people at the reactor site were admitted to hospital, 134 of whom were diagnosed as having acute radiation sickness, 31 of these died within three months and one-third of the remainder suffered various disorders.
- Psychological effects, believed to be unrelated to direct radiation exposure, resulted from the lack of information immediately after the accident, the stress and trauma of compulsory relocation to less contaminated areas, the break in social ties, and the fear that radiation exposure could cause health damage in the future.
- An increase in the incidence of childhood thyroid cancer has been one of the major health consequences of the accident, particularly in Belarus.
- Ultimately it is estimated that the after effects of this nuclear disaster will cause 6600 deaths from cancer and leukaemia.

The newest and most threatening environmental hazards are global warming and the depletion of the stratospheric ozone layer by pollution and by the release of chemicals, particularly chlorofluorocarbons used in refrigeration fluids into the environment[2]. Ironically, it was the accumulation of stratospheric ozone that shielded the earth from damaging ultraviolet light and thus enabled the evolution of species[38]. Most of the ozone-destroying chemicals and greenhouse gases come from wealthy countries. Ozone layer depletion will lead to greater exposure to incoming solar ultraviolet radiation. The direct health effects of ozone depletion include an increase in the risk of skin cancer and cataract. Greater indirect effects, however, could result through damage to the food chain.

The 'greenhouse' effect or global warming is caused by carbon dioxide and other gases that trap heat radiation from the earth's surface and lead to global warming. The effects of global warming are more long term, more damaging, and more difficult to prevent than ozone depletion. The health impact of climatic and other environmental changes includes an increase in the global population exposed to vector-borne diseases[68]. There is some evidence of an increased occurrence of tick borne encephalitis in Sweden, which is attributed to changing climate as evidenced by warmer winters[69]. Global warming may also raise ocean levels and have a variety of effects on crop production[70]. In addition, there are already at least 25 million people who can no longer gain a secure livelihood in their homelands because of drought, soil erosion, desertification, deforestation and other environmental problems. These environmental refugees will increase dramatically unless the motivation to migrate is reduced by supplying them with acceptable lifestyles[71].

These global environmental changes have generated much debate, including at the 1992 Earth Summit which produced Agenda 21, an environmental agenda for the next century (see Box 3.4). In part, this debate was a result of inadequate and often conflicting information. The follow-up to this Summit was held in South Africa in 2002[72, 73] but with little progress made on the major health issues[74]. Since the Summit, the attention of the major donor countries has been diverted from the promises made at the Summit by the war in Iraq and by the economic downturn in the USA.

Box 3.4 Agenda 21: a strategy for change[13]

Areas in which international commitment to change is needed:

- allocating international aid to programmes directed at poverty alleviation and environmental health;
- investing in efforts to reduce soil erosion and to put agricultural practices on a sustainable footing;
- allocating more resources for family planning and education, especially for girls;
- supporting governments in their attempts to remove distortions and macroeconomic imbalances that damage the environment;
- providing finance to protect natural habitat and biodiversity;
- investing in research and development of non-carbon energy alternatives to respond to climate change.

Calls for action have come mainly from wealthy countries, although the environmental effects ultimately will be experienced globally. Epidemiological data are sparse in this area. Interdisciplinary collaboration and methods for estimating long-term effects on the basis of theoretical models require development. Predictions made over the last few years on the basis of global warming have been accurate. In 1995, the Inter-governmental Panel on Climate Change confirmed that the warming of the past few years 'is unlikely to be entirely due to natural causes' and that 'a pattern of climate response to human activities is identifiable in the climatological record'[75]. The 2001 third report of this Panel was even stronger and concluded that most of the warming observed over the last 50 years is attributable to human activities and estimated that between 1900 and 2100, average global temperatures will rise by at least 1.4 °C, and perhaps by as much as 5.4 °C – even a 1 °C rise would be greater than any change that has occurred in a single century of the past 10 000 years. The report also noted that the increased occurrence of extreme weather events and their adverse effects on humans over the past decade is probably a reflection of climatic instability due to global climate change[55].

The solution to these global environmental changes includes population control and a reduced dependence on cheap fossil fuels as a source of energy. Of more fundamental importance is sustainable development and the redistribution of global wealth to prevent the further destruction of the environment, especially in poor countries. However, the global response has been low key, and preventive actions on a scale to conserve the environment have not yet matched the rhetoric, apart from a few exceptions. In 1987, 36 nations signed the Montreal Protocol and agreed to restrict their release, but not production, of ozone-damaging chemicals with the aim of halving the release of chlorofluorocarbons by the year 2000. This Protocol was noteworthy because the evidence linking ozone depletion to adverse health effects was theoretical, and the empirical evidence non-existent. The decision was taken even before the ozone-damaging effect of these chemicals was confirmed.

The Montreal Protocol was revised and strengthened in 1990 and again in 1992. A halving of the peak 1988 emission levels of chlorofluorocarbons has been achieved in a few years as a result of this concerted global effort[38]. This positive development indicates that, where political will is strong, progress is possible. The Montreal Protocol is now faced with its first cases of defaulters and some evasion of the controls is occurring with the rapid growth of the black market[76]. The proposals of the 1997 Kyoto Protocol on global warming highlight the problems faced by public health practitioners when dealing with global issues. The rather modest goal of the Protocol is to limit the emission of greenhouse gases worldwide by an average of 5% of 1990 levels by 2012. The USA, a major contributor to the global problem, has declined to ratify the treaty which addresses the projected impact of global warming. The US prefers to protect national economic growth, even though this sustained growth will further exacerbate the environmental problem and its public health consequences[77].

3.4 Population growth and over-consumption

3.4.1 Population growth

Underlying the adverse global environmental changes are two fundamental issues: rapidly increasing population in poor countries and over-consumption in rich countries. The exponential population growth of the last ten generations will lead to either a levelling off because of actions taken now, or a dramatic reduction because of environmental disaster, if no action is taken. Population growth is indisputably a public health issue[78]. Public health programmes are a central means for stabilising or reducing population growth.

Globally, world population growth slowed from an annual rate of increase of 2.1% in the late 1960s to about 1.6% in the 1990s, reflecting the substantial decline in total fertility rate[11]. Growth rates are expected to continue declining to reach an average annual rate of population increase of about 1% by about the year 2020. Population growth is still considerably higher in the low income countries (2.2% per year between 1975 and 2000) compared with the wealthy countries (0.7% per year in the same period)[10].

The world's population is growing at approximately 70 million a year with 90% of this growth occurring in poor countries[79]. It is estimated that there are between 65 and 110 million females of all ages 'missing' as a result of higher than expected (or 'excess') female mortality in parts of the developing world, most notably in South Asia, China, West Asia, and parts of North Africa. Although the number of missing women has risen in absolute terms over the past decade, the share of missing women in relation to overall population has fallen, suggesting that the phenomenon has stabilised at a high level[80].

The Indian population contributes almost one in five of the world's total increase in population each year. A new policy to control population growth proposed by an expert group in India is said to be 'pro-nature, pro-poor and pro-women'[81]. The policy aims to replace vertically structured and target-oriented family planning welfare systems with people-oriented, decentralised and democratic planning involving village and city councils as well as state legislatures. Not all aspects of the proposed policy have been supported by members of women's organisations who have been the recipients of coercive programmes in the past.

Several countries in sub-Saharan Africa may already have entered the demographic trap where rapid population growth, as a result of falling death rates and sustained high birth rates, results in increasing pressure on resources, a rapidly deteriorating environment and ultimately an increase in infant death rates[82]. This has been called 'demographic entrapment'[83,84] (see Box 3.5). One essential requirement for preventing this process is a radical reduction of fertility.

The alternative, external reliance on provision of food, can at best, be only a short-term solution and runs the risk of encouraging starvation or warfare, as is the case in Rwanda[85].

Box 3.5   Demographic entrapment[82]

'A local population is demographically trapped if it has exceeded, or is projected to exceed, the combination of:

* the carrying capacity of its own ecosystem;
* its ability to obtain the products, and particularly the food, produced by other ecosystems except as food aid;
* its ability to migrate to other ecosystems in a manner which preserves (or improves) its standard of living.

The first two conditions describe the links that a population has with other ecosystems, and are crucial. They are most easily thought of as 'connectedness', and its opposite 'disconnectedness'. A severely trapped population faces the four tragedies of entrapment in varying combinations. Depending on local cultural, political and ecological factors it can starve, die from disease, slaughter itself or its neighbours, or be supported indefinitely by food aid'.

A critical feature is the ultimate size of a population at the end of its demographic transition in relation to its carrying capacity and its connection. The central importance of child survival instead of family planning and development poses important ethical questions that have not yet been adequately addressed at an international level[86–88]. For example, while UNICEF has emphasised the close interaction between poverty, population growth and environmental degradation[42], it disputes the poverty trap and is reluctant to recognise that aid directed towards reducing child death rates may be aggravating the effects of population growth, especially in the absence of fertility reduction, which requires substantial social and economic resources[81].

China provides an example of what has been done in one poor country to avoid entrapment. Population growth has been limited with the official one child-per-family policy announced in 1979. There are a number of unexpected outcomes of this policy in the short term, and in the long term it means that China will age sooner and more quickly than most other poor countries. The policy was easier to implement in urban areas than in rural China and, in general, the policy has 'reduced' the population by at least 250 million. One unanticipated outcome of the policy has been its stimulus to sex discrimination[89].

There is controversy on the nature of the relationship between poverty and population growth. Some biologists suggest the central problem is high birth rates. Others suggest that poverty is the force behind high birth rates, either because parents need more children for their own (economic) survival in later life, or because of a real sense of despair and lack of control. These two competing explanations have profoundly different policy implications. From a practical point of view, evidence favours the importance of making contraception available because there is general agreement that rapid population growth impedes social and economic progress[90]. Ultimately, of course, the solution must lie in the integration of both approaches – more equitable distribution of wealth and the provision of reproductive health care (Box 3.6).

Box 3.6 The reproductive revolution

Bangladesh is a good example of the so-called 'reproductive revolution'[91]. Despite being one of the world's poorest nations with high child mortality, and a society where most families depend on children for labour and support in old age, fertility rates declined from 7 to 5.5 children per woman between 1970 and 1990 and to 3.8 in the period 1995–2000[10]. During the same period, the use of contraception increased from 3% to over 50%. Bangladesh still has a low literacy rate; basic literacy and women's education are important factors in increasing the use of contraceptives. The availability of contraceptives in the context of quality integrated health care and real freedom of choice are essential.

In many parts of the world religion and politics all too often have taken precedence over public health concerns. Women in much of Central and Eastern Europe, particularly in Romania, have relied heavily on unsafe abortion because of the enforced scarcity of suitable contraception and safe abortion services. In the United States of America and elsewhere, women's legal right to safe abortion services is constantly under threat.

At present, only about 1% of all foreign aid is devoted to international family planning. Double this amount would be sufficient to make contraceptive choices available universally before the end of the century. About 100 million couples around the world want to limit the size of their families but cannot gain access to family planning services[92]. Cultural and religious beliefs hinder progress in this area. In 1996 the budget for the US Agency for International Development, a long-term leader in international family planning, was cut by almost seven-eighths; this cut will have major adverse effects on the health of women and families worldwide[93]. The current US administration has again enforced the so-called 'gag rule', which prohibits foreign aid to agencies that support abortion[94].

As we have seen in Chapter 2, diseases and deaths related to pregnancy complications cause substantial preventable mortality and morbidity. Births to very young women, closely spaced births and frequent pregnancies, inadequate prenatal and natal care, unwanted pregnancies that lead to unsafe and often illegal abortion, and malnutrition, all increase the risks of pregnancy. Women in some poor countries spend over half their childbearing years either pregnant or breast feeding[95]. Clearly maternal mortality is responsive to social and political changes. For most of these women, reproductive health is inseparable from general health.

In 2002 the world's population was approximately six billion people. The highest projection by the United Nations Population Fund suggests that, by the year 2050, there will be a staggering 12.5 billion; the mid-range estimate is for 9 billion. At the 1994 United Nations Conference in Cairo on Population and Development, guidelines were adopted to contain the world's population at about 7.3 billion by the year 2015, and at 7.8 billion in the year 2050. The conference polarised secular liberals and religious conservatives, who had serious reservations about references to abortion, the family, and sex education in the 20-year draft programme of action. Fortunately, a positive compromise was reached and a programme of action endorsed. The programme is farsighted and, apart from birth control, acknowledges the importance of the status of women, education, sexually transmitted diseases, health care, population distribution and migration[90]. The recommendations of the conference are non-binding, and the impact on population growth, as well as the more general targets, may be limited. Regrettably, at the 2002 Summit in South Africa little concrete action was agreed to further the goals of the earlier Cairo Summit[72].

3.4.2 Over-consumption

Over-consumption of energy, the other fundamental cause of global environmental degradation, is a defining feature of the rich world[96], and is growing at a faster rate than the population. As energy consumption increases because of population growth and as poor people become richer, economic growth has the potential of dramatically increasing energy consumption in poor countries, even with only a modest rise in the standard of living. This rise in energy consumption, and the associated rise in carbon dioxide concentrations, will contribute further to global warming. A narrow focus on economic growth is short-sighted and unhealthy consumption patterns threatens sustainable development[73].

Both the rich and the poor worlds have a role to play. The rich world needs to limit its carbon dioxide production and share its food and other resources. The poor world needs to limit its population. Both rich and poor have to adopt a sustainable life-style[81, 97]. Logically, however, given that 20% of the world's population consumes 80% of the resources, the initiatives must come from the rich world. Unfortunately, the prospects for this leadership are slim: it may take a global crisis of huge proportions for wealthy countries to take seriously their responsibility for the future of the world's poor. It has been speculated widely that the war in Iraq in 2003 was motivated in part by the need by the USA to control the huge oil reserves in this region.

3.5 Personal behaviours and health

Epidemiological research over the last five decades has focused on the association of personal behaviours with non-communicable disease, epitomising the rise of individually focused public health – at the expense of research focusing on the broader environmental determinants of health behaviour[98]. This research has been enormously productive, although it has often led to preventive programmes that blame individuals for their unhealthy habits (or lifestyles), rather than the powerful social and economic forces which drive these behaviours. Research on the role of individual human behaviours undoubtedly has been of great value in identifying specific risk factors. This information has been of primary benefit to privileged groups within wealthy countries. A focus on individual risk factors identifies only one of the pathways to disease. A major challenge is the integration of epidemiological research with research from other disciplines to clarify the other important influences on pathways to health (see Chapter 6).

3.5.1 Tobacco smoking

The products of the tobacco industry are the most readily preventable modern cause of premature death and disease. Tobacco has been used for centuries, although it was not until the development of mass production and marketing techniques that the habit became widespread. There are more than one billion smokers in the world today – one billion men and 215 million women; the

Table 3.2. *Number and percentage of adult smokers (15 years and older) by level of development*[100]

	Men		Women		Total	
	(millions)	%	(millions)	%	(millions)	%
Developed countries	115	34	76	21	191	27
Developing countries	810	50	115	7	925	29
Transition countries	83	54	24	14	107	33
World	1008	48	215	10	1223	29

majority of smokers, 925 million, live in poor countries (Table 3.2)[99, 100]. Men are almost five times as likely to use tobacco as women, yet almost 1 in 5 women are smokers in the Americas and Europe.

The per capita consumption of tobacco peaked in some countries of Western Europe, North America and Australasia over three decades ago and has been declining in many of these countries, although the decline may have stopped in the 1990s. A feature of the tobacco market in wealthy countries is the growth in the consumption by young people, especially women, even where consumption is declining in men and older people[101]. Lung cancer has already overtaken breast cancer as the leading cause of cancer death in women in the United States of America, and the worldwide lung cancer epidemic is still evolving.

*Another important aspect of smoking trends in wealthy countries is the widening social class gradients in cigarette smoking. Although smoking used to be a habit of wealthy people, this has not been the case over the last few decades. Since the first authoritative public health campaigns of the early 1960s, privileged groups increasingly have given up smoking and overall smoking prevalence has declined. This widening inequality by social class gradients is one example of the unintended effects of a health policy, which does not consider the complexity of the social circumstances in which individuals make personal health choices.

The epidemiological data on smoking point to a more general paradox: people whose health is already at risk through the cumulative effects of social and economic disadvantage are the most likely to pursue unhealthy patterns of behaviour[102]. This is paradoxical only if health behaviours are considered in individualistic terms without considering the social context; nor is this approach helpful in understanding why people, often women, pursue lifestyles that damage their health. Women and poor people generally develop routines that reflect a daily struggle to meet a set of conflicting health needs that are related to the welfare of an entire household. Health choices reflect a compromise that maintains household routines[101]. In this context, smoking by young and disadvantaged women is one means by which the welfare of the family is promoted, despite its long-term adverse health effects on the individual. Among many low-income families, smoking is one of the few luxuries and remains the norm[103].

  ＊A great concern is the steady rise in consumption in poor countries stimulated by the profit-seeking multi-national tobacco industry[104]. Even WHO has suffered from the malign influence of the tobacco industries[105]. The poor world is particularly vulnerable to the tactics of the tobacco industry[106]. In many poor countries tobacco is considered an 'affordable luxury' for people with few educational or employment opportunities. In a Chinese survey more than two-thirds of men and especially young men, were smokers (but only 2% of women) and smokers spent a substantial proportion of their income on cigarettes; there was a low rate of quitting and a low desire to quit[107]. The main increase in cigarette consumption in China took place only in the 1990s so tobacco mortality will increase substantially over the next few decades[108]. Reprehensively, the government of the United States of America has used the threat of trade sanctions to open up domestic cigarette markets in many countries to multi-national tobacco companies. For example, Thailand was forced to open its markets to multinational companies. However, because of strong government action, at least in part as a response to powerful anti-tobacco groups, the prevalence of smoking has actually declined in Thailand[109]. Unfortunately, most countries do not have such a strong response and the usual outcome of increasing exposure to foreign products and marketing techniques is an increase in consumption[110]. In many countries tobacco is an important cash crop and a source of export earnings. It is the most widely grown non-food crop in many African countries[111]. Zimbabwe, for example, is the second largest exporter of tobacco leaf in the world and derives more than a quarter of its export earnings from the crop[112]. Tobacco tax revenue is attractive to all governments, especially those of impoverished and indebted countries.

  Tobacco production is directly responsible for other important adverse consequences apart from health effects. For most countries, tobacco is responsible for a deficit in the balance of trade. Some of the poorest nations use precious capital to purchase tobacco, and deforestation is a serious and rapidly growing problem.

  Tobacco advertising is widespread and subject to few controls. There is evidence from at least one poor county, Papua New Guinea, that a systematic price policy not only reduces consumption but also increases national tax receipts for many years before a point of diminishing return is reached[113]. This relationship is well described for rich countries, although the point of diminishing returns to government revenue may be reached soon. There is conflicting evidence as to whether an increase in the price of cigarettes only makes poor families poorer or encourages them to stop smoking[107, 114]. The long-term solution is to deal with the underlying poverty and the lack of esteem amongst poor families. In the short term, the development and the evaluation of smoking cessation programmes of relevance to disadvantaged people is a priority.

The adverse health consequences of tobacco have been documented endlessly over the last 50 years by epidemiologists. This evidence is accepted by all but the tobacco industry and its special consultants[115]. The impact of tobacco on health is staggering. Worldwide, over four million adults die each year from tobacco-caused diseases[5]. About ten million people (mostly in China and India) will die from tobacco each year by the year 2025. It is useful to note that these ten million people are now alive (and smoking) and could be prevented from dying prematurely. To put it another way, tobacco will kill approximately 500 million of the six billion people alive today. The epidemic of smoking-caused deaths in women has not yet reached its peak anywhere. Death from smoking has become common in women in only a few countries. The proportion of women killed eventually by tobacco will be similar to the proportion of men if they continue to smoke, as has happened in Denmark[116]. The influential Queen of Denmark – a public smoker – may have had an adverse effect on death rates in women in her country[117] (Fig. 3.3).

The decline in consumption in wealthy countries is a result of public health campaigns and comprehensive tobacco control policies, which have evolved through the efforts of coalitions of special interest groups and the support of some governments, although the battle is not yet over in these countries[118]. Most efforts, however, have been directed towards regulating the behaviour of individuals, rather than controlling the tobacco industry. The biennial World Conferences on Tobacco and Health continue to encourage all nations to implement the comprehensive international strategies for tobacco control. A regional example is shown in Box 3.7. At long last it appears that the European Union is taking a firmer stance on tobacco smoking, though progress has been slowed by the resistance of Germany and other countries to support stronger control measures[119], and the European Union continues to spend much more on tobacco crop subsidies than it does on control measures[44].

The rise of passive smoking as a health issue in the 1980s gave a new environmental dimension to the previous focus on individual responsibility for health and expanded the arena for policy action[96]. Litigation, at least in wealthy countries, may have a major impact on future consumption trends. To date, tobacco companies have been successful in winning law suits claiming damages

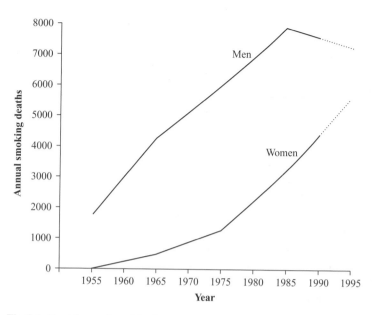

Fig. 3.3. Smoking-attributed deaths per year in Denmark, 1955–95. Estimated . . .
Source: Peto *et al*[116].

for smoking-caused illnesses, although the tide has turned as the emphasis shifts from individual law suits to class action suits. For example, US states have reached agreement from tobacco manufacturers for a huge settlement to compensate them for the costs of providing health care to patients with smoking-related diseases. Unfortunately, in many states much of this money has been used to fund budget deficits rather than tobacco control programmes. A positive side effect of the US litigation will be the need for tobacco companies to increase the price of cigarettes and this in turn will deter young smokers. A possible negative effect would be an increasing dependence of state governments on tobacco revenue. Another positive outcome of the US litigation has been the court-ordered release of a huge amount of industry documents which are now available publicly[120]. These documents have provided extraordinarily useful information to tobacco control groups and clarify the long-standing tactics of deception used by the industry to protect and expand its markets[105].

In summary, despite the enormous success of epidemiology in identifying the extent of the tobacco-induced epidemics, from a global perspective prevention policies have had only limited success. The lesson from wealthy countries is that changing addictive behaviour requires intensive effort to build a social movement at a non-governmental level which, when strong, will lead to government policy changes[121]. Public health practitioners have failed so far to deal comprehensively with this most preventable cause of premature death and disease largely because of the focus on individual behaviours and their associated risks rather than on the economic, social and cultural determinants of the tobacco epidemics. Local and national tobacco control efforts will be complemented by the acceptance by the World Health Assembly in May 2003 of the Framework Convention on Tobacco Control. This treaty represents the global legal response to the global epidemics of tobacco deaths and is described in more detail in Chapter 10.

3.5.2 Alcohol

The consumption of alcohol, especially by men, is widespread in most societies. The adverse health effects of alcohol consumption are many and varied, although in contrast to tobacco there are some beneficial effects. In most countries, important health problems stem from the excessive consumption of alcohol by a small proportion of the population. In New Zealand, for example, 11% of the population drink over half the total alcohol consumed, and young men make up most of this high-risk group[122]. Excessive consumption is dangerous. Combined with other activities such as driving, it becomes even more dangerous, both to the drinker and to others. Although alcohol-related problems are more frequent in heavy drinkers, the moderate drinking segment of the population, a much larger group, contributes the greater proportion of the problems. Effective strategies for the prevention and control of alcohol-induced health and social problems must therefore focus on all drinkers, not just on the small segment of the population at most risk[123]. The alcohol industry would prefer to focus on the so-called problem drinkers, which would require a much more restricted set of policies and programmes.

Alcohol-related diseases affect 5% to 10% of the world's population and was estimated to account for about 4% of the global burden of disease[5], although this is probably an underestimate. There is still much to be learnt about the balance between the adverse and beneficial social and health consequences of alcohol consumption. The protective effects against coronary heart disease, for example, appear real but are only of public health importance in older people who are at an increased risk of cardiovascular disease[124]. In some countries alcohol is responsible for about 20% of all deaths among 15–34 year old people. On balance, it is likely that alcohol is responsible for about 500 000 excess deaths worldwide, mostly from injury. The adverse disease effects are equal to the preventive effects on cardiovascular disease.

Average alcohol consumption increased between 1950 and 1980, particularly in poor countries which started from low levels of consumption. Since then, per capita consumption has levelled off, especially in wealthy countries. Consumption is increasing in many developing countries – especially in men – and in the countries of Central and Eastern Europe[125,126]. A particularly worrying feature of the alcohol scene is the young age at which many people begin drinking. Heavy consumption by young people is, to a large extent, a response to social ostracism and the despair resulting from unemployment and the lack of prospects. It appears that excess alcohol consumption in the form of binge drinking is a major cause of the striking increase in mortality rates in men in the former Soviet Union[127].

The alcohol industry is powerful and pervasive. Alcohol advertising has established the industry firmly as an important and accepted sponsor of many sporting events. It is not surprising that attempts to control alcohol advertising have met with little success. The alcohol industry remains the main barrier to the prevention of alcohol-related mortality and morbidity. A range of strategies are available to prevent alcohol problems, though more research is required concerning the effectiveness of policies in developing countries[125]. Strong community and government leadership is required to implement these policies.

3.5.3 Dietary imbalance: underconsumption and overconsumption

Malnutrition resulting from lack of food is the major dietary problem worldwide and is responsible for a significant part of the global burden of disease[5]. As countries become richer, consumption of animal fat replaces traditional foods, which generally contain less fat and more carbohydrates – the nutrition transition as described in Chapter 1. The relationship between diet and non-communicable disease is complex, but the increased consumption of saturated and *trans*-fatty acids is the major underlying cause of the modern epidemic of coronary heart disease[128]. Vegetarians have lower mortality largely because of their low intake of animal fat and the protective effect of fruit and vegetables. More generally, the affluent, high meat-eating quarter of the world's population is not desirable ecologically at a global level, because of the large amount of edible energy required to produce animal products[47].

Increased salt intake, along with excessive body weight and alcohol intake, is responsible for the high average levels of blood pressure in wealthy countries[129]. An imbalance between intake of calories and levels of activity, results in the striking increase in the prevalence of obesity observed in many countries over the last two decades. In the USA approximately 64% of the adult population is overweight (Body Mass Index (BMI) over 25) and 31% is obese (BMI over 30)[130]. Decreasing levels of physical activity have made an important contribution to the epidemics of obesity[131]. Obesity has a variety of adverse health effects including raised blood pressure, diabetes, heart disease and joint problems. A range of other dietary components are implicated in a variety of modern diseases, for example, calcium intake and osteoporosis, but collectively their public health significance is much less than the major non-communicable diseases such as heart disease, stroke and cancer. Public health practitioners in wealthy countries are concerned rightly about the health effects of over-nutrition, but from a global perspective hunger is a much more important problem. In many poor populations there is now an unfortunate tendency for obesity to co-exist with underweight in the same household, with adult men tending to be overweight and children underweight[132].

3.5.4 Physical inactivity

The increasing prevalence of physical inactivity in wealthy countries illustrates the manner in which socio-economic development influences health adversely. Traditionally, most people were physically active[133] and in a few societies this pattern is still widespread. Physical activity has now become a leisure time activity undertaken in wealthy countries by only a small (and usually the most advantaged) proportion of the population. The publication of the influential report of the US Surgeon General on physical activity and health[134] provided a platform for the recognition of physical activity as a major public health issue. Since then, the emerging epidemiological evidence has shown unequivocal relationships between the adverse effects of physical inactivity on health and the health-promoting effects of activity[135, 136]. Physical inactivity is associated strongly with increased risks of various conditions including heart disease, ischaemic stroke, breast cancer, colon cancer and Type 2 diabetes. The relationship between inactivity and these conditions has been shown to be causal, and biologically plausible pathways exist to explain the association. Estimates of the global burden of disease in 2000 revealed that physical inactivity accounted for 22% of heart disease, 11% of ischaemic stroke, 14% of diabetes, 16% of colon cancer and 10% of breast cancer[5]. Overall, physical inactivity was responsible for between 3% and 4% of the total global burden of disease due to these conditions.

Evidence is less clear for the association between participation in physical activity and osteoporosis and the incidence of falls among the elderly, but physical activity can increase quality of life and independent living among older people[137]. Physical activity can also reduce the severity of symptoms among those suffering depression and anxiety[138] and, along with diet, it is an important factor in the maintenance of healthy weight.

Current public health guidelines reflect epidemiological evidence that, to obtain health benefits, moderate intensity physical activity must be done for at least 30 minutes on most days of the week. Despite this seemingly modest level of activity required for health, available prevalence data suggest that, for most adults, it is still too demanding. In most developed countries, less than 50% of adults undertake physical activity at levels sufficient to confer health benefits[135]. Incorporating even this small amount of activity into daily life in wealthy countries is surprisingly difficult and not made easier by dependence on personalised transport, the lack of recreational facilities, the move away from physical activity as part of school curricula, and increased working hours. Participation rates in some countries have stabilised[139] or declined despite public awareness campaigns to increase activity. These campaigns have reiterated public health guidelines, which emphasise the importance of walking and participation in moderate intensity activities rather than the less feasible goal of vigorous activity. Successful interventions tend to reflect an integrated approach where awareness campaigns have broad-based community support and infrastructures in place[140].

3.5.5 Unsafe sex

Sexually transmitted diseases are a major public health problem. The advent of the human immunodeficiency virus (HIV), responsible for AIDS, however, added a new and cruel dimension to sexual activity. HIV/AIDS indicates our vulnerability to emerging microbes. HIV infection is transmitted by three means: contact with contaminated blood, sexual transmission and mother to child transmission. The major mode of transmission worldwide is by sexual contact, but in some geographical areas injecting drug use is the predominant mode of transmission.

Approximately 50% of HIV-infected people develop AIDS within 9 years and the average survival after AIDS is 12 months without modern treatment. Only a very small proportion of HIV infected people do not progress to AIDS and these people may ultimately provide the clues for the development of effective vaccines against HIV. Although there is no cure or preventive immunisation, the availability of a range of new, and expensive, pharmaceutical agents have increased survival of AIDS patients dramatically. However, in the absence of effective treatment, as is the case in most of the world, the majority of AIDS patients will die. Without treatment, the case fatality at 1 year from AIDS diagnosis is approximately 95%. The lack of access to effective drugs because of their cost and because of the continued lack of support to the health sector in many countries is a continuing public health tragedy. The current interpretation of patent rules and regulations under the World Trade Organization's (WTO) Multilateral Agreement on Trade Related Aspects of Intellectual Property Rights (TRIPS) is widely perceived as a serious barrier to wider access, particularly in countries without pharmaceutical manufacturing capacity. Considerable pressure is being directed to the WTO and the pharmaceutical companies to ensure wider and cheaper access to drugs, and progress is being made with the increasing availability of cheap generic products and through differential pricing.

The first case of AIDS was diagnosed in 1981. The AIDS epidemic began at a time when wealthy countries were becoming complacent about infectious diseases. Not since the 1918 influenza pandemic had such a devastating epidemic appeared. By the end of 2002, it was estimated that almost 42 million people were living with HIV/AIDS including 3.2 million children under the age of 15 years. In 2002, 5 million people were newly infected with HIV alone, and about 17 million adults and 1.5 million children were infected with HIV/AIDS[141]. There is a large discrepancy between the reported and estimated number of AIDS cases because of under diagnosis, incomplete reporting, and reporting delay. In 2002, approximately three million AIDS deaths occurred, including 1.2 million women and 600 000 children with four out of five deaths occurring in sub-Saharan Africa (Fig. 3.4).

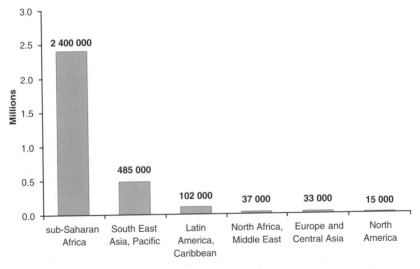

Fig. 3.4. Estimated adult and child deaths due to HIV–AIDS during 2002.[141]

The public health impact of the AIDS epidemic is chilling. For example, AIDS has lowered the life expectancy in Zambia and Zimbabwe by several decades with life expectancy now around 40 years. The highest prevalence rates of HIV infection are in Botswana where the prevalence is approaching 40% in the adult population, threatening the very survival of the country. The world was not ready, either politically or socially, to confront the public health crises which rapidly developed in the 1980s as the epidemic spread. The epidemic was categorised initially as a disease specific to homosexual men, who consequently suffered stigmatisation and additional discrimination. It took time to reduce the prejudice and bureaucratic inertia that characterised the initial response of most governments It is especially tragic that the lessons learnt in the United States of America and Europe have been applied so slowly in other regions.

The rate of development of new HIV infections has levelled off in Western Europe, the United States and other Western countries, possibly because of changing behaviour and secure blood supplies. Where antiretroviral drugs are available for treatment of HIV/AIDS, largely in developed countries, there has been a dramatic decline in new AIDS cases and AIDS deaths. Unfortunately, this is not the case in Eastern Europe and Central Asia; the virus continues to ravage sub-Saharan Africa. Uganda has successfully slowed the epidemic at least in part because of the strong public leadership from the President and a comprehensive mobilisation campaign involving a wide range of local agencies focusing on abstinence, condom use, support for people with AIDS and action against discrimination. In contrast, 4 years after single dose nevirapine was shown to reduce perinatal HIV infection by 50%, less than 4% of pregnant women with HIV infection receive treatment[142]. The epidemic is now spreading rapidly through Asia. India and China seem particularly vulnerable although they have now stepped up their anti-HIV programmes[143, 144]. Cambodia provides another example of an effective national response that has turned the epidemic around. The opportunity for bringing the HIV/AIDS epidemic under control is narrowing rapidly in Asia[142, 145].

In many countries of sub-Saharan Africa, AIDS is the most common cause of death in young men and women, and this is now also the case in parts of the United States in certain population groups. In many poor countries, up to 50% of all new HIV infections occur in people aged 15–24 years. An expanding HIV epidemic continues in India. The consequences could be catastrophic. An estimated four million people were living with HIV at the end of 2001 – the second-highest figure in the world, after South Africa[142]. One estimate puts the number of potential cases of AIDS in India at 20 million by 2010[144]. A depressing feature of the epidemic is the rapidly growing number of AIDS orphans, i.e. children whose parents have died of AIDS[146]; by the end of 2001 it was estimated that 14 million children aged under 15 years had lost one or both parents to AIDS.

Epidemiologists have played primary roles in identifying HIV and tracking the spread of the AIDS pandemic and more recently in the trials which have demonstrated the effectiveness of anti-retroviral drugs. There are three broad epidemiological patterns to this epidemic: low prevalence, concentrated and generalised, although there are also a range of sub-regional epidemics (Table 3.3). In the United States, Canada, Central and Western Europe, Australia, North Africa and parts of South America, HIV has spread mainly among homosexual and bisexual men and injecting drug users. Prevalence remains low and concentrated in specific population groups. In the remainder of sub-Saharan Africa, where multiple sexual partners are common, most infections have been acquired heterosexually and the epidemics are more generalised. Eastern European countries such as Russia and Estonia now have the most rapidly developing epidemics driven by injecting drug use.

Social and demographic factors affect the spread of HIV greatly. In many poor countries, male migration to more wealthy countries in search of work is common, and economically impoverished women are forced to move to urban areas and become sex workers to earn money for their poor rural families. The task of convincing apparently healthy young men and women to abstain or practise safe sex by using condoms and barrier methods is difficult, especially given the lack of availability and unacceptability of family planning in many parts of the world and culturally entrenched imbalances in gender and power relationships in many societies.

An important change in the international campaign against AIDS was the establishment of the Joint United Nations Programme on HIV/AIDS in 1995, initially bringing together six United Nations agencies, which has since expanded to eight, with significant HIV/AIDS-related activities. The rationale for such a development was the need to promote an expanded response, recognising the need for a multi-sectoral response, complementing the health sector response and better coordination of the work of different agencies. Equally important is the recognition that the AIDS epidemic is now at a critical juncture. In many countries, boredom and complacency have compromised the commitment in countries to act, and resources have not been adequate for the sustained prevention and education programmes that are required. In some countries the epidemics previously confined to specific vulnerable populations (such as injecting drug users) and geographic areas (such as large urban areas), are now spreading into general populations and areas. As a consequence, targeted

Table 3.3. *Regional HIV/AIDS statistics and features, end of 2002*[142]

	Epidemic Started	Adults and children living with HIV/AIDS	Adults and children newly infected with HIV	Adult prevalence rate	% of HIV-positive adults who are women	Main mode(s) of transmission for those living with HIV/AIDS*
Sub-Saharan Africa	Late 1970s Early 1980s	29.4 million	3.5 million	8.8%	58%	Hetero
North Africa and Middle East	Late 1980s	550 000	83 000	0.3%	55%	Hetero, IDU
South and South-East Asia	Late 1980s	6.0 million	700 000	0.6%	36%	Hetero, IDU
East Asia & Pacific	Late 1980s	1.2 million	270 000	0.1%	24%	IDU, Hetero, MSM
Latin America	Late 1970s Early 1980s	1.5 million	150 000	0.6%	30%	MSM, IDU, Hetero
Caribbean	Late 1970s Early 1980s	440 000	60 000	2.4%	50%	Hetero, MSM
Eastern Europe and Central Asia	Early 1990s	1.2 million	250 000	0.6%	27%	IDU
Western Europe	Late 1970s Early 1980s	570 000	30 000	0.3%	25%	MSM, IDU
North America	Late 1970s Early 1980s	980 000	45 000	0.6%	20%	MSM, IDU, Hetero
Australia and New Zealand	Late 1970s Early 1980s	15 000	500	0.1%	7%	MSM
Total		42 million	5 million	1.2%	50%	

* Hetero, heterosexual transmission; IDU, injecting drug users; MSM, men who have sex with men.

prevention efforts for such groups as men who have sex with men and injecting drug users risk being neglected. In China, ignoring these factors has provided the foothold for a major epidemic in less than a decade[147]. In some countries where prevention efforts had been very effective among these vulnerable populations, increasing risk behaviours and HIV transmission rates are now being witnessed. Few communities have achieved a level of behaviour change sufficient to halt the spread of HIV. The demonstration that treatment of other sexually transmitted diseases with relatively cheap interventions also slows the transmission of HIV, is another source of hope for the future.

An important insight from almost two decades of prevention and control efforts is the critical relationship between social discrimination and vulnerability to HIV[148]. This discrimination interferes with every aspect of prevention and control programmes. The Global AIDS Policy Coalition has prepared a new strategy to reduce the widening gap between the pandemic and the response[149]. This strategy is based on the recognition that social forces shape personal and collective vulnerability to HIV/AIDS and provides an excellent outline of an appropriate response to a global problem.

A pressing challenge in most countries is the need to build the health service infrastructure to facilitate the delivery of the effective anti-retroviral drugs and to provide the counselling and support services needed by patients and their families. A very encouraging development was the UN General Assembly Special Session on AIDS in July 2001. In an unprecedented move – the General Assembly had never before devoted a session to a specific disease – the leaders of all nations agreed to support the fight against HIV using a comprehensive approach that mobilises all sectors of society and in which both prevention and care are given detailed attention. They also committed to specific action targets for 2003 and 2005 (3 million on treatment by 2005). Other positive developments include new global resources (e.g. hundreds of millions of dollars available through The Global Fund to Fight AIDS, TB and Malaria and World Bank loans and grants), and new international and local partnerships, which are bringing together governments, the private sector, affected communities and civil society. The challenge now for the public health community is to hold governments accountable for their pledges and support their actions against the epidemic.

3.6 Injury: unintentional and intentional

Injuries are a major and increasing cause of death and disability in all countries. Although individuals are often blamed for their injuries, in most cases there are powerful environmental forces responsible for the incident leading to the injury.

3.6.1 Car crashes

In many rich countries, cars are an indispensable aspect of daily life for much of the population. These societies are organised on the assumption that personal transport is readily available. The widespread use of motor cars is a mixed blessing and the adverse health consequences affect most of the population, not just the car users[150]. Car crashes are an important cause of death, responsible for over 1.2 million deaths worldwide in 2000 with 50% of the deaths occurring between the ages of 15 and 44 years; 90% of all road traffic deaths occur in low and middle income countries and, globally, the mortality rates of males is almost three times higher than that for females[5]. The highest burden of injuries and fatalities is borne disproportionately by poor people in developing countries, as pedestrians, passengers of buses and minibuses, and cyclists[151]. The numbers killed in car crashes is not high compared to heart disease, but the people killed are usually young. As the number of cars increases, so does the number of deaths[152]. The reunification of Germany apparently led to a dramatic increase in the rate of traffic-related mortality as a result of the economic changes and the greater availability of cars in conjunction with an increase in the number of inexperienced drivers on relatively poor roads[153].

The type of injury varies according to the type of vehicle used most commonly. In countries with a high proportion of motorcycles, for example, Southeast Asia, the risks are greater for drivers or passengers, but lower for pedestrians. In wealthy countries, the highest crash death rate is among young men, reflecting car ownership patterns and high risk behaviours such as drinking and driving.

Future trends in motor vehicle crash death rates in poor countries will depend on traffic densities and on the initiation and effectiveness of preventive measures including the use of cycling and pedestrian routes and greater access to reliable and free-moving public transport systems. In many rich countries, death rates are declining, despite increasing traffic densities, because of the gradual introduction of safety measures and the general economic slowdown which reduces road travel. Public health campaigns and legislation, for example, pre-licence training, drink–driving laws including random breath tests, control of speeding, compulsory wearing of seat belts, vehicle design requirements, road improvements and better management of injuries, have all been effective. So even with an increasing exposure to motor vehicles, the risk of death can be reduced. It remains to be seen whether the same methods will control the expected increase in road death rates in poor countries as motorised transport becomes increasingly available.

3.6.2 Occupational hazards

Occupational hazards are an under-appreciated cause of death and of economic costs, particularly in poor countries where workers do not have the benefit of occupational health and safety standards. Worldwide, at least two million fatalities occur each year due to occupational disease or injuries[154]. These figures are likely to be serious underestimates because of the limited data from most countries.

WHO evaluated the contribution of six occupational risk factors to the global burden of disease in its recent Comparative Risk Analysis[5]. More than 300 000 fatal injuries were found to occur each year, primarily in the occupations associated with agriculture, transportation, construction, and primary industries such as mining. In wealthy countries, occupational dangers and the high cost of accidents to productivity have been recognised, and this, together with strong unions, has made the work place relatively more safe. The WHO analysis found that occupational exposure to carcinogens is responsible for 10% of global lung cancer and 2% of leukaemia[5]. This problem is exacerbated by the selective transfer of hazardous industries and chemicals to poor countries, often in the absence of adequate safety measures[6]. Some risks have their impact on morbidity rather than mortality. Low back pain is associated with many ergonomic stressors at work, including lifting and carrying heavy loads, forceful movements and frequent bending. Occupational noise exposures often exceed standards. WHO found that 37% of global back pain is due to work routine and 16% of hearing loss is due to workplace exposures[5].

The impact of many new occupational risks is not measurable due to inadequate data. Disorders in this group include stress-related cardiovascular disease and occupational overuse syndrome (or repetitive strain injury), and they continue to emerge and reflect the changing patterns of employment. In poor countries, the rapid industrialisation has permitted little time for adjustment and workforce training, resulting in considerably higher rates of industrial injuries and occupational diseases than in wealthy countries. The problem is exacerbated by the selective transfer of hazardous industries and chemicals to poor countries, often in the absence of adequate safety measures. Most of the time, work-related disorders are preventable and the burden of occupational risk factors can be diminished by improving work conditions.

3.6.3 Violence: personal, civil and international

Violent death is a very common feature of daily life. In 2000, violence caused approximately 700 000 deaths worldwide[5]. Violence takes many forms, and may be self-directed (suicide), family-directed (child or spouse abuse and murder), random (drive-by killings), or directed at ethnic, cultural or national enemies. Suicide is an important cause of death, especially among young men, and is responsible for about 50% of all violent deaths. The causes are complex and the preventive remedies elusive. In many countries, suicide rates are increasing. Homicide in many societies usually involves family members, although the pattern varies. In general, rates are highest in young men, especially black men in the United States, but rates vary by income, residence and ethnicity and relate closely to the availability of firearms[155]. Gun violence is the second leading cause of death among people aged 4–19 years in the United States[156]. Violence against women is pervasive in all societies (see Box 3.8).

The impact of war on health has a depressingly long history. Even more appalling is the continuing resort to warfare to solve territorial, ethnic or cultural conflict. Between 1945 and 1992, there were 149 major wars, killing more than 23 million people. On an average yearly basis, the number of war deaths in this period was more than double the deaths in the nineteenth century, and seven times greater than in the eighteenth century[161]. Collective violence which includes war and genocide, was responsible for about 20% of all violent deaths estimated to have occurred worldwide in 2000[157]. The 'risk factors' for collective violence include the widespread availability of small arms, inequalities in access to educational, economic and political opportunities, and human rights abuses[162]. Collective violence mediates health effects both through direct death and injury related to violence, and indirectly, through degradation of the social environment, disruption to basic health services and health care systems, population displacement, severe food shortages, and widespread destruction of public water and sanitation systems[163, 164].

In terms of direct health effects, it has been estimated that conflicts accounted for over 230 000 deaths in 2001 (0.4% of all deaths) with over half of these occurring in sub-Saharan Africa[165]. Men aged 15–44 accounted for well over a third of these deaths.

A wide variety of different effects on health arise from the disruptive social changes accompanying collective violence. Collective violence typically creates population displacement and a substantial degradation of social infrastructure such as health care systems and food production and distribution networks[162, 163]. Not frequently, life-sustaining infrastructure of civilian populations is specifically targeted in conflicts through acts such as execution of health

Box 3.8   Violence against women: a violation of human rights[157]

Violence against women is a pervasive, but little recognised, human rights
abuse. It ranges from wife or partner abuse to mutilation of girls' genitals
to ensure virginity until marriage, to murder of young brides when parents
fail to provide expected dowries. The key feature in all of these cases is
that women are targets for violence simply because they are female.

Assaults on women by their husbands or male partners are the most
common form of violence. Intimate partner violence occurs in all
countries, irrespective of social, economic, religious or cultural group[158].
It is estimated that about a quarter of the world's women are abused
within their own homes, and that physical violence in intimate
relationships is often accompanied by psychological abuse, and in
one-third to over one-half of cases by sexual abuse[159]. The health
consequences of violence include not just physical injury, but psychiatric
disturbance and major depression often leading to attempted suicide.
Pregnant mothers are prime targets for abuse, and women battered during
pregnancy have a twofold risk of miscarriage and a fourfold risk of
having a low birthweight baby compared with women who are not
beaten[160].

Violence (or the threat to violence) is all too common a dimension of
sexual decision-making, including the use of family planning. The
international initiative on safe pregnancy and childbirth, Safe
Motherhood, could well extend its brief to include the physical safety of
the mother and her child. Similarly, UNICEF and other agencies involved
with child survival initiatives could place family violence higher on the
international agenda. Ultimately, this would place value on the quality of
women's lives.

care workers, and destruction of food and water distribution complexes[164, 166].
Research in these settings has shown a significant reduction in indicators such
as vaccination status, which accompany collective violence. The high rates of
associated civilian mortality are also a reflection of pre-existing fragility of the
population and a failure of international development aid pre-conflict[167].

While it is difficult to estimate the burden of health effects that are attributable
to these changes with precision, available evidence suggests they are substantial.
Non-fatal injuries related to conflict are substantial. Crude mortality rates in
displaced populations fleeing collective violence have been reported at 5 to 12

times above baseline rates[168], and were substantially higher among those fleeing the Rwandan genocide[169]. The primary causes of death in these circumstances are communicable diseases and malnutrition. The incidence of AIDS in Africa has also increased considerably as a direct result of civil wars[170].

The ratio of people wounded to those killed during conflicts spanning the twentieth century have been estimated to range from 1.9 to 13.0 with an average of around three people wounded for every individual killed[171]. The use of anti-personnel mines in many recent conflicts has meant that the after-effects of active warfare continue for years[172, 173]. The traditional tools of public health can mitigate a number of the direct and indirect effects of collective violence, and draw attention to some of the determinants of collective violence. True progress towards preventing collective violence can only be made through broad based efforts that extend into the political sphere and make genuine progress in addressing root causes of conflict[162, 174].

3.7 Summary

The most important causes of ill health in all countries are the underlying social and economic characteristics of a society. Unfortunately, these factors are poorly defined and, from a policy perspective, difficult to deal with and too often neglected. A basic and surprisingly low level of wealth is an essential requirement for health. Income distribution within a country seems to be an important determinant of overall health status. The negative effects of globalisation and the specific long-term effects of global environmental degradation, caused by over-population and over-consumption, present a special challenge for epidemiologists and public health practitioners.

The pathways between the social and economic characteristics of a society and health and disease status are complex and require further multi-disciplinary study. Much more attention has been directed towards the role of individual health behaviours. The most readily preventable of these is tobacco consumption. Unfortunately, the tobacco epidemic is spreading rapidly in poor countries, due to the effective and unscrupulous marketing and promotion campaigns of the multinational tobacco companies and the weakness of the government responses. Although much is known about the general and specific causes of health and disease, this information is integrated into public health policy and practice insufficiently. As a consequence, the burden of preventable death and disease remains high in all countries and the benefits of the impressive amount of new knowledge on risks to health have been utilised disproportionately by the more privileged groups within society[175].

Chapter 3   Key points

- The major global public health problem is poverty. The absolute number of people living in poverty is increasing.
- Other important socio-economic determinants of health status are: poor housing, unsafe water supply, lack of sanitation, malnutrition and illiteracy.
- A major new public health hazard is the global environment change: global warming and ozone depletion.
- Rapid population growth, especially in poor countries, and over-consumption in wealthy countries, are inter-related issues which require a global response.
- Tobacco smoking, the major personal behaviour affecting health, has received much epidemiological attention; the tobacco-induced epidemics continue unabated.
- HIV/AIDS, the most devastating of the new communicable diseases, is having a major effect on public health, especially in poor countries of Africa, and increasingly in Asia.

References

1. Evans, R.G., Barer, M.L. & Marmor, T.R. *Why Are Some People Healthy and Others Not?* New York: de Gruyter, 1994.
2. McMichael, A.J. *Human Frontiers, Environments and Disease.* Cambridge: Cambridge University Press, 2001.
3. Rose, G. *The Strategy of Preventive Medicine.* Oxford: Oxford University Press, 1992.
4. Axelsson, G., Liljeqvist, T., Andersson, L., Bergman, B. & Rylander, R. Dietary factors and lung cancer among men in West Sweden. *Int. J. Epidemiol.* 1996; **25**: 32–9.
5. World Health Organization. *World Health Report 2002. Reducing Risks, Promoting Healthy Life.* Geneva; World Health Organization, 2002.
6. Pearce, N., Matos, E., Vainio, H., Boffetta, P. & Kogevinas, M. *Occupational Cancer in Developing Countries.* Lyon: IARC Scientific Publications, 1994.
7. Powles, J. Changes in disease patterns and related social trends. *Soc. Sci. Med.* 1992; **35**: 377–87.
8. World Health Organization. *Report of the Commission on Macroeconomics and Health. Macroeconomics and Health: Investing in Health for Economic Development.* Geneva: WHO, 2001.
9. World Development Report, 1993. *Investing in Health, World Development Indicators.* New York: Oxford University Press, 1993.

10. United Nations Development Programme. *Human Development Report 2002. Deepening Democracy in a Fragmented World*. New York: Oxford University Press, 2002.

11. United Nations Development Programme. *Human Development Report*. New York: Oxford University Press, 1994.

12. Integrated Regional Information Network. Ethiopia: *Campaign to Eradicate Polio Suffers Setback*, 13 December 2001. Nairobi: UNOCHA, 2001.

13. World Development Report. *Development and the Environment*. Oxford: Oxford University Press, 1992.

14. Moore, P. Young people's health affected by relative poverty. *Lancet* 1997; **349**: 1152.

15. Dean, M. Absolute effective of relative poverty. *Lancet* 1994; **344**: 463.

16. Najman, J.M. Health and poverty: past, present and prospects for the future. *Soc. Sci. Med.* 1993; **36**: 157–66.

17. Quick, A. & Wilkinson, R.G. *Income and Health*. London: Socialist Health Association, 1991.

18. United Nations Development Programme, Arab Fund for Economic and Social Development. *Arab Human Development Report 2002: Creating Opportunities for Future Generations*. New York: United Nations Development Programme, Regional Bureau for Arab States, 2002.

19. Murray, C.J.L. & Chen, L.C. In search of a contemporary theory for understanding mortality change. *Soc. Sci. Med.* 1993; **36**: 143–55.

20. Grosse, R.N. Interrelation between health and population: observations derived from field experiences. *Soc. Sci. Med.* 1980; **14C**: 99–120.

21. Wilkinson, R.G. Income distribution and life expectancy. *Br. Med. J.* 1992; **304**: 165–8.

22. Wilkinson, R.G. *Unhealthy Societies. The Afflictions of Inequality.* London: Routledge, 1999.

23. Watt, G.C.M. Health implications of putting value added tax on fuel: time to combat fuel poverty. *Br. Med. J.* 1994; **309**: 1030–1.

24. Kawachi, I., Levine, S., Miller, S.M., Lasch, K. & Amick, B. *Income inequality and life expectancy: theory, research and policies.* (Working paper no. 94–2). The Health Institute, New England Medical Center, 1994.

25. Marmot, M.G. & Davey-Smith, G. Why are the Japanese living longer? *Br. Med. J.* 1989; **299**: 1547–51.

26. Evans, R.G. & Stoddart, G.L. Producing health, consuming health care. *Soc. Sci. Med.* 1990; **31**: 1347–63.

27. Kawachi, I. & Kennedy, B. *The Health of Nations: Why Inequality is Harmful to Health*. New York: The New Press, 2002.

28. Mackenbach, J.P. Income inequality and population health. *Br. Med. J.* 2002; **324**: 1–2.

29. Marmot, M.G., Davey Smith, G., Stansfeld, S. *et al.* Health inequalities among British civil servants: the Whitehall II study. *Lancet* 1991; **337**: 1387–93.

30. Wennemo, I. Infant mortality, public policy and inequality – a comparison of 18 industrialised countries 1950–85. *Soc. Hlth Illness* 1993; **15**: 429–45.

31. Smith, R. *Unemployment and Health: a Disaster and a Challenge*. Oxford: Oxford University Press, 1987.

32. World Health Organization. *The World Health Report 1995. Bridging the Gaps.* Geneva: WHO, 1995.
33. Watkins, K. *The Oxfam Poverty Report.* Oxford: Oxfam, 1995.
34. Department of Economic and Social Affairs, Population Division. *World Urbanization Prospects. The 1999 Revision.* New York: United Nations, 2001.
35. Wang'ombe, J.K. Public health crisis of cities in developing countries. *Soc. Sci. Med.* 1995; **41**: 857–62.
36. Heath, I. The poor man at his gate. Homelessness is an avoidable cause of ill health. *Br. Med. J.* 1994; **309**: 1675–6.
37. Bartram, J. New water forum will repeat old message. *Bull. WHO* 2003; **81**: 158.
38. McMichael, A.J. *Planetary Overload. Global Environmental Change and the Health of the Human Species.* Cambridge: Cambridge University Press, 1993.
39. Vidal, J. Ready to fight to the last drop. *Guardian Weekly*, August 20th, 1995.
40. World Health Organization. *Diet, Nutrition and the Prevention of Chronic Disease.* Technical Report Series No. 916. Geneva:WHO/FAO, 2003.
41. UNICEF. *The State of the World's Children.* New York: Oxford University Press, 1995.
42. Editorial. Foie gras, fine words, and failure – just another UN summit. *Lancet* 2002; **359**: 2047.
43. Barker, D.J.P. *Fetal and Infant Orgins of Adult Disease.* London: British Medical Journal, 1992.
44. Beaglehole, R. & Yach, D. Globalization and the prevention of noncommunicable disease: the neglected chronic diseases of adults. *Lancet* 2003; **362**: 903–8.
45. Dyson, T. Prospects for feeding the world. *Br. Med. J.* 1999; **319**: 988–91.
46. Conway, G. & Toenniessen, G. Feeding the world in the twenty-first century. *Nature* 1999; **402** Suppl: C55–8.
47. McMichael, A.J. Impact of climatic and other environmental changes on food production and population health in the coming decades. *Proc. Nutr. Soc.* 2001; **60**: 195–201.
48. Conway, G. *The Doubly Green Revolution: Food for All in the 21st Century.* New York: Penguin Books, 1997.
49. Vitti, P., Delange, F., Pinchera, A. *et al.* Europe is iodine deficient. *Lancet* 2002; **361**: 1226.
50. Hetzel, B.S. From Papua New Guinea to the United Nations: the prevention of mental defect due to iodine deficiency. *Aust. J. Publ. Hlth* 1995; **19**: 231–4.
51. Adams, T.A.I. International Council for Control of Iodine Deficiency Disorders, and the Hetzel phenomenon. *Aust. J. Publ. Hlth* 1995; **19**: 225.
52. Evans, I. SAPping maternal health. *Lancet* 1995; **346**: 1046.
53. Caldwell, C. Health transition: the cultural, social and behavioural determinants of health in the third world. *Soc. Sci. Med.* 1993; **36**: 125–35.
54. Costanza, R., d'Arge, R., de Groot, R. *et al.* The value of the world's ecosystem services and natural capital. *Nature* 1997; **387**: 253–60.
55. Intergovernmental Panel on Climate Change. Climate Change 2000, *Third Assessment Report.* Cambridge: Cambridge University Press, 2001.
56. Lomberg, B. How healthy is the world? *Br. Med. J.* 2002; **325**: 1461–4.
57. McMichael, A.J. Population, environment, disease, and survival: past patterns, uncertain futures. *Lancet* 2002; **359**: 1145–8.

58. Rees, W.E. & Wackernagel, M. Urban ecological footprints: why cities cannot be sustainable and why they are a key to sustainability. *Environ. Impact Assess. Rev.* 1996; **16**: 223–48.
59. McMichael, A.J. Gilding the global lily. *Br. Med. J.* 2002; **325**: 1461–6.
60. McMichael, P. The impact of globalisation, free trade and technology on food and nutrition in the new millennium. *Proc. Nutr. Soc.* 2001; **60**: 215–20.
61. Brunekreef, B. & Holgate, S.T. Air pollution and health. *Lancet* 2002; **360**: 1233–42.
62. Bobak, M. & Feachem, R.G.A. Air pollution and mortality in Central and Eastern Europe. *Eur. J. Pub. Hlth* 1995; **5**: 82–6.
63. Kumar, S. Independent assessment at Bhopal. *Lancet* 1994; **343**: 283–4.
64. Jasanoff, S. *Learning from Disaster: Risk Management after Bhopal.* Philadelphia: University of Pennsylvania Press, 1995.
65. Lapierre, D. & Moro, J. *Five Past Midnight in Bhopal.* New York: Scribner, 2002.
66. Bhopal website www.bhopal.net.
67. Nuclear Energy Agency. *Chernobyl Assessment of Radiological and Health Impacts. 2002 Update of Chernobyl: Ten Years On.* Paris: OECD, 2002.
68. Patz, J.A., Epstein, P.R., Burke, T.A., Balbus, J. M. & Kornfeld, J.M. Global climate change and emerging infectious diseases. *J. Am. Med. Assoc.* 1996; **275**: 217–23.
69. Lindgren, E. & Gustafson, R. Tick-borne encephalitis in Sweden and climate change. *Lancet* 2001; **358**: 16–18.
70. McMichael, A.J., Haines, A., Slooff, R. & Kovat, S. (eds.). *Climate Change and Human Health.* Geneva: World Health Organization, 1996.
71. Myers, N. & Kent, J. *Environmental Exodus: An Emergent Crisis In The Global Arena.* Washington: Project of the Climate Institute, June 1995.
72. Editorial. A check list for Johannesburg. *Lancet* 2002; **360**: 581.
73. Von Schirnding, Y.V. & Yach, D. Unhealthy consumption threatens sustainable development. *Rev. Saude Publica* 2002; **36**: 379–82.
74. Vidal, J. Ten years on – slow progress on sustainable development. *Lancet* 2002; **360**: 737.
75. Dyer, G. Global warming: it scares the hell out of you. *New Zealand Herald*, December 27th 1995:6.
76. Brack, D. Developed world takes the pledge. *Guardian Weekly*, December 31st, 1995:15.
77. Editorial. Climate change – the new bioterrorism. *Lancet* 2001: **358**: 2119.
78. McMichael, A.J. Contemplating a one child world. *Br. Med. J.* 1995: **311**: 1651–2.
79. www.worldbank.org/depweb/english/modules/social.
80. Klasen, S. & Wink, C. A turning point in gender bias in mortality? An update on the number of missing women. *Pop. Dev. Rev.* 2002; **28**: 285–312.
81. Kumar, S. India's proposed population policy. *Lancet* 1994; **344**: 533.
82. King, M. Health is a sustainable state. *Lancet* 1990; **336**: 664–7.
83. King, M. & Elliot, C. Double think – a reply. *World Health Forum* 1995; **16**: 293–8.
84. King, M. & Morley, D. Demographic entrapment and demons. *Lancet* 2002; **361**: 5992.
85. Bonneux, L. Rwanda: a case of demographic entrapment. *Lancet* 1994; **344**: 1689–90.
86. UNICEF. *The State of the World's Children.* Oxford: Oxford University Press, 1992.

87. King, M., Elliott, C., Hellberg, H. & Lilford, R. Does demographic entrapment challenge the two-child paradigm? *Hlth Pol. Planning* 1995; **10**: 376–83.
88. Claeson, M., Hogan, R.C., Torres, A. & Waldman, R.J. Double think and double talk. *World Health Forum* 1994; **15**: 382–5.
89. Kane, P. & Choi, C.Y. China's one child family policy. *Br. Med. J.* 1999; **319**: 992–4.
90. McIntosh, C.A. & Finkle, J.L. The Cairo Conference on population and development: a new paradigm? *Pop. Dev. Rev.* 1995; **21**: 223–60.
91. Porritt, J. Birth of a brave new world order. Guardian Weekly, September 11, 1994.
92. Anon. Cairo: a matter of choice. *Lancet* 1994; **344**: 557–8.
93. Potts, M. USA aborts international family planning. *Lancet* 1996; **347**: 556.
94. Editorial. Undermining international family-planning programmes. *Lancet* 2002; **359**: 539.
95. World Health Organization. *Women, Health and Development. Progress Report by the Director-General.* Geneva: WHO, 1992.
96. Smith, R. Overpopulation and overconsumption: combating the two main drivers of global destruction. *Br. Med. J.* 1993; **306**: 1285–6.
97. King, M. & Elliott, C. Cairo: damp squib or Roman candle? *Lancet* 1994; **344**: 528.
98. Berridge, V. Passive smoking and its pre-history in Britain: policy speaks to science? *Soc. Sci. Med.* 1999; **49**: 1183–95.
99. Mackay, J. & Eriksen, M. *The Tobacco Atlas.* Geneva: World Health Organization, 2002.
100. Guindon, G.E. & Boisclair, D. Past, current and future trends in tobacco use. *HNP Discussion Paper – Economics of Tobacco Control Paper No 6.* World Bank: Washington, 2003.
101. Greaves, L. *Smoke Screen. Women's Smoking and Social Control.* London: Scarlet Press, 1996.
102. Graham, H. Behaving well: women's health behaviour in context. In: Roberts, H. (ed.). *Women's Health Counts.* London: Routledge, 1990.
103. Marsh, A. & McKay, S. *Poor Smokers.* Bournemouth: Bourne Press, 1994.
104. Jha, P. & Chaloupka, F. (eds.). *Tobacco Control in Developing Countries.* Oxford: Oxford University Press, 2000.
105. Zeltner, T., Kessler, D.A., Martiny, A. & Randera, F. Tobacco industry strategies to undermine tobacco control activities at the World Health Organization. *Report of the Committee of Experts on Tobacco Industry Documents.* Geneva: World Health Organization, July 2000.
106. Yach, D. & Bettcher, D. Globalisation of tobacco industry influence and new global responses. *Tob. Control* 2000; **9**: 206–16.
107. Gong, Y.L., Koplan, J.P., Feng, W. *et al.* Cigarette smoking in China: prevalence, characteristics, and attitudes in Minhang District. *J. Am. Med. Assoc.* 1995; **274**: 1232–4.
108. Niu, S.-R., Yang, G.-H., Chen, Z.-M. *et al.* Emerging tobacco hazards in China: 2. Early mortality results from a prospective study. *Br. Med. J.* 1998; **317**: 1423–4.
109. Taylor, A.L., Chaloupka, F., Guindon, G.E. & Corbett, M. Trade policy and tobacco control. In: Jha, P. & Chaloupka, F. (eds.). *Tobacco Control in Developing Countries.* Oxford: Oxford University Press, 2000.

110. Bettcher, D., Subramaniam, C., Guindon, E. *et al. Confronting the Tobacco Epidemic in an Era of Trade Liberalization.* Geneva: World Health Organization, 2001.

111. Yach, D. Tobacco in Africa. *World Hlth Forum* 1996; **17**: 29–36.

112. Chapman, S. All Africa conference on tobacco control. *Br. Med. J.* 1994; **308**: 189–91.

113. Chapman, S. & Richardson, J. Tobacco excise and declining tobacco consumption: the case of Papua New Guinea. *Am. J. Pub. Hlth* 1990; **80**: 537–40.

114. Townsend, J., Roderick, P. & Cooper, J. Cigarette smoking by socioeconomic group, sex, and age: effects of price, income, and health publicity. *Br. Med. J.* 1994; **309**: 923–7.

115. Yach, D. & Bialous, S.A. Tobacco lawyers and public health. Junking science to promote tobacco. *Am. J. Pub. Hlth* 2001; **91**: 1745–8.

116. Peto, R., Lopez, A.D., Boreham, J., Thun, M. & Heath, C. *Mortality from Smoking in Developed Countries 1950–2000: Indirect Estimates from National Vital Statistics.* Oxford: Oxford University Press, 1994.

117. Kesteloot, H. Queen Margrethe II and mortality in Danish women. *Lancet* 2001; **357**: 871–2.

118. Kluger, R. *Ashes to Ashes. America's Hundred-year Cigarette War, the Public Health and the Unabashed Triumph of Philip Morris.* New York: Knopf, 1996.

119. Neuman, M., Bitton, A. & Glantz, S. Tobacco industry strategies for influencing European Community tobacco advertising legislation. *Lancet* 2002; **359**: 1323–30.

120. Ciresi, M.V., Walburn, R.B. & Sutton, T.D. Decades of deceit: document discovery in the Minnesota tobacco litigation. *William Mitchel Law Rev.* 1999; **25**: 478–564.

121. Beaglehole, R. Science, advocacy and public health: lessons from New Zealand's tobacco wars. *J. Pub. Hlth Pol.* 1991; **12**: 175–83.

122. Scragg, R. A quantification of alcohol-related mortality in New Zealand. *Aust. NZ J. Med.* 1995; **25**: 5–12.

123. Rose, G. & Day, S. The population mean predicts the number of deviant individuals. *Br. Med. J.* 1990; **301**: 1031–4.

124. Beaglehole, R. & Jackson, R. Alcohol, cardiovascular diseases and all causes of death: a review of the epidemiological evidence. *Drug Alcohol Rev.* 1992; **11**: 275–90.

125. Room, R., Jernigan, D., Carlini-Marlatt, B. *et al. Alcohol in Developing Societies: A Public Health Approach. Summary.* Geneva: Finnish Foundation for Alcohol Studies in collaboration with the World Health Organization, 2002.

126. World Health Organization. *Global Status Report on Alcohol.* Geneva: WHO, 1999.

127. McKee, M. & Shkolnikov, V. Understanding the toll of premature death among men in eastern Europe. *Br. Med. J.* 2001; **323**: 1051–5.

128. Hu, F.B. & Willett, W.C. Optimal diets for prevention of coronary heart disease. *J. Am. Med. Assoc.* 2002; **288**: 2569–78.

129. MacGregor, G.A. & de Wardener, H.E. *Salt, Diet and Health: Neptune's Poisoned Chalice: The Origins of High Blood Pressure.* Cambridge: Cambridge University Press, 1998.

130. NCHS 1999 – U.S. Department of Health and Human Services – http.//www.cdc.gov/nchs/products/pubs/pubd/hestats/obese/obse99t2.htm.
131. Prentice, A.M. & Jebb, S.A. Obesity in Britain: gluttony or sloth? *Br. Med. J.* 1995; **311**: 437–9.
132. Popkin, B.M. An overview on the nutrition transition and its health implications: the Bellagio meeting. *Pub. Hlth Nutr.* 2002; **5**: 93–103.
133. Booth, F.W., Chakravarthy, M.V., Gordon, S.V. & Spangenburg, E.E. Waging war on physical inactivity: using modern molecular ammunition against an ancient enemy *J. Appl. Physiol.* 2002; **93**: 3–30.
134. United States Department of Health and Human Services (USDHHS) 1996. *Physical Activity and Health: A Report of the Surgeon General.* Atlanta, GA:U.S. Department of Health and Human Services, Centers for Disease Control and Prevention, National Center for Chronic Disease Prevention and Health Promotion, 1996.
135. Kasaniemi, Y.A., Fanforth, E.J., Jensen, M.D. *et al.* Dose-response issues concerning physical activity and health: an evidence-based symposium. *Med. Sci. Sports Exercise* 2001; **33**: S351–8.
136. Bull, F.C., Armstrong, T., Dixon, T. *et al.* Physical inactivity. In: Ezzati, M., Lopez, A., Rogers, A. & Murray, C. (eds.) *Comparative Quantification of Health Risks: Global and Regional Burden of Disease due to Selected Major Risk Factors 2003.* Geneva: World Health Organization (in press).
137. Spirduso, W.W. & Cronin, L. Exercise dose–response effects on quality of life and independent living in older adults. *Med. Sci. Sports Exercise* 2001; **33**: S598–S610.
138. Dunn, A.L., Trivedi, M.H. & O'Neal, H. Physical activity dose–response effects on outcomes of depression and anxiety. *Med. Sci. Sports Exercise* 2001; **33**: S587–S597.
139. Physical activity trends – United States, 1990–1998. *MMWR* 2001; **500**: 166–9.
140. Increasing physical activity: a report on recommendations of the Task Force on Community Preventive Services; *MMWR* 2001; **500**: 1–16.
141. UNAIDS/ WHO. *AIDS Epidemic Update* December 2002. Geneva: UN-AIDS/WHO, 2002.
142. Guay, L.A., Musoke, P., Fleming, T. *et al.* Intrapartum and neonatal single dose nevirapine compared with zidovudine for prevention of mother-to-child transmission of HIV-1 in Kampala, Uganda: HIVNET 012 randomised trial. *Lancet* 1999; **354**: 795–802.
143. Zhang, K. & Ma, S.J. Epidemiology of HIV in China. *Br. Med. J.* 2002; **324**: 803–4.
144. Potts, M. & Walsh, J. Tackling India's HIV epidemic: lessons from Africa. *Br. Med. J.* 2003; **326**: 1389–92.
145. Ammann, A.J. Preventing HIV. Time to get serious about changing behaviour. *Br. Med. J.* 2003; **326**: 1342–3.
146. Bhargava, A. & Bigombe, B. Public policies and the orphans of AIDS in Africa. *Br. Med. J.* 2003; **326**: 1387–9.
147. Choi, K.-H., Liu, H., Han, L., Mandel, J. & Rutherford, G.W. Emerging HIV-epidemic in China in men who have sex with men. *Lancet* 2003; **361**: 2125–6.
148. Mann, J.M. Human rights and the new public health. *Hlth Human Rights* 1995; **1**: 229–33.
149. Global AIDS Policy Commission. *Towards a New Health Strategy for AIDS.* Cambridge, USA, 1993.

150. Dora C. A different route to health: implications of transport polices. *Br. Med. J.* 1999; **318**: 1686–8.

151. Nantulya, V.M. & Reich, M.R. The neglected epidemic: road traffic injuries in developing countries. *Br. Med. J.* 2002; **324**: 1139–41.

152. World Health Organization. *World Health Organization Report on Road Crashes.* Geneva: WHO, 1989.

153. Winston, F.K., Rineer, C., Menon, R. *et al.* The carnage wrought by major economic change: ecological study of traffic related mortality and the reunification of Germany. *Br. Med. J.* 1999; **318**: 1647–50.

154. International Labour Organization. *Global Estimates of Occupational Accidents and Work-related Diseases, 2002.* www.ilo.org/safework.

155. Fontanarosa, P.B. The unrelenting epidemic of violence in America: truths and consequences. *J. Am. Med. Assoc.* 1995; **273**: 1792–3.

156. Anon. Child deaths from gunfire. *New Zealand Herald,* 10 April, 1996.

157. World Health Organization. *World Violence Report.* Geneva: WHO, 2002.

158. World Health Organization. *Violence Against Women: a Priority Health Issue.* Geneva: World Health Organization, 1997.

159. Ellsberg, M.C., Pena, R., Herrera, A., Liljestrand, J. & Winkvist, A. Candies in hell: women's experience of violence in Nicaragua. *Soc. Sci. Med.* 2000, **51**: 1595–610.

160. Bullock, L.F. & McFarlane, J. The birth-weight/battering connection. *Am. J. Nursing.* 1989; **89**: 1153–5.

161. UNICEF. *The State of the World's Children.* New York: Oxford University Press, 1996.

162. Stewart, F. War and underdevelopment: Can economic analysis help reduce the costs? *J. Int. Dev.* 1993; **5**: 357–80.

163. Collier, P. On the economic consequences of civil war. *Oxford Economic Papers* 1999; **51**: 168–83.

164. Toole, M.J. 2000. Displaced persons and war. In: Levy B.S. & Sidel, V.W. (eds.) *War and Public Health,* updated edition. Washington, DC: American Public Health Association.

165. World Health Organisation. *Mental Health; New Understanding, New Hope.* Geneva. World Health Organization, 2001.

166. Fitzsimmons, D.W. & Whiteside, A.W. *Conflict, War, and Public Health.* Conflict Studies 276. London: Research Institute for the Study of Conflict and Terrorism, 1994.

167. Guha-Sapir, D. & von Panhuis, G. The importance of conflict-related mortality in civilian populations. *Lancet* 2003; **361**: 2126–8.

168. Ghobarah, H., Huth, P. & Russett, B. Civil wars kill and maim people – long after the shooting stops (Draft 29 Aug 2001). Center for Basic Research in the Social Sciences. www.cbrss.harvard.edu/programs/hsecurity/papers/civilwar.pdf (accessed 30 June 2002).

169. Meddings, D.R. Civilians and War: a review and historical overview of the involvement of non-combatant populations in conflict situations. *Med. Confl. and Survival,* 2001, **17**: 6–16.

170. Reid, E. A future, if one is still alive: The challenge of the HIV epidemic. In: Moore, J. (ed.). *Hard Choices: Moral Dilemmas in Humanitarian Intervention.* Lanham, MD: Roman & Littlefield: 269–86, 1998.

171. Coupland, R.M. & Meddings, D.R. Mortality associated with use of weapons in armed conflicts, wartime atrocities, and civilian mass shootings: literature review. *Br. Med. J.* 1999; **319**: 407–10.
172. Anon. Antipersonnel mines, the all-too-conventional weapon. *Lancet* 1995; **346**: 715.
173. Ascherio, A., Biellik, R., Epstein, A. *et al.* Deaths and injuries caused by land mines in Mozambique. *Lancet* 1995; **346**: 721–4.
174. Guha-Sapir, D. & van Panhuis, W.G. *Armed Conflict and Public Health.* WHO Collaborating Centre for Research on the Epidemiology of Disasters, Université Catholique de Louvain, Brussels, 2002.
175. World Health Organization. *The World Health Report 2003: Shaping the Future.* Geneva: World Health Organization, 2003.

PART II

Epidemiology

Epidemiology is the study of the distribution and determinants of health-related states or events in human populations and the application of this study to the control of health problems. The word '*epidemiology*' is derived from the Greek: *epi* (upon); *demos* (the people); *logos* (to study). In this part of the book we trace the evolution of epidemiological ideas and methods, assess the achievements and failures of modern epidemiology, and outline the challenges epidemiology must confront to have a more central and constructive position in the health endeavour. An historical focus clarifies the development of epidemiological reasoning and serves as a reminder of the early and close connection between epidemiology and the practice of public health – a relationship that needs to be strengthened.

4

Evolution of epidemiology: ideas and methods

4.1 Introduction

Epidemiology in its modern form is a relatively new discipline. The core of epidemiology is the use of quantitative methods to study diseases in human populations so that they might be prevented and controlled. Some of the central ideas of epidemiology extend as far back as the works of the Hippocratic school which emphasised the influence of the physical environment on health over 2000 years ago.

The origins of modern epidemiology can be traced to the work of the English sanitary reformers and French scientists in the first half of the nineteenth century. It emerged as a distinct discipline in the period 1840–70. After a quiescent period at the end of the nineteenth century, a revival began in the first half of the twentieth century. The 'modern age' of epidemiology started after the Second World War and since then epidemiology has passed through several phases. It developed in close association with clinical medicine, but this relationship has often been a source of tension because of epidemiology's population-wide focus. The links between epidemiology and other population sciences, such as demography and the social and political sciences, have been less developed.

4.2 The origins of epidemiology

4.2.1 Early origins

Hippocrates, a Greek physician, lived from about 460 to 375 BC. His writings covered a broad range of topics, but most of the works attributed to him were written by other members of the Hippocratic School. These works are known collectively as the Corpus Hippocraticum. The prime contribution of this school to the evolution of epidemiology was the idea that the environment plays a crucial role in causing disease. Unfortunately, the environment was seen then in cosmic, astrological or theological terms, which remain outside the scope of prevention[1]. The Hippocratic school stressed the influence of physical factors on health and disease. For example, variations in weather patterns and the character of the seasons were thought to determine the rise and fall of epidemics[2]. *Air, Places and Waters* was the first systematic presentation of the relationship between the environment and disease. For more than 2000 years, this was a basic text and provided the theoretical background for understanding disease occurrence (see Box 4.1).

Box 4.1   Hippocrates on 'mode of life'

Hippocrates' comments on the importance of a clean water supply and 'mode of life' are as relevant today as they were 2400 years ago:
  Whoever wishes to investigate medicine properly . . . must consider . . . the waters which the inhabitants use, whether they be marshy and soft, or hard, and running from elevated and rocky situations. . . . and the mode in which the inhabitants live, and what are their pursuits, whether they are fond of drinking and eating to excess, and given to indolence, or are fond of exercise and labor, and not given to excess in eating and drinking . . . [3]

In his own time, Hippocrates had a strong reputation as a physician and a teacher and the ideas of the Hippocratic School influenced the Greek personal hygiene movement[4], although some practical hygiene measures date from an earlier period – one of the earliest known water-flushed toilets belonged to the Queen of Knossos who lived approximately 3500 years ago in the Minoan palace in what is now Crete. The Romans also placed great emphasis on public sanitation[5] and many of the conduits built by the Romans remained in use until the early twentieth century. Aqueducts became a symbol of the Roman way of life, as well as a symbol of power. Despite the Greco-Roman emphasis on personal hygiene, life expectancy in this period was only about 25 years and an enormous gap separated the rich and the poor[6]. The ideals promoted by the wealthy citizens had little impact on the general public's health and indeed this was not their purpose.

Following the decline of the Roman Empire in the fifth century, little attention was paid to the science of hygiene, either personal or public. The introduction of Germanic customs in Europe interrupted the Greco-Roman public health tradition until the Christian Mediterranean cities began to expand in the eleventh and twelfth centuries. The physical and economic deterioration and widespread poverty, which followed the decline of the classical civilisations, led to the pandemics of the Middle Ages. This period has been described as a 'universe of hunger' and a 'universe of disease'[7], with a life expectancy of between 30 and 35 years, reducing to about 20 years by the plague pandemic of the year 1348 (Box 4.2).

Box 4.2   Impact of the plague

It was the appearance of the plague in the fourteenth century, and its periodic return throughout the next two centuries, that crystallised the interest in public health that had begun with the isolation of lepers in the thirteenth century[7]. Some cities compiled 'books of the dead' which were comprehensive mortality records used to identify epidemics and follow their course. Mortality rates in the early epidemics were staggering, with up to half of the population dying in cities during the plague pandemic. In response to the first plague pandemic, Northern Italian city-states instituted a series of public health measures designed to protect the health of the elite. For example, the authorities isolated ships suspected of carrying disease; the quarantine lasted for 40 days.

Two main theories of disease – the miasma theory and the contagious theory – competed for centuries[8]. The miasma theory had its origins in the work of the Hippocratic School and was formally developed in the early eighteenth century. A 'miasma', composed of malodorous and poisonous particles generated by the decomposition of organic matter, was thought to be responsible for many diseases. This theory was supported strongly by political and economic groups that sought to avert the imposition of costly quarantine measures justified by the contagious theory of disease. From a practical point of view, the miasma theory, although eventually discredited, led to important public health interventions.

The contagious theory was expressed ultimately as the germ theory just over 100 years ago. This theory had its origin in the ancient practice of isolating diseased people and was stated first explicitly by Girolamo Fracastoro (1478–1553) in 1546. He attributed the spread of epidemics to small 'seeds' that carried the disease. The discovery of micro-organisms with the microscope, invented in 1683, contributed to the development of this theory.

Natural and *Political*

OBSERVATIONS

Mentioned in a following INDEX,

and made upon the

Bills of Mortality.

By *JOHN GRAUNT*,

Citizen of

LONDON.

With reference to the *Government*, *Religion*, *Trade*,
Growth, *Ayre*, *Difeafes*, and the feveral Changes of the
faid C I T Y.

———— *Non, me ut miretur Turba, laboro,*
Contentus paucis Lectoribus ————

LONDON,
Printed by *Tho: Roycroft*, for *John Martin*, *James Alleftry,*
and *Tho: Dicas*, at the Sign of the *Bell* in St. *Paul's*
Church-yard, MDCLXII.

Fig. 4.1. Weekly Bills of Mortality (see PHC, 1997).

4.2.2 Seventeenth- and eighteenth-century influences

In the seventeenth century, the foundations of modern clinical medicine were laid by William Harvey and Thomas Sydenham, who emphasised the importance of direct observation and experimentation. In parallel, Graunt was laying the basis of health statistics and epidemiology with his analyses of the Weekly Bills of Mortality[9] (Fig. 4.1).

The Bills of Mortality were initiated in the late sixteenth century by the parish clerks in London to warn, or reassure, the population about the extent of an epidemic. Using these data, Graunt described patterns of mortality and fertility, for example, the excess of male births, the high infant mortality, and seasonal variations in mortality. Graunt also developed the first life table and proposed that comparisons between countries could be made using this technique. Graunt recognised the limitations of the available data and stressed the need for better data, a continuing concern even today.

Graunt's friend and colleague, William Petty, coined the phrase 'political arithmetic'. This involved the coordination of political, economic, social and health surveys to inform public choices and collective action[10, 11]. Petty believed that it was in the interests of an economically strong state to have the largest possible number of healthy (and therefore productive) subjects. He wanted to contribute to increasing the power and prestige of England and, as an essential part of this process, he stressed the need for statistical data on population, trade, manufacture and disease, amongst other topics. Petty's ideas had no immediate effect, in part because of the absence of an effective local civil administration operating under central direction. Modern parallels are not hard to identify.

In 1747 James Lind, a British naval surgeon, undertook one of the forerunners of the clinical trial by developing a hypothesis concerning the cause and treatment of scurvy, a debilitating disease not known then to be caused by vitamin C deficiency[12]. Lind took 12 seamen with scurvy and, in addition to a common diet, gave each of six pairs of seamen a different dietary supplement for 6 days. The two seamen given oranges and lemons made an almost complete recovery. Lind inferred that citric acid fruits cured scurvy and would probably also prevent it. He published his results in 1753, a long delay even by modern publication standards, but it was not until 1795 that the British naval authorities accepted his results and included limes in the diet of sailors. The delay between the original research and its formal application was not simply due to the slowness of the Naval bureaucracy, but by the difficulties in establishing causality and the general lack of knowledge. Lind's results were not replicated, in part because of competing theories. It was not until 1920 that alternative theories were discredited and agreement reached that scurvy was a dietary deficiency.

In the eighteenth century there was a strong French influence on the development of epidemiology through the work of mathematicians such as Laplace. The repressive political climate resulted in a reluctance in France to link statistical theory with social and political reality as advocated by Petty[10]. The dominant theory of disease in eighteenth-century France stressed the importance of natural phenomena such as climate[13]. The French Revolution stimulated a general interest in public health, initiated the Parisian School of Medicine, and encouraged the epidemiological approach to disease by symbolising a break with past traditions[14, 15]. This approach was also used in China following the 1949 revolution. The rallying cry of the French Revolution – 'liberty, fraternity, equality' – is still relevant to modern public health practice[16].

4.2.3 The nineteenth-century blossoming of epidemiology

The Industrial Revolution had a profound effect on the health of populations. The squalor and poverty associated with urbanisation was a direct threat to the health of the labour force and therefore an economic and political threat to industrialists and politicians. The appalling social conditions and the resulting increased mortality, stimulated the interest of reformers who gradually realised the power and importance of statistical data for their various causes.

The growth of statistical ideas during the nineteenth century was closely related to the growth of epidemiology. Major epidemiological developments occurred as a result of the tutelage of Pierre Charles Alexander Louis in Paris in the middle years of the nineteenth century. Louis' ideas were spread to England by Farr, Budd and Guy (the author of the first book on public health)[17], and to the United States by many clinicians, including Holmes and members of the Shattuck family.

Louis was the first to introduce statistics to medicine and he did more than anyone else in the nineteenth century to develop the central concepts of epidemiological methods and reasoning. He also integrated philosophical and quantitative concepts and applied them to the study of disease, the so-called *methode numérique*. He initiated the period of 'statistical enlightenment', although there was strong opposition from many of his colleagues who feared that statistical methods would obscure the importance of individual variations[18]. A well-known contribution by Louis was the demonstration of the harmful effects of routine bleeding. Ironically, Louis' ideas, although enthusiastically taken up by public health practitioners, had little impact on medical practice until the development of clinical epidemiology over a century later[19].

The early years of the nineteenth century in France were also the creative period of the French Hygienist's movement[15]. The climatic theory on the cause of disease yielded to a theory based on the importance of social and economic causes of disease. This approach was epitomised by the work of René Villerme, who extensively studied the living conditions and health of Parisians. As the Industrial Revolution developed, this led to the investigation of occupational diseases[13]. Occupational studies have continued as a major focus of epidemiology, especially of the occupational risks for cancer[20].

One hundred years after Lind's experiment, an important series of comparative studies were conducted by Semmelweiss on mortality from puerperal fever in two Divisions of the Lying-In hospital in Vienna (see Box 4.3).

Ironically, after 1850, French epidemiology declined at the time that it was growing vigorously in England on the basis of the work of Louis' students. The decline of epidemiology in France has been attributed to not using vital statistics, which in England date back to the Bills of Mortality[14]. The development of epidemiology in the United States, 40 years later than in England, was due partly to the time it took Louis' students to develop vital statistical systems in the United States.

The other ingredients necessary for the growth of epidemiology were present in all three countries: an identifiable philosophy of epidemiology; a familiarity with statistics; and a well-organised hygienic movement. It is interesting to draw parallels with the continuing poor state of epidemiology in some affluent European countries, such as Germany, which is due, in part, to the lack of access

Box 4.3   An early clinical trial

Semmelweiss identified the contagious nature of puerperal fever by comparing mortality rates between 1841 and 1846 in the Division staffed by physicians and their assistants, who came to the maternity wards after attending autopsies, and in the Division used for training midwives. Semmelweiss hypothesised that the high maternal mortality in the Division staffed by physicians resulted from the transmission of infectious particles from the autopsy room to the maternity ward. In 1847 he introduced handwashing with a chlorinated solution by the physicians and their assistants before they performed deliveries; the death rate fell immediately to the level of that in the Division staffed by midwives (Table 4.1)[12]

Table 4.1.

Year	Physician's division			Midwive's division		
		Deaths			Deaths	
	Births *n*	*n*	%	Births *n*	*n*	%
1842	3287	518	15.8	2659	202	7.5
1844	3157	260	8.2	2956	68	2.3
1846	4010	459	11.4	3754	105	2.7
Introduction of intervention (handwashing) in May 1847						
1848	3556	45	1.3	3219	43	1.3

by epidemiologists to vital statistics. A worrying trend in many countries is the conflict between 'individual rights' and the 'common good', which is reflected in the development of privacy laws to restrict this access further.

In both England and France there was a close connection between epidemiology and the public health movement in the nineteenth century. This connection provided a major stimulus to epidemiology[21]. The work of the sanitary physicians (so called because they earned their livelihood by clinical practice) and the organisations they founded such as the London Epidemiological Society, led to the formal creation of the discipline of epidemiology. In 1863, the term 'scientific epidemiologists' was used. This was the first known reference to 'epidemiologists'[22].

The credit for institutionalising epidemiology in England is due to William Farr, who built on the ideas of Graunt and Petty[23]. Farr acquired an interest in health statistics while studying with Louis in Paris. In 1839, he was appointed to the newly established General Register Office where he initiated an anatomically based system of vital statistics which is the basis of the International Classification of Diseases, now in its tenth revision. Over the next 40 years, Farr developed methods for studying the distribution and determinants of human diseases.

Box 4.4   Weekly reports in the 'spirit of Farr'

In 1960 the 'spirit of Farr' was revived in the *Morbidity and Mortality Weekly Reports* published by the Communicable Disease Center in Atlanta, Georgia[27]. Many countries are now issuing regular surveillance reports, all of which bear some resemblance to Farr's reports, and the World Health Organization publishes the *Weekly Epidemiological Record*. A recent example from WHO shows the pattern of cases due to Sudden Acute Respiratory Syndrome (SARS) in Vietnam.

Figure 4.2 traces the rise and fall of probable cases from SARS worldwide in 2002–3.

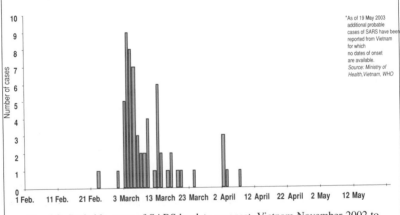

Fig. 4.2. Probable cases of SARS by date on onset. Vietnam November 2002 to July 2003 $n = 59.0$ cases excluding 2527 probable cases of SARS for which no dates of onset are available.

Farr's contributions cover the broadest range of epidemiological methods and many are still in use (see Box 4.4). He was not only one of the founders of modern epidemiology, he was also one of the leaders of the public health movement. Farr had a firm commitment to environmental reform using medical and political ideals to reinforce each other[24]. Farr built an advanced public health surveillance system, which provided some of the evidence later used by John Snow in his studies on cholera[25]. Farr saw statistics as the science of social reform, a science that gave reformists a focus and a platform for a limited range of social reforms, mainly educational and sanitary[26]. In many respects, epidemiologists have lost this commitment to ensuring that epidemiological data is used for reform purposes.

For Farr, human health was a prerequisite to social advancement. He believed that the State had a responsibility to prevent poverty, but he also reflected the ambivalence of many middle-class reformers towards poverty. The moralistic view of poverty blamed the poor for their own misery and opposed public support for the poor. However, Farr had a genuine sympathy for the 'worthy' poor. In this view, relief to the poor was necessary, both to protect the poor and to secure social order. Despite the complexity and often contradictory nature of Farr's views about the nature and causes of poverty, he concluded that public intervention was part of the solution[26]. His vision was broad: 'No variation in the health of the states of Europe is the result of chance; it is the direct result of the physical and political conditions in which nations live' – a statement that remains as true today as it was in 1866.

Farr stressed the need for economic, environmental and social reforms to improve health. Chadwick, one of Farr's contemporaries, reached different conclusions. He believed that disease aggravated poverty and increased the costs of supporting the poor. Chadwick brought together a mass of information in 1842 in the 'Report on an Inquiry into the Sanitary Conditions of the Labouring Population of Great Britain'. As a result, the General Board of Health was created in 1848 with responsibility for public health, but it lasted only 7 years[23].

The broad approach of the sanitary movement was replaced gradually by more specific ideas concerning such things as the importance of clean water. Notable studies were carried out by John Snow, one of the founders of modern epidemiology and a contemporary of Farr. He investigated, in an integrated series of studies, the causes of the cholera epidemics of 1848–49 and 1853–54. Snow, a London doctor and anaesthetist, who famously administered chloroform during Queen Victoria's eighth delivery, is most remembered epidemiologically for his identification of the Broad Street pump as the vehicle for an explosive epidemic in Soho in August–September 1854[28], even though the removal of the pump handle occurred well after the peak of the epidemic[29]. Snow's investigations were brilliant, systematic, thorough and wideranging, and his later studies were based on a clear prior hypothesis concerning the contagious nature of cholera[30]. He described the epidemiology of the cholera epidemic in a social and economic context and was much more than a narrowly focused quantitative epidemiologist, as he usually is portrayed in epidemiological texts[31]. Snow's work was only one part of the body of research which led to the general acceptance of the contaminated drinking water theory of the origin of cholera[29]. Snow's work did not achieve the status of a 'classic' until after the reprint of his original work in 1936 assisted by the use of his studies for teaching purposes. The John Snow so revered today seems to be a construct of several contrasting ideas from the history of epidemiology[32].

Guy and Farr became associated closely with the Statistical Society of London, which had been founded in 1834. By the mid-nineteenth century, this Society was the centre of biostatistics and epidemiology and was involved with five major statistical areas, including medical statistics. During the 1840s, epidemiology began to emerge as a separate discipline, but the application of epidemiological approaches to disease control remained uncoordinated until 1850[22]. In this year, the London Epidemiological Society was founded to inform the medical profession, the public and politicians about the raging epidemic of cholera. The meetings of the London Epidemiological Society marked the foundation of modern epidemiology and the society flourished during the next 20 years (Box 4.5).

Box 4.5   The London Epidemiological Society[22].

The purposes of the London Epidemiological Society were:

To institute rigid examination into the causes and conditions which influence the origin, propagation, mitigation, and prevention of epidemic disease ... to institute ... original and comprehensive researches into the nature and laws of disease ... to communicate with government and legislature on matters connected with the prevention of epidemic diseases ... to publish original papers; to issue queries; to publish reports; to form statistical tables; to prepare illustrative maps; and to collect works relative to epidemic disease.

Comparative mortality studies, evaluations of smallpox inoculation and vaccination, and morbidity surveys were carried out frequently. Most of the work was performed by clinicians acting as epidemiologists in a part-time and unpaid capacity. *The Journal of Public Health* was founded in 1855 and published the transactions of the London Epidemiological Society until 1859, when it was discontinued for financial reasons.

The Society withered with the death of its founding members. Its demise marked the end of the first epidemiological era and was replaced by the bacteriological era from about 1870. For the next half century, epidemiology was overshadowed by the bacteriological paradigm. Laboratory-based criteria for judging causal relationships, the Henle–Koch postulates, replaced the population-based inferences of the mid-nineteenth-century epidemiologists, even though these postulates were rarely fulfilled in causal judgements for infectious diseases[24]. It was only in the early decades of the twentieth century, when it became apparent that bacteria were not responsible for all diseases, that epidemiology gradually reappeared. In comparison with other health sciences, the consolidation of epidemiology as a growing discipline was delayed by almost a century. Initially, epidemiology was very concerned with promoting and protecting the public's health. Unfortunately, modern epidemiologists have neglected this tradition, to the detriment of the public's health. This tradition needs to be reclaimed[33,34].

4.3 The twentieth-century resurgence

4.3.1 Non-communicable disease epidemiology

During the period dominated by bacteriology, biostatistics continued to develop under the leadership of Galton and Pearson, and departments of statistics nourished the next generation of epidemiologists. Foremost among them were Major Greenwood and Percy Stocks in England, and Wade Hampton Frost in the United States, all of whom combined the disciplines of biostatistics and epidemiology and were concerned with both infectious and non-infectious diseases. In 1935, Greenwood published *Epidemics and Crowd Disease*, with chapters not only on tuberculosis and other infectious diseases, but also on cancer and psychological causes of illness[35]. The appointment of Ryle as the first Professor of Social Medicine at Oxford University in 1943, symbolised the emerging importance of non-infectious disease epidemiology and the recognition of the importance of the social determinants of disease[36]. Bradford Hill, initially a colleague of Greenwood, introduced the numerically naive medical profession to the facts of statistical life in a series of articles which were subsequently reprinted in book form[37].

Research in non-communicable disease epidemiology in Great Britain developed primarily as an academic discipline, whereas in the United States of America it was based, at least initially, in Departments of Health – federal, state and local. In both countries, occupational studies remained an important focus of epidemiology. The Hygienic Laboratory, established by the United

States Public Health Service in 1887, was involved in both infectious and non-communicable disease epidemiology. Goldberger, working for the Hygienic Laboratory, identified the cause of pellagra through an elegant series of studies conducted between 1914 and 1930. He demonstrated that pellagra was not an infectious disease, as was generally believed, but the result of a dietary deficiency later found to be nicotinic acid, part of the vitamin B complex. In the 1930s, important epidemiological studies of fluoride and dental disease were conducted, culminating in a community-based experiment in Grand Rapids, Michigan. In 1946, the Communicable Disease Center was founded by conversion of the agency for Malaria Control in War Areas and provided federal support and leadership for epidemiology; later it became the Centers for Disease Control[38]. The Epidemiologic Intelligence Service of the Centers for Disease Control trained many physicians in the methods of infectious disease epidemiology and led to many similar training programmes in both field epidemiology and public health[39].

The influence of the health transition theory – despite its limitations – in refocusing the task of epidemiology towards non-communicable disease cannot be over-emphasised. The increase in death rates from age-related diseases, such as heart disease and cancer, caught the attention of epidemiologists. Initially, these diseases were thought to be degenerative in origin, an inevitable consequence of the ageing process. A major outcome of the early studies of lung cancer and heart disease was to shift attention to the role of potentially preventable environmental causes. This marked a dramatic shift from the dominance of the early infectious disease paradigm, although the environmental causes were conceptualised at the level of the individual and not at the broader socio-economic level. Infectious disease epidemiology remains important in wealthy countries because of the emergence of new infectious diseases, such as AIDS, and the re-emergence of 'old' diseases such as tuberculosis, and in poor countries because of the continuing epidemics of infectious diseases – both old and new.

Evidence for the emergence of a new epidemiological paradigm is to be found in the systematisation of the epidemiological literature, the concentration in wealthy countries on non-communicable diseases, the development of graduate training programmes, and the availability of research funds[40]. The shift in focus from a search for specific infectious agents to the search for multiple causes led, in the space of a few decades after the Second World War, to the development of a wide range of methods and to the maturation of epidemiology[40]. The practice of epidemiology encouraged the development of epidemiological theory and methods, mostly by statisticians.

The transition from infectious to non-communicable disease epidemiology occurred smoothly, partly because the technical differences between the divisions are minor and arbitrary[41]. Although the natural histories of the two broad groups of disease are often different, both infectious and non-infectious diseases can be acute or chronic. Tuberculosis was the bridging condition for many epidemiologists, who made the transition from the study of infectious to non-communicable diseases; for example, Frost chose tuberculosis as the springboard for his early venture into the field of chronic diseases in the 1930s and this work directed attention to the method of cohort analysis[42].

There are several reasons for the early emergence of non-communicable disease epidemiology in Great Britain and the United States, but not in Germany, Scandinavia, France or Eastern Europe. The central role of a system of vital statistics was critical, although such systems were well developed in Scandinavia. The strong tradition of an independent epidemiological discipline in Great Britain was also important. The establishment of public health institutions, such as the London School of Hygiene and Tropical Medicine and the schools of public health and research institutes in the United States, fostered interdisciplinary groups of epidemiologists and biostatisticians and, in the United States, provided a major new source of research funding. Many of these new institutions were established with the support of the Rockefeller Foundation and played a role in supporting the process of colonisation in Africa and Asia[43].

The success of the new paradigm was ensured by the outcome of two research endeavours begun in the late 1940s. Firstly, of greatest importance were the results of case control studies in the United States and Britain, which confirmed early German studies[29] linking cigarette smoking with lung cancer[44, 45] even if not all scientists, let alone politicians, accepted the findings[46]. Secondly, the Framingham study developed the cohort study methods, initially of heart disease, but soon expanded to study a wide range of non-communicable diseases and now includes the children and grandchildren of the original cohort[47].

4.3.2 Phases of modern epidemiology

Since 1946 there have been several phases in the development of epidemiology. The whole period has been called the 'second epidemiologic revolution' or the conquest of non-communicable diseases, in contrast to the 'first epidemiologic revolution', which focused on the conquest of infectious diseases[48]. It is now apparent that the conquest of infectious diseases is far from complete and is unlikely ever to finish[49–51]. What is now required is a third 'epidemiological revolution', which integrates methods for the study and control of infectious and non-communicable diseases and examines their common causes and solutions from a global perspective.

The first phase of modern epidemiology, from 1946 to the mid-1960s, saw the creation of epidemiological methods necessary for the study of non-communicable diseases, including methods for estimating various measures of risk. The publication in the late 1950s and early 1960s of the first texts on modern epidemiology was a critical point in the evolution of epidemiology[52,53]. These texts contained the first systematic discussion of epidemiological study designs, and their application to chronic diseases, and the first explicit mention of the multi-causal web of causation that has dominated epidemiology[54].

Another early textbook listed the 'personal characteristics' with which the epidemiologist is primarily concerned: demographic, biological, socio-economic, and personal living habits[55]. By focusing on the agent, host and environment as the principal determinants of disease occurrence, the social system became sidelined and it has largely remained outside the consideration of epidemiologists.

The second phase from the mid-1960s to the early 1980s covered the development of more sophisticated methods including the clarification of bias[56] and confounding[57], interaction, and the practical development of the case control study design. The development of computers enhanced methods of analysis, especially of large data sets. The publication in 1983 of the first edition of Last's *Dictionary of Epidemiology*[58] represented an important consensus on epidemiological terminology, including a widely accepted definition of epidemiology itself, something that had eluded previous generations of epidemiologists[59]. The dictionary is now in its fourth edition[60], indicating the continuing evolution of epidemiological terminology, and over 50 introductory textbooks on epidemiology have been published.

The third phase, over the last decade, has emphasised the coherence of epidemiological study designs and the unitary nature of epidemiological methods, irrespective of the subject matter[61]. Greater attention has been given to the measurement of exposure, which had previously taken second place to the measurement of outcomes. A large range of exposures is now studied in the epidemiology of non-communicable diseases. In the 1980s, and judging from papers published in the *American Journal of Epidemiology*, aspects of diet, use of tobacco and alcohol, occupation, past medical history, and use of medications were the most commonly studied exposures[62].

'Molecular epidemiology', the use of biological markers as more precise indicators of exposure effect, susceptibility or outcome, has generated considerable interest, especially in cancer epidemiology[63]. Molecular techniques may overcome the limited ability of epidemiology to elucidate mechanisms; molecular epidemiology holds the promise of opening the 'black box' of epidemiology and exploring intervening pathways and causal processes[19,64]. The demonstration of the person-to-person tracking of HIV and tuberculosis are good examples of the potential contribution of molecular epidemiologists[65]. This approach, however, has so far yielded few new hypotheses and has contributed little substantial benefit to the public's health[66]. There is a real danger that the molecular paradigm will come to dominate epidemiology in the same way as the germ theory achieved dominance at the end of the nineteenth century[34]. The expectations that the sequencing of the human genome will lead to rapid advances in the control of many diseases are unlikely to be met, although undoubtedly it will improve understanding of the mechanisms of disease development and may advance many therapeutic areas[29]. It remains true, however, that although genetic factors may influence individual susceptibility to disease, they cannot explain rapid changes in the occurrence at the population level[67].

Experimental epidemiology has, over the last decade, gained greater status, and methods of aggregating and summarising data from numerous small studies are now common. The most recent topic to engage epidemiologists has been the impact of global environmental changes on health[68]. This area will make fundamentally new demands on the practice of epidemiology, as we shall see in Chapter 6.

A feature of epidemiological practice has been the subdivision of the discipline into various branches which describe the type of exposure (e.g. nutritional, environmental or occupational epidemiology), or disease (e.g. cancer, cardiovascular disease or injury epidemiology), or group of participants under study (e.g. paediatric or clinical epidemiology), and even more inappropriately, the technique used (e.g. molecular epidemiology). It would be more appropriate for the sub-specialities to become united under the label of 'public health epidemiology', as distinct from 'clinical epidemiology'[69]. There has also been a division among epidemiologists in their sphere of interest, between those interested in the health problems of wealthy countries and those more interested in poor countries[70]. There is some evidence of regional diversity in the development of epidemiology; in Latin America, for example, there has been a much closer connection between epidemiology and the practice of public health[71].

4.4 Ideas and methods

Epidemiology is unique because of its way of looking at problems, its theories and methods, and the problems it studies – states of health and disease in human populations. The central ideas of epidemiology are relatively simple, and many have been known since the time of Farr in England and Louis in France 150 years ago[22].

There are two fundamental types of epidemiological ideas:

• causal inference, that is, the identification of causal pathways; and
• theoretical and methodological issues related to study design and analysis.

The major recent improvements in epidemiology have been in the areas of study design and analysis.

4.4.1 Causal inference

The early literature on causal inference was systematised by Hill in 1965[72]. The origin of Hill's criteria can be traced back to the eighteenth-century Scottish philosopher, David Hume[73]. The United States Surgeon General, in assessing the association of smoking with lung cancer in 1964, described five criteria for judging the causality of a given association. This early literature emphasised that causal inference required qualitative judgements, based on the available quantitative evidence. This necessity for exercising judgement is held against epidemiologists often by other biomedical scientists and politicians with both groups, when it suits them, requiring 'certainty'.

The criteria proposed by Hill (see Box 4.6) were neither all necessary, apart from temporality, nor sufficient, and have continued to generate much criticism,

---

Box 4.6 Criteria for causation as proposed by Hill[72].

Strength	What is the strength (relative risk) of this association?
Consistency	Has the association been 'repeatedly observed by different persons, in different places, circumstances, and times'?
Specificity	Is this association limited to 'specific workers and to particular sites and types of disease'?
Temporality	'Which is the cart and which the horse'?
Biological gradient	Is there a dose–response curve?
Plausibility	Is the association biologically plausible?
Coherence	'The cause-and-effect interpretation should not seriously conflict with the generally known facts of the natural history and biology of the disease'.
Experiment	Is there experimental, or semi-experimental, evidence?
Analogy	Is it 'fair to judge by analogy'?

especially from scientists more familiar with laboratory techniques. Hill cautioned against the dogmatic use of hard rules, and while appreciating that all scientific work is incomplete, recognised the need to act on existing knowledge. The criteria, which have since been revised, are mutually supportive and complementary[74].

Over the last two decades a more formal approach to causality has been encouraged by Popper's view of the central role of falsifiability in science[75]. In this view, causal inference results in a much more tentative conclusion because it is based on the exclusion of other causes for the observed association. This view, however, can lead to a retreat into purity and away from reality. Discussions over the value and meaning of Popper's ideas continued for over a decade and contributed to a broader philosophical inquiry on the nature of the discipline. One important outcome of the Popperian debate is the recognition that epidemiology is concerned with much more than data gathering and is not simply a set of methods.

In part, the usefulness of Popper's ideas depends on the purpose of epidemiology. As pure scientists, epidemiologists can remain tentative about the nature of associations. As public health specialists, however, judgements must be made in the absence of final proof in order to reduce the health risks to the public. Unfortunately, this distinction sets up a dichotomy and can lead to the divorce of epidemiology from its purpose – the prevention and control of disease. The Popperian debate has now faded without having left much impact on the practice of epidemiologists. Epidemiologists are now free to rediscover again the social context of their work.

4.4.2 Study design

The development of epidemiological study designs and methods went hand in hand. The unified nature of epidemiological study designs is now recognised increasingly with the randomised controlled trial promoted as the 'gold standard'[61]. When modern epidemiology began to mature at the end of the 1940s, the cross-sectional survey, adapted from the social sciences, was the major study design. As the weaknesses of the survey become apparent, particularly as a tool in the search for causation, more complex and robust designs become popular. Surveys continue to have an important role in assessing the health status of populations and have become institutionalised in many countries. In general, surveys remain more popular with other social scientists than with epidemiologists.

Cohort studies

The Framingham Study was the prototype of the longitudinal or cohort study[47]. It was established to measure incidence rates of heart disease in the general population, but soon expanded to examine factors influencing the development of heart disease. The Framingham Study has been very influential, but given the way it was originally conceived, it would not have received funding support through the current peer review system. The aims were poorly addressed, the required sample size was not specified, data collection methods were not described, and the reliability of the data was not assessed. Despite the weaknesses that are so apparent in retrospect, the study was a powerful force in shaping the development of epidemiology.

The Framingham Study led to other cohort studies, both of cardiovascular and other non-communicable diseases, and to long-term community studies. The classic cohort study is more expensive and more time consuming than other study designs. The historical cohort study and the nested case control study have been developed to make economical use of the advantages of the cohort designs.

The modern form of the cohort study combines two features: simplicity of design and large size, often in specific and convenient occupational groups. The Nurses' Health Study, for example, collected baseline information by mailed self-administered questionnaires from approximately 120 000 married nurses in the north-eastern states of the United States[76]. Mortality is assessed from the national vital registration system and self-reported morbidity is validated on a subsample. The generalisability of results from this type of 'convenience' cohort is dependent on confirmation by other studies. New cohort studies have been promoted recently in several poor countries mainly to document the number of deaths attributed to tobacco use[77,78], although this is a questionable use of limited research resources.

Case control studies

Case control studies now dominate epidemiology, especially in North America. This design was treated for many years with disdain by epidemiologists familiar with cohort design. Case control studies are relatively cheap to perform in comparison with cohort studies and large randomised controlled trials. They also have advantages when there is a long interval between exposure to the possible cause and the onset of disease; the starting point for this study design is cases with established disease. This design avoids the need for the long periods of follow-up required in all but the largest cohort studies.

The antecedents of the case control study lie in the clinical case series, and several of these early studies included information on non-cases to provide a reference for comparison of various exposures[79]. Gregg, for example, compared the frequency of a history of rubella in cases of congenital cataract and in 100 other patients attending his clinic in the early 1940s[80].

The modern use of the case control design began with the studies on smoking and lung cancer in the United States and Britain[44,45], the latter, in particular, laying out the essential features and potential problems of the design. Remarkable developments and extensions of the case control design have occurred and texts are now devoted solely to this design[81]. There is now a sound appreciation for the potential sources of bias to which this method is prone, especially in the selection of controls, and of methods for its avoidance. This study design has been used to assess the efficacy of health service interventions such as screening. In 'case crossover study', the case acts as its own control where short-term exposures are under investigation.

Experimental studies

The best study design for hypothesis testing is the experimental design. Because of the time and effort involved as well as ethical issues, the use of this design is limited. It is particularly suited to the assessment of the value of medical treatment where clear hypotheses can be tested. It is particularly unsuited to the evaluation of complex public health or policy interventions. The antecedents of experimental studies in epidemiology can be traced back to Lind's study of treatment for scurvy in 1753[12]. The importance of comparative studies of medical therapies has long been recognised. Although Fisher introduced randomisation into agricultural research in the 1920s, random allocation of participants was introduced into medical research by Bradford Hill only in 1946. Prior to the initial Medical Research Council trials, various other forms of allocation had been used including alternation, whereby alternative participants were allocated to different arms of the trial[82]. Hill was also responsible for stressing the importance of the analysis of randomised controlled trials on the basis of 'intention to treat'.

The modern era of clinical trials began with the multi-centre trial of streptomycin in the treatment of tuberculosis conducted for the Medical Research Council in Britain in the late 1940s[83]. Streptomycin, a new drug for the treatment of tuberculosis, was available in sufficient quantities for only about 50 patients. The trial gave impressive results. After 6 months of treatment with streptomycin and bed rest, seven of 55 patients were dead, compared with 27 of

52 patients who received only bed rest. On the basis of this trial, streptomycin was accepted as standard treatment for tuberculosis, although the problem of drug resistance was soon recognised. The experimental design has also been used effectively in the study of preventive interventions. An early randomised controlled trial tested the value of a pertussis vaccine[84]. Other examples include the assessment of the BCG vaccine for tuberculosis and the poliomyelitis vaccine.

The Cochrane controlled trial register now contains more than 300 000 records[85]. Increasingly, randomised controlled trials are undertaken in poor countries or in poor populations with high mortality and morbidity and occasionally in the absence of appropriate ethical oversight[86]. Unfortunately, the results of intervention studies are not always applicable to the populations from which the study participants are drawn. Health services in poor countries may not be suitable for the delivery of the intervention if, in fact, it is shown to be useful. In most of the world, health budgets are inadequate and may not be sufficient or flexible enough to include new interventions or treatments. These considerations should be explored well before studies are conducted in all settings, but they are especially important in poor countries.

Major experimental studies have not always produced clear answers and the results have often generated controversy, particularly when behaviour modification has been the focus. For example, the Multiple Risk Factor Intervention Trial failed to demonstrate an effect on total mortality of several interventions against coronary heart disease in high risk middle-aged men in the United States[87]. The outcome of this trial is open to several interpretations and its policy implications are not clear. A particular difficulty faced by this trial, and the more recent large-scale cardiovascular disease community intervention projects, is the striking decline in cardiovascular disease mortality in the United States[88]. This decline has reduced the chance of detecting a reduction in mortality in the treatment group (or community) because of the general reduction in risk factor levels reflecting the success of population-wide prevention efforts.

In contrast, large-scale, simple and collaborative randomised controlled trials of the treatment of common conditions have on occasions influenced physician behaviour in a relatively short time. For example, the ISIS-2 study of the separate effects of streptokinase and aspirin on survival after acute myocardial infarction involved over 17 000 patients in Western Europe, North America and Australasia[89]. Each drug was found to reduce the case fatality by about 20% and the two combined reduced it by about 40%. Prior to this massive study, many small trials had been completed with mixed results and only about 5% of cardiologists in the United Kingdom were routinely using streptokinase. After the results of the ISIS-2 trial and another similar trial in Italy[90] were published, it was shown that 95% of cardiologists were using both streptokinase and aspirin routinely in appropriate patients[91].

The mega-trials of necessity do not always adhere to all the principles of good study design. For example, they are not always double-blind and informed consent from participants is not always possible. Furthermore, huge trials on poorly defined groups of patients may not provide the detailed information required in clinical practice to ensure the best therapy for specific groups of patients[92]. The results of trials on highly selected patients may also be of little use to practising physicians dealing with a wide range of patients under routine conditions. At the other end of the spectrum, randomised controlled trials in single patients, so-called 'n of 1 trials', have been used when there is doubt about the best treatment for a stable condition in individual patients[93].

Ecological studies

The emphasis on study designs within populations has led to the neglect of studies focusing on the major, and largely unexplained, differences between populations in disease rates[94]. Ecological studies address these population differences by examining the relationship between average disease rates and average exposure levels among populations that often are defined geographically. This design is simple and easy to apply and has been used effectively in exploring inter-population differences in health status. Because of the population-wide focus, this design offers much potential for public health and the results of many ecological studies have endured[95]. Unfortunately, this design has, until recently, been a relatively unsophisticated tool prone to bias. The ecologic study design does not link outcome events to individual exposure at the level of the individual, and this is the source of their special biases; the 'ecologic fallacy' results from the fact that the average exposure of a group of people does not necessarily reflect their individual risk[96]. The evaluation of bias in ecologic studies is especially difficult because of the many potentially interacting variables that may differ across geographical regions. This study design has been very useful for identifying hypotheses, which can be tested with more robust designs, and recent methodological work has greatly increased the value of this type of study[95,97]. It remains the most practical study design for investigating cross-county patterns of disease[94].

4.4.3 Epidemiological analyses

A critical development, which began with a paper published in 1946[98], has been the attention given to systematic sources of error (bias) in epidemiology. In 1979, Sackett identified over 35 potential sources of bias[99]. For practical purposes they can be grouped into three major categories: selection, misclassification, and confounding, although confounding is not now generally regarded as a bias, but as a particular feature of the data under investigation.

Risk estimates, both relative and absolute, are central to epidemiology and were first discussed formally in 1951[100]. Methods of adjusting estimates of risk for possible confounding were developed[101] and have become increasingly sophisticated. Furthermore, the crude risk rate has been broken down into two components, one reflecting confounding and the other reflecting the effect of the exposure[102]. The central importance of obtaining valid results for all studies, irrespective of their design, is now appreciated, as is the fact that even randomised controlled trials are subject to bias.

An unfortunate legacy of the input of statisticians into the development of epidemiological methods has been the dominance of statistical hypothesis testing in data analysis, at the cost of meaningful interpretation. Fortunately, this approach is being replaced increasingly by alternative methods that emphasise estimates as the strength of associations. Statisticians also developed multivariate models in epidemiology to overcome the problems generated by limited data in the ordinary stratified analysis. The first multivariate model was used by Cornfield in his analysis of data from the Framingham study[103]. The multiple logistic model method has now become a primary tool of epidemiology. The rapid advance in computers has encouraged the practical and, often unthinking, application of a range of multiple logistic methods; there is still much to be gained from simpler methods of cross-classification, a point often lost on those influenced by powerful computer programmes.

The important effect of sample size on statistical power is now recognised and, in retrospect many early studies, especially clinical trials, produced false-negative results as a consequence of insufficient sample size. This recognition has led to large and rather simple randomised controlled trials (the 'mega-trials') and to systematic reviews and meta-analyses (statistical pooling) of data from numerous small trials investigating the same issue. Guidelines for improving systematic reviews and meta-analyses have been developed[104]. Systematic reviews and meta-analyses are gradually replacing reviews based on the opinions of experts. Their essential feature is that they are undertaken according to strict and pre-formulated criteria. The procedure requires that all properly conducted trials are included, irrespective of whether they have been published and irrespective of the language of publication. However, the quality of trials appears to be a more important source of bias than the reporting and dissemination of trials except when the meta-analyses are based on few trials[105]. Usually, meta-analyses are based on the summary statistical results of the studies but occasionally use data from individual participants in the studies. A major impediment to systematic overviews is that about half of the 40 000 trials published in the decade after 1985 were not retrievable by expert Medline searches[106, 107]. The quantitative results of the overview provide a good indication of the effect that could be expected in a similar group of patients. Many useful overviews are now influencing clinical practice. The Cochrane Collaboration has been initiated to further the practice of meta-analysis and the dissemination of its results[106]. An interesting recent meta-analysis summarised the data on the value of fluoridation for the prevention of dental disease[108]. Two findings emerged, firstly the poor quality of the evidence and secondly, the rather weak association between fluoridation and oral health – despite the conventional public health wisdom on the value of fluoridation.

4.5 Conclusions

The basic notions of epidemiology have their origin in the works of the Hippocratic School which, over 2000 years ago, stressed the importance of the environment for health. The origins of modern epidemiology go back only to the early decades of the nineteenth century. Two historical themes are of continuing importance: the strong statistical contribution to the development of epidemiology and the original and close connection between epidemiology and public health practice.

Non-communicable disease epidemiology had its origins in the years following the Second World War when studies were initiated into the causes of two modern epidemics: heart disease and lung cancer. Over the last four decades, epidemiology has made important contributions to understanding the causes of both communicable and non-communicable diseases. Few of these advances rival the contribution of the early, and in retrospect, rather simple studies of the adverse health effects of tobacco. Technical aspects of epidemiology have developed remarkably over the last two decades and the discipline has concentrated more on methods, rather than on public health ends.

Epidemiology has contributed greatly to improving the health of populations worldwide. If epidemiology is to fulfil its potential, however, it will need to address several challenges which are described in the next two chapters.

Chapter 4   Key points

- Epidemiology in its modern form developed over the last half century in response to the emergency of non-communicable disease epidemics.
- Recent developments include mega-trials and meta-analyses.
- Epidemiology has concentrated on studies of individuals and has neglected the largely unexplained differences in disease rates between populations.
- Epidemiology has concentrated increasingly on technique and is losing its connection with public health practice.

References

1. Stallones, R.A. To advance epidemiology. *Ann. Rev. Pub. Hlth* 1980; **1**: 69–82.
2. Rosen, G. *A History of Public Health*. Baltimore and London: Johns Hopkins University Press, 1958.
3. Hippocrates. *The Genuine Works of Hippocrates*. Translated from Greek by Francis Adams. Baltimore: Williams and Wilkins, 1939.
4. Nutton, V. Healers in the medical market place: towards a social history of Graeco-Roman medicine. In: Wear, A. (ed.). *Medicine in Society*. Cambridge: Cambridge University Press, 1992.
5. Winslow, C.E.A. *Man and Epidemics*. Princeton: Princeton University Press, 1952.
6. Carmichael, A.G. History of public health and sanitation in the West before 1700. In: Kiple, K.F. (ed.). *The Cambridge World History of Human Disease*. Cambridge: Cambridge University Press, 1993.
7. Park, K. Medicine and society in Medieval Europe, 500–1500. In: Wear, A. (ed.). *Medicine in Society*. Cambridge: Cambridge University Press, 1992.
8. Porter, D. *Health, Civilization and the State. A History of Public Health from Ancient to Modern Times*. London: Routledge, 1999.
9. Rothman, K.J. Lessons from John Graunt. *Lancet* 1996; **347**: 37–9.
10. White, K.L. *Healing the Schism. Epidemiology, Medicine, and the Public's Health*. New York: Springer, 1991.
11. Banta, J.E. Sir William Petty: modern epidemiologist (1623–1687). *J. Commun. Hlth* 1987; **12**: 185–98.
12. Lilienfeld, A.M. *Ceteris paribus*: the evolution of the clinical trial. *Bull. Hist. Med.* 1982; **56**: 1–18.
13. Hannaway, C. Discussion (The French influence on the development of epidemiology – Lilienfeld, D.E. and A.M.). In: Lilienfeld, A.M. (ed.). *Times, Places, and Persons: Aspects of the History of Epidemiology*. Baltimore: Johns Hopkins University Press, 1980.
14. Lilienfeld, A.M. & Lilienfeld, D.E. *Foundations of Epidemiology*. New York: Oxford University Press, 1980.

15. Ramsey, M. Public health in France. In Porter, D. (ed.). *The History of Public Health and the Modern State*. Amsterdam: Editions Rodopi B.V., 1994.

16. Wilkinson, R. Commentary. Liberty, fraternity, equality. *Int. J. Epidemiol.* 2002; **31**: 538-43.

17. Guy, W.A. *Public Health: A Popular Introduction*. London: Renshaw, 1874.

18. Lilienfeld, D.E. & Lilienfeld, A.M. The French influence on the development of epidemiology. In: Lilienfeld, A.M. (ed.). *Times, Places, and Persons: Aspects of the History of Epidemiology*. Baltimore: Johns Hopkins University Press, 1980.

19. Vandenbroucke, J.P. Epidemiology in transition: a historial hypothesis. *Epidemiology* 1990; **1**: 164–7.

20. Pearce, N., Matos, E., Vainio, H., Boffetta, P. & Kogevinas, M. *Occupational Cancer in Developing Countries*. Lyon: International Agency for Research on Cancer, 1994.

21. Lilienfeld, A.M. & Lilienfeld, D.E. Epidemiology and the public health movement: a historical perspective. *J. Pub. Hlth Pol.* 1982; **3**: 140–9.

22. Lilienfeld, D.E. The greening of epidemiology: sanitary physicians and the London Epidemiological Society (1830–1870). *Bull. Hist. Med.* 1979; **52**: 503–28.

23. Hamlin, C. State medicine in Great Britain. In: Porter, D. (ed.). *The History of Public Health and the Modern State*. Amsterdam: Editions Rodopi B.V., 1994.

24. Susser, M. & Adelstein, A. The work of William Farr. In: Susser, M. (ed.) *Epidemiology, Health and Society*. New York: Oxford University Press, 1987.

25. Morabia, A. Snow and Farr: a scientific duet. *Soz. Praventiv. Med.* 2001; **46**: 223–4.

26. Eyler, J.M. The conceptual origins of William Farr's epidemiology: numerical methods and social thought in the 1830s. In: Lilienfeld, A.M. (ed.). *Times, Places, and Persons. Aspects of the History of Epidemiology*. Baltimore: Johns Hopkins University Press, 1980.

27. Langmuir, A.D. William Farrö: founder of modern concepts of surveillance. *Int. J. Epidemiol.* 1976; **15**: 13–18.

28. Winkelstein, W. A new perspective on John Snow's communicable disease theory. *Am. J. Epidemiol.* 1995; **142**: S3–S9.

29. Davey Smith, G. & Ebrahim, S. Epidemiology – is it time to call it a day? *Int. J. Epidemiol.* 2001; **30**: 1–11.

30. Vandenbroucke, J.P. Which John Snow should set the example for clinical epidemiology? *J. Clin. Epidemiol.* 1988; **41**: 1215–16.

31. Cameron, D. & Jones, I.G. John Snow, the Broad Street pump and modern epidemiology. *Int. J. Epidemiol.* 1983; **12**: 393–6.

32. Vandenbroucke, J.P. Changing images of John Snow in the history of epidemiology. *Soz. Praventiv. Med.* 2001; **46**: 288–93.

33. Pearce, N. Traditional epidemiology, modern epidemiology, and public health. *Am. J. Pub. Hlth* 1996; **86**: 678–83.

34. McMichael, A.J. Prisoners of the proximate: loosening the constraints on epidemiology in an age of change. *Am. J. Epidemiol.* 1999; **149**: 887–97.

35. Greenwood, M. *Epidemics and Crowd Diseases: An Introduction to the Study of Epidemiology*. London: Williams and Northgate, 1935.

36. Porter, D. Changing disciplines: John Ryle and the making of social medicine in twentieth century Britain. *Hist. Sci.* 1992; **30**: 119–47.

37. Hill, A.B. *Principles of Medical Statistics*. London: Lancet, 1937.
38. Terris, M. Healthy lifestyles: the perspective of epidemiology. *J. Pub. Hlth Pol.* 1992; **13**:186–94.
39. Cardenas, V.C., Roces, M.C., Wattanasri, S. *et al.* Improving global public health leadership through training in epidemiology and public health: the experience of TEPHINET. *Am. J. Pub. Hlth* 2002; **92**: 196–7.
40. Susser, M. Epidemiology in the United States after World War II: the evolution of technique. *Epidemiol. Rev.* 1985; **7**: 147–77.
41. Barrett-Connor E. Infectious and chronic disease epidemiology: separate and unequal? *Am. J. Epidemiol.* 1979; **109**: 245–9.
42. Comstock, G.W. Cohort analysis: W.H. Frost's contribution to the epidemiology of tuberculosis and chronic disease. *Soz. Präventiv. Med.* 2001; **46**: 7–12.
43. Brown, E.R. *Rockefeller Medicine Men*. Berkeley: University of California Press, 1980.
44. Wynder, E.L. & Graham, E.A. Tobacco smoke as a possible etiologic factor in bronchiogenic carcinoma: a study of 654 proved cases. *J. Am. Med. Assoc.* 1950; **143**: 329–36.
45. Doll, R. & Hill, A.B. Smoking and carcinoma of the lung: preliminary report. *Br. Med. J.* 1950; **ii**: 739–48.
46. Vandenbroucke, J.P. Those who were wrong. *Am. J. Epidemiol.* 1989; **130**: 3–5.
47. Dawber, T. *The Framingham Study*. Cambridge: Harvard University Press, 1980.
48. Terris, M. The complex tasks of the second epidemiologic revolution: the Joseph W. Mountin Lecture. *J. Pub. Hlth Pol.* 1983; **4**: 8–24.
49. Berkelman, R.L. & Hughes, J.M. The conquest of infectious diseases: who are we kidding? *Ann. Intern. Med.* 1993; **119**: 426–7.
50. Hughes, J.M. & La Montagne, J.R. Emerging infectious diseases. *J. Infect. Dis.* 1994; **170**: 263–4.
51. Epstein, P.R. Emerging diseases and ecosystem instability: new threats to public health. *Am. J. Pub. Hlth* 1995; **85**: 168–72.
52. Morris, J.N. *Uses of Epidemiology*. Edinburgh: Livingstone, 1957.
53. MacMahon, B., Pugh, T.F. & Ipsen, J. *Epidemiologic Methods*. Boston: Little Brown and Co, 1960.
54. Krieger, N. Epidemiology and the web of causation: has anyone seen the spider? *Soc. Sci. Med.* 1994; **39**: 887–902.
55. Lilienfeld, A.M. *Foundations of Epidemiology*. New York: Oxford University Press, 1976.
56. Vineis, P. History of bias. *Soz. Praventiv. Med.* 2002; **47**: 156–61.
57. Vandenbroucke, J.P. The history of confounding. *Soz. Präventiv. Med.* 2002; **47**: 216–24.
58. Last, J.M. *A Dictionary of Epidemiology*. New York: Oxford University Press, 1983.
59. Lilienfeld, D.E. Definitions of epidemiology. *Am. J. Epidemiol.* 1978; **107**: 87–90.
60. Last, J.M. *A Dictionary of Epidemiology*, 4th edn New York: Oxford University Press, 2000.
61. Rothman, K. *Modern Epidemiology*. Boston: Little Brown & Co, 1986.
62. Armstrong, B.K., White, E. & Saracci, R. *Principles of Exposure Measurement in Epidemiology*. Oxford: Oxford University Press, 1992.

63. McMichael, A.J. 'Molecular epidemiology': new pathway or new travelling companion?'. *Am. J. Epidemiol.* 1994; **140**: 1–11.
64. Susser, M. & Susser, E. Choosing a future for epidemiology: 1. Eras and paradigms. *Am. J. Pub. Hlth* 1996; **86**: 668–73.
65. Wilcox, A.J. Molecular epidemiology: collision of two cultures. *Epidemiology* 1995; **6**: 561–2.
66. Pearce, N., de Sanjose, S., Boffetta, P., Kogevinas, M., Saracci, R. & Savitz, D. Limitations of biomarkers of exposure in cancer epidemiology. *Epidemiology* 1995; **6**: 190–4.
67. Rose, G. *The Strategy of Preventive Medicine.* Oxford: Oxford University Press, 1992.
68. McMichael, A.J. *Human Frontiers, Environments and Disease.* Cambridge: Cambridge University Press, 2001.
69. Mackenbach, J.P. Public health epidemiology. *J. Epidemiol. Commun. Hlth* 1995; **49**: 333–4.
70. Wall, S.G.I. Epidemiology in developing countries. *Scand. J. Soc. Med.* 1990; **Suppl. 46**: 25–32.
71. Waitzkin, H., Iriart, C., Estrada, A. & Lamadrid, S. Social medicine in Latin America: productivity and dangers facing the major national groups. *Lancet* 2001; **358**: 315–23.
72. Hill, A.B. The environment and disease: association or causation? *Proc. R. Soc. Med.* 1965; **58**: 295–9.
73. Morabia, A. On the origin of Hill's causal criteria. *Epidemiology* 1991; **2**: 367–9.
74. Susser, M. What is a cause and how do we know one? A grammar for pragmatic epidemiology. *Am. J. Epidemiol.* 1991; **133**: 635–48.
75. Susser, M. The logic of Sir Karl Popper and the practice of epidemiology. *Am. J. Epidemiol.* 1986; **124**: 711–18.
76. Colditz, G.A., Bonita, R., Stampfer, M.J. *et al.* Cigarette smoking and risk of stroke in middle-aged women. *New Engl. J. Med.* 1988; **318**: 937–41.
77. World Health Organization. *Tobacco Alert.* Geneva: WHO, 1995.
78. Niu, S.-R., Yang, G.-H., Chen, Z.-M. *et al.* Emerging tobacco hazards in China: 2. Early mortality results from a prospective study. *Br. Med. J.* 1998; **317**: 1423–4.
79. Armenian, H.K. & Lilienfeld, D.E. Overview and historical perspective. *Epidemiol. Rev.* 1994; **16**: 1–5.
80. Gregg, N.M. Congenital cataract following German measles in the mother. *Trans. Ophthalmol. Soc. Aust.* 1941; **3**: 35–46.
81. Schlesselman, J.J. *Case-Control Studies: Design, Conduct, Analysis.* New York: Oxford University Press, 1982.
82. Doll, R. Sir Austin Bradford Hill and the progress of medical science. *Br. Med. J.* 1992; **305**: 1521–6.
83. Medical Research Council Streptomycin in Tuberculosis Trials Committee. Streptomycin treatment for pulmonary tuberculosis. *Br. Med. J.* 1948; **ii:** 769–82.
84. Medical Research Council Whooping-cough Immunisation Committee. The prevention of whooping-cough by vaccination. *Br. Med. J.* 1950; **i**: 1463–71.

85. Clarke, M. & Langhorne, P. Revisiting the Cochrane Collaboration. *Br. Med. J.* 2001; **323**: 821.
86. Wikler, D. & Cash, R. Ethical issues in global public health. In: Beaglehole, R. (ed.). *Global Public Health*: A New Era. Oxford: Oxford University Press, 2003.
87. MRFIT (Multiple Risk Factor Intervention Trial Research Group). Mortality rates after 10.5 years for participants in the Multiple Risk Factor Intervention Trial. Findings related to a prior hypothesis of the Trial. *Circulation* 1990; **82**: 1616–28.
88. Sellers, D.E., Crawford, S.L., Bullock, K. & McKinlay, J.B. Understanding the variability in the effectiveness of community heart health programs; a meta-analysis. *Soc. Sci. Med.* 1997; **44**: 1325-39.
89. ISIS-2 Collaborative Group. Randomised trial of intravenous streptokinase, oral aspirin, both, or neither among 17187 cases of suspected acute myocardial infarction. *Lancet* 1988; **ii**: 349–60.
90. GISSI. Effectiveness of intravenous thrombolytic therapy in acute myocardial infarction. *Lancet* 1986; **i**: 397–401.
91. Doll, R. Development of controlled trials in preventive and therapeutic medicine. *J. Biosoc. Sci.* 1991; **23**: 365–78.
92. Ertl, G. & Jugdutt, B. ACE inhibition after myocardial infarction: can megatrials provide answers? *Lancet* 1994; **344**: 1068–9.
93. Guyatt, G., Sackett, D., Adachi, J. *et al.* A clincan's guide for conducting randomised trials in individual patients. *Can. Med. Assoc. J.* 1988; **139**: 497–503.
94. Pearce, N. The ecological study strikes back. *J. Epidemiol. Commun. Hlth* 2000; **54**: 326–7.
95. Susser, M. The logic in ecological: II. The logic of design. *Am. J. Pub. Hlth* 1994; **84**: 830–5.
96. Greenland, S. & Robins, J. Ecologic studies: biases, misconceptions, and counterexamples. *Am. J. Epidemiol.* 1993; **139**: 747–60.
97. Susser, M. The logic in ecological: I. The logic of analysis. *Am. J. Pub. Hlth* 1994; **84**: 825–9.
98. Berkson, J. Limitations of the application of fourfold table analysis to hospital data. *Biometrics* 1946; **2**: 47–53.
99. Sackett, D.L. Bias in analytic research. *J. Chron. Dis.* 1979; **32**: 51–63.
100. Cornfield, J. A method of estimating comparative rates from clinical data. Applications to cancer of the lung, breast, and cervix. *J. Natl Cancer Inst.* 1951; **11**: 1269–75.
101. Mantel, N. & Haenszel, W. Statistical aspects of the analysis of data from retrospective studies of disease. *J. Natl Cancer Inst.* 1959; **22**: 719–48.
102. Miettinen, O.S. Components of the crude risk ratio. *Am. J. Epidemiol.* 1972; **96**: 168–72.
103. Cornfield, J. Joint dependence of risk of coronary heart disease on serum cholesterol and systolic blood pressure: a discriminant function analysis. *Fed. Proc.* 1962; **2**: 58–61.
104. Sackett, D.L. & Spitzer, W.O. Guidelines for improving meta-analysis. *Lancet* 1994; **343**: 910.

105. Egger, M., Ebrahim, S. & Davey Smith, G. Where now for meta-analysis? *Int. J. Epidemiol.* 2002; **31**: 1–5.

106. Godlee, F. The Cochrane Collaboration. *Br. Med. J.* 1994; **309**: 969–70.

107. Dickersin, K., Scherer, R. & Lefebvre, R. Identifying relevant studies for systematic reviews. *Br. Med. J.* 1994; **309**: 1286–91.

108. McDonagh, M., Whiting. P.F., Wilson, P.M. *et al.* Systematic review of water fluoridation. *Br. Med. J.* 2000; **321**: 855–9.

5

The current state of epidemiology: achievements and limitations

5.1 Introduction

Many of the historical epidemiological achievements have been referred to in earlier chapters. In this chapter we review the current state of epidemiology, summarise some of the recent achievements and discuss the limitations of epidemiological methods and outlook. The chapter also reviews some of the main criticisms of epidemiology. The next chapter continues this theme and identifies the main challenges facing epidemiology. Some epidemiological achievements can also be viewed as failures, and many achievements are not the sole responsibility of the epidemiologists involved. Nevertheless, it is useful to attempt to summarise the state of epidemiology, fully recognising that other reviewers might come up with different conclusions – a timely warning on the perils of subjective reviews!

5.2 Achievements

5.2.1 The growth of epidemiology

Epidemiology is flourishing in many countries. The 'fall' of epidemiology by the year 2000, predicted by Rothman in 1981[1] was, in retrospect, an absurd prediction. Judging by the proliferation of peer-reviewed journals, the lively discussion of epidemiological methods and results in medical journals, and its popularity with the media, epidemiology is in good heart. There are, however, worrying trends, It has been suggested that, at least in the United States of America, young epidemiologists are withdrawing from the field[2].

Despite the overall growth of epidemiology, there is both a global shortage and a maldistribution of epidemiologists, reflecting poor workforce planning and lack of satisfactory career development options[3]. There is also the tendency

136

for epidemiologists to migrate, along with other professionals, to wealthy countries; there are, for example, more Indian epidemiologists in the USA than in India. It is difficult to estimate the required number of epidemiologists. Should they rank on a per capita basis with general practitioners, brain surgeons or sociologists? A feature of the discipline, especially in North America, has been the increase in non-physician epidemiologists. In 1975 there were no more than 500 fully trained epidemiologists in the United States of America, 300 of whom were physicians[4]; by 1985 there were an estimated 4600 epidemiologists, 54% of whom were physicians[5]. It was suggested that by 2000 the United States of America would require about five times the 1990 number of medically trained epidemiologists[4]. In now appears that there are approximately 3000 epidemiologists in the USA (personal communication from Betsy Foxman, 12 May 2003), far fewer than the number estimated in 1985, suggesting that epidemiologists are not yet very good at counting themselves.

There is still little information on the gender and ethnic composition of the epidemiological workforce. A 1992 study by the American College of Epidemiology found a severe under-representation of minority groups in epidemiology, especially in relation to the severity of the ethnic morbidity and mortality gap. For example, in 1992, African–Americans, who made up 12% of the population, constituted only 2% of epidemiology faculty members in epidemiology degree programmes. There was also a marked deficit of students from minority population groups[6] and a need for more active recruitment plans[7]. This situation also exists in Australia and New Zealand, although the gender balance is more equal in these countries. Within Europe, there is a wide variation in the number of epidemiologists per million population, ranging from a high of almost 100 in the Netherlands and Denmark, to a low of about 5 in Germany[8].

When compared with other public health disciplines within the United States of America (biostatistics, health services administration, health education and environmental sciences), epidemiology had the second lowest level of minority representation amongst faculty and the lowest among students[9]. Faculty representation of minority groups in public health in the United States of America was virtually unchanged between 1985 and 1992, although the percentages of students from minority groups increased by more than one-third during this period, largely because of increases in Hispanic and Asian students[9].

It is a sad irony that epidemiology, which has exposed the health impact of social disadvantage, now finds its own ranks less socially representative than other public health disciplines. Recommendations have been made to improve the participation of under-represented minority group in epidemiology[6]. It is to be hoped that epidemiology can rapidly improve its own 'health'; to this end, the American College of Epidemiology has produced a statement of principles, which recognises the importance of achieving racial and ethnic diversity in the profession[10].

The situation of epidemiology in poor countries is even more difficult to assess. In 2002 the International Epidemiological Association had a total of approximately 2000 members, including 80 in Africa, 90 in South East Asia, 203 in the Eastern Mediterranean region and almost 200 in South America[11]. It is not known how well these numbers reflect the active epidemiological workforce, although the IEA estimates that its members account for only about 10% of all epidemiologists. Many epidemiological studies in poor countries are conducted, at least in part, by epidemiologists based in wealthy countries; this type of epidemiology produces its own challenges, both practical[12, 13] and ethical[14], and its own rewards[15].

In summary, epidemiology has flourished in some countries; however, there is a global shortage of epidemiologists, an under-representation of minority groups, and a maldistribution of the available workforce, which is particularly deficient in the poorer regions.

5.2.2 Epidemiology and health status improvement: essential but not sufficient

Epidemiology undoubtedly has contributed directly to global improvements in health. For example, without the contribution of epidemiologists, smallpox would not have been eradicated or the health hazards of tobacco identified in such (excruciating) detail. Epidemiology has identified the causes of many non-communicable diseases and has contributed to their prevention, including heart disease and stroke, many cancers and dietary deficiency diseases such as iodine deficiency. Two recent contributions are the identification of the probable causes of an iatrogenic epidemic of death from asthma[16] and of sudden infant deaths[17]. Infectious disease epidemiologists have made many contributions and can take credit, most recently, for our understanding of the HIV/AIDS epidemic, despite our failure to act on this knowledge to prevent the global spread of HIV/AIDS.

With regard to cancer there has been debate as to whether the so-called 'war against cancer' is being won or lost. A decline in mortality has been noted for most, but not all, cancers. An important exception is lung cancer in women, which has already outstripped breast cancer mortality in women in the United States of America. For most cancers in children and young adults, mortality rates are declining[18]. Of those cancers for which incidence rates have increased substantially since the early 1970s, one is associated with the spread of AIDS (Kaposi's sarcoma) and two may be due to more frequent screening (breast and prostate). Only for lung cancer in women and until recently, for testicular cancer in men, and melanoma are the increases in incidence rates independent and genuine. These favourable trends in cancer incidence and mortality indicate the importance of epidemiology and prevention; only a small proportion of these improvements is due to specific treatments, for example, leukaemia, especially in young people – the treatment of lung cancer is almost completely ineffective still.

Unfortunately, the relationship between epidemiological endeavour and health improvements is not always clear. Although it is relatively easy to identify the contribution of epidemiology to the control of specific diseases over the last few decades, it is much more difficult to assess the contribution of epidemiology to the dramatic overall improvement in health status over the last century. As epidemiology is only one part of public health, and public health interventions are only one of the factors contributing to health improvement, this is not surprising.

In assessing the value of epidemiology to health improvements, the case of tobacco consumption is both instructive and depressing. The case control studies published in 1950, now viewed as epidemiological classics, built on earlier German studies and were the first of literally thousands of studies of this association. In the absence of epidemiological data, the cause of the epidemics of lung cancer and other tobacco induced diseases would not have been identified. Indeed, the early investigations in Great Britain were established to examine the role of air pollution and other environmental factors. The accumulated epidemiological knowledge has been an essential stimulus for public health action. By itself, however, knowledge is not sufficient to promote adequate control measures. The identification of the role of smoking in the aetiology of lung cancer led to the focus on personal responsibility for smoking control, which was politically much more acceptable than discussion of the environmental causes of air pollution; this in turn supported public health 'individualism', which remained the dominant paradigm for about two decades[19]. Where progress has occurred, a constellation of forces has acted together[20]. Despite over five decades of research and public health intervention, more people are now exposed to, and die from, tobacco than ever before. This depressing fact testifies to the success of the marketing and promotion campaigns of the multinational tobacco companies which continue to exploit new markets in poor countries ruthlessly[21]. Interventions in wealthy countries, which have focused on consumption and not production, have only added to the inequalities in health between the poor and rich within wealthy countries, and between poor and wealthy countries.

A similar focus on the adverse effect of consumption of a high fat diet on cardiovascular disease and educational efforts directed towards encouraging knowledge of personal cholesterol levels, has also contributed to widening social class differentials in coronary heart disease occurrence in wealthy countries. Health education strategies have focused too often on modification of individual risk factors to the neglect of the commercial forces that encourage consumption of fat. As a consequence, while educated and relatively wealthy people have been able to reduce their cardiovascular disease risk status, poor people have been less successful. Furthermore, the consequences of the animal-oriented agriculture business which supports the mass consumption of saturated fat has been neglected almost entirely[22]. Only recently has the public health community begun to discuss the role of food producers in the aetiology of the non-communicable disease epidemics[23,24].

5.2.3 Contributions to medical care

Epidemiology has also made important contributions to the medical care of individuals through the application of the randomised controlled trial to medical care issues[25], studies of the effectiveness and efficiency of health services, and the development of 'clinical epidemiology' and 'evidence-based medicine'[26].

The Cochrane Centre was established in Oxford in 1993 to facilitate systematic and up-to-date reviews of randomised controlled trials of health care. Information from the Centre, which maintains a register of systematic reviews and randomised controlled trials (both published and unpublished), is disseminated through seminars, workshops and electronic media including the 'Online Journal of Current Clinical Trials'. The Centre encourages the formation of collaborative review groups which may be problem-based (e.g. coronary heart disease, stroke, breast cancer, pregnancy and childbirth), intervention based (e.g. nutrition, neonatal care), or speciality based (e.g. public health, primary care). The main focus of the Collaboration was randomised studies and this, of course, was not useful for the many areas which are not appropriate for randomised trials, for example, many preventive interventions such as suicide prevention[26]. The Cochrane Health Promotion and Public Health Field now represent the needs and concerns of health promotion and public health practitioners in the Collaboration and recognises that many important interventions, which are not appropriate for controlled trials, can benefit from systematic reviews[27]. Newer collaborations, such as the Campbell Collaboration, are summarising the effects of interventions based on the results from research in the social sciences[28].

The importance of systematic overviews and dissemination of results is illustrated readily. The first trial of the use of corticosteroids by women for the prevention of respiratory disease in potentially premature babies was published in 1972[29]. It was not until 1989, however, that a systematic review of the many, usually small, randomised controlled trials in this area demonstrated that corticosteroids reduced the risk of babies dying from the complications of immaturity by 30 to 50%[30]. Many obstetricians would not have been aware of the benefits of this form of care until the 1989 review was published. In retrospect, enough information was available 10 years earlier for the evidence to change practice. Another excellent example of the contribution of epidemiology to health care is the accumulation of evidence over the last two decades on effective interventions for established cardiovascular disease and for patients at high risk of these diseases[31]. Large-scale trials have been central to this success, even if these therapies still do not reach a high proportion of people who would benefit – even in wealthy countries[32]; the situation is probably much worse in poor countries, although the data are limited[33].

Clinical epidemiology has generated controversy. Some saw it as a contradiction in terms[34]; others viewed it as outdated, a threat to health, or as a part of a movement serving the interests of pharmaceutical companies[35, 36]. There is no doubt that the application of epidemiological methods and principles to medical practice has been of enormous benefit, despite the slow progress. Advice contained in medical textbooks and review articles often fails to reflect the strong evidence available from randomised controlled trials, thus delaying implementation of some life-saving therapies[37]; other treatments continue to be recommended long after controlled trials have shown them to be either ineffective or even harmful.

Regrettably, epidemiology, and public health more generally, have had little impact on debates on the reorganisation of health services, which are occurring in most countries. Powerful vested interests and ideological considerations are much more influential in directing or resisting changes to the organisation and delivery of health services. For example, the ongoing debate about the reform of health care in the United States of America has not been led by public health practitioners[38]. It is thus not surprising that, when health services are re-organised (or 'redisorganised'), the focus is not on public health and reforms are driven primarily by hospital concerns, for example, surgical waiting lists, and not by the need for accountability for trends in population health status, especially growing health inequalities.

5.3 Limitations

Epidemiology has been criticised from two different perspectives representing different philosophies and different conceptions of health and disease: the individualistic and the collectivist[39]. The individualistic view emphasises the primacy of the individual; society, in this view, is the outcome of the actions and motives of distinct individuals. In the collectivist view, the emphasis is on society as a whole. The individualistic philosophy has its counterpart in the natural science or mechanistic view of health, which underpins modern medicine and considers health as the absence of disease. The contrasting broad view of health is enshrined in the original WHO definition of health.

Most of the criticism of epidemiology is based on the mechanistic view of health and concentrates on the supposed failure of epidemiology to reach the standards of other natural sciences. Concern has been expressed at the epidemiological emphasis on risk factors for multi-factorial diseases, on the poor quality of epidemiological data, and on a general failure to adhere to 'scientific standards'. More challenging criticisms of epidemiology have been expressed from the broad population perspective[22,40,41]. The most immediate threat to epidemiology is that posed by the mechanistic critics as they challenge the ability of epidemiology to meet 'scientific' criteria.

5.3.1 'Risk factor' epidemiology

Critics are justified when they point to the loose use of the term 'risk factor', and the equation of risk factors with causes[42,43]. Unfortunately, many of the critics are unable to separate important risk factors from the trivial associations that delight the mass media so much, and do not use the techniques and criteria available for exactly this purpose. While it is counterproductive to dismiss all risk factors, it is equally inappropriate to condemn all epidemiological studies of risk factors as unscientific because of a few poor studies. Too often the contributions of this type of epidemiology to our understanding of the causes of the cardiovascular disease and cancer epidemics are ignored; furthermore, epidemiological studies of high quality often lead to appropriate biological research[44]. A major, and perhaps wilful, misunderstanding of the contribution of epidemiology is the continuing assertion that the major risk factors for coronary heart disease only explain about half the new events within populations[45]. The reality is that a small number of well-established risk factors explain over 75% of new events; the only 50% myth has been perpetuated, it seems, by investigators trying to strengthen their requests for research funding for studies searching for new risk factors[46].

The multi-factorial concept of disease is a fair and useful reflection of the real world. Some critics are convinced that non-communicable disease epidemiology is stagnating and believe that further understanding of coronary heart disease, for example, will come from laboratory studies and not from epidemiology, despite the impressive gains from prevention over the last two decades[47]. The causes of the major differences in disease experience within and between countries, however, will not be discovered in a laboratory; the ecological study design is a useful, and the only, means of exploring these intriguing differences[48].

One persistent critic of 'risk factor' epidemiology (also referred to as 'black box' epidemiology) went further and questioned the *raison d'être* of epidemiology[42,49–51]. Skrabanek asserted that epidemiologists turned their attention away from infectious diseases (because these diseases were becoming less prevalent), leaving an epidemic of epidemiologists who were short of diseases suitable for study[42]. In part this is true; of much more importance, however, was the rise in death rates from non-communicable diseases. Skrabanek believed that the preoccupation with causes and prevention of disease encouraged epidemiologists to become moralists, preaching the 'good life'[42].

Two examples used to illustrate the 'poverty of epidemiology' are amylnitrate as a cause of AIDS and the association of oestrogen replacement therapy with heart disease in women[49]. To the credit of epidemiology, the amylnitrate and AIDS relationship was soon discarded as a hypothesis when HIV was discovered[52]. The conflicting results of two studies published in the same issue of the *New England Journal of Medicine* on the associations of oestrogen replacement therapy with heart disease in women generated controversy and, more importantly, further study[53]. The association of hormone replacement therapy (HRT) with a reduced risk of heart disease was identified in many observational studies. Active promotion by a variety of interest groups encouraged a large number of women, especially in the USA, to use these products at least in part on the expectation that their risks of heart and other diseases would be reduced. Only with evidence from randomised controlled trials has it become apparent that there is no protective effect and the observational associations were probably due largely to a healthy women effect, i.e. low risk women being more likely to take these preparations[54]. So, far from indicating epidemiological ineptitude, these studies illustrate the progressive nature of epidemiological research and the importance of waiting for the strongest possible evidence before advising on clinical interventions, especially when they are for healthy people.

5.3.2 Data quality and scientific standards

Epidemiologists have been accused repeatedly of ignoring the common criticisms of epidemiology. These include the use of poor quality data, a lack of precision in measurement, invalid extrapolation, inappropriate use of terminology, bias in the interpretation of data, and an undue emphasis on statistical inference at the expense of causal inference[55–57]. Feinstein is correct in calling for further improvement in the quality of epidemiological data, but there is nothing in this challenge that would not be accepted by most epidemiologists. Indeed, it has been identified repeatedly as a major issue[58]. There is also support for his call for less dependence on mathematical modelling and the need for epidemiology to become more integrated with other scientific disciplines.

The limitations of their data are all well recognised by most epidemiologists and are addressed through a variety of approaches including the preparation of detailed protocols and manuals of operation. The difficulties in studying human populations explain some of the problems in the science of epidemiology. There is, of course, a need for continuing attention to the scientific quality of the evidence as well as to the appropriate statistical methods of analysis and adjustment for possible biases and confounding variables[52, 59].

5.3.3 Asocial epidemiology

The most challenging criticisms of epidemiology stem from its individualistic philosophical underpinning and its reluctance to place individuals in their social context[60, 61]. In particular, the risk factor approach to epidemiology and prevention does not give adequate weight to the role of social and economic factors in explaining population differences in the distribution of health problems[62]. This individualistic approach also runs the risk of blaming the victim and of encouraging health education strategies at the expense of social, economic and environmental changes. The result is the medicalisation of prevention rather than its socialisation. This criticism of epidemiology recognises that the ethics and purpose of epidemiology must be broadened to include the health impact of social, economic and environmental conditions on a range of outcomes, not just death and disease.

It has also been suggested that epidemiology, as it cannot easily tap into the experiences and perceptions of people, is unlikely to be effective when it comes to prevention and control[63]. Epidemiology should combine qualitative studies of the concerns and views expressed by people about the disease or injury under investigation with quantitative information, data gathering and interpretation. Interpretation of both qualitative and quantitative data is critical in understanding what is happening and what can be done[64]. The aim of epidemiology is to understand the causes of disease so that health status is improved. From this perspective, epidemiology cannot be practised in isolation from the people who make up the study population. Epidemiological studies of the future need to integrate fully qualitative and quantitative research methods in the context of people's lives. The application of this rounded approach is most easily envisaged in occupational health epidemiology. It is more difficult to apply in the context of large-scale studies of randomly chosen population samples.

Much of the controversy generated by epidemiology is due to the intrinsic imprecision of epidemiology; also of importance is the recent epidemiological emphasis on methods, to the neglect of purpose[22,40]. Ironically, although the distinguishing feature of epidemiology as a science is its population focus, much of modern epidemiology ignores the unique features of populations and, instead, isolates individual characteristics and risk factors from their social context[65]. The impact of modern epidemiology on public health has been limited severely by this focus on specific individual exposures. Not surprisingly, the recommended public health interventions have focused on these exposures (risk factors) to the neglect of their social and economic determinants.

The current lack of interest in social factors and in the population perspective has been attributed to the personal and professional isolation of epidemiologists, who are usually dependent on funding by government or voluntary agencies[66]. The prevailing ideology in most countries still favours individual responsibility over collective responsibility[67]. Furthermore, the current interest of epidemiologists with the role of social capital as a major socioeconomic determinant of health[68] runs the risk of deflecting attention from broader macrolevel social and economic processes that influence health across the life course[69]. Unfortunately, for many epidemiologists the study of social factors is considered usually both too difficult and too political to address, despite the fact that it is also an implicit 'political' decision not to address the broader issues[70].

5.4 Conclusions

To its credit, epidemiology survived long neglect at the expense of the bacteriological paradigm. Over the last half century, epidemiology has grown and flourished in many wealthy countries, although there remains an overall shortage of epidemiologists, and the workforce is both maldistributed and unrepresentative in ethnic composition. Epidemiology has made many important contributions to the prevention and control of disease, although epidemiology alone cannot claim responsibility for either specific or general health improvements. Epidemiology has contributed to establishing the scientific basis of clinical medicine and has much to offer the health services in the identification of effective and efficient services.

Epidemiology has been criticised from two opposing perspectives. Biomedical scientists are concerned by the inability of epidemiologists to replicate the strict methods of laboratory based science. Social scientists are concerned by exactly this reductionist basis to modern epidemiology; in this view, epidemiology neglects the social context in which people live and work and concentrates on individual attributes at the expense of the characteristics of populations. The 'scientific' criticisms are the most threatening, at least from a funding viewpoint, because the agencies responsible for allocating research funds generally reflect this view. From a public health perspective, the most serious challenge for epidemiology is to re-establish its social responsibility and its connection with public health practice. This is one of several challenges addressed in the next chapter.

Chapter 5   Key points

- Epidemiology is flourishing, although there is a global shortage of epidemiologists and a maldistribution of the workforce.
- Epidemiology has contributed to the improvements in health status of populations worldwide and to the increased efficiency and effectiveness of medical care.
- Epidemiology has been criticised as being too closely allied with both medicine and the natural sciences and, from another perspective, of ignoring the social and economic determinants of health and disease.

References

1. Rothman, K.J. The rise and fall of epidemiology, AD 1950–2000. *New Engl. J. Med.* 1981; **304**: 600–2.
2. Harlow, B.L. Coping with the personal and professional frustrations of epidemiologic research. *Am. J. Epidemiol.* 1995; **142**: 785–7.
3. Greenberg, R.S. The future of epidemiology. *Ann. Epidemiol.* 1990; **1**: 213–4.
4. White, K.L. Healing the Schism. *Epidemiology, Medicine, and the Public's Health.* New York: Springer, 1991.
5. Williams, S.J., Tyler, C.W., Clark, L., Coleman, L. & Curran, P. Epidemiologists in the United States: an assessment of the current supply and the anticipated need. *Prev. Med.* 1988; **4**: 231–8.
6. Schoenbach, V.J., Reynolds, G.H. & Kumanyika, S.K. For the committee on minority affairs of the American College of Epidemiology. Racial and ethnic distribution of faculty, students and fellows in US epidemiology degree programs, 1992. *Ann. Epidemiol.* 1994; **4**: 259–65.
7. St George, D.M.M., Schoenbach, V.J. & Reynolds, G.H. *et al.* Recruitment of minority students to US epidemiology degree programs. *Ann. Epidemiol.* 1997; **7**: 304–10.

8. Ben-Shlomo, Y. & Hense, H.-W. *European Epidemiology Federation News Letter.* Spring 2003.

9. Greenberg, R.S. Is epidemiology broken down by race and ethnicity? *Ann. Epidemiol.* 1994; **4**: 337.

10. American College of Epidemiology. Statement of Principles. *Ann. Epidemiol.* 1995; **5**: 505–8.

11. Mandil, A. *IEA Database*, Personal communication, 4 May 2003.

12. Fortney, J.A. Reproductive epidemiologic research in developing countries. *Ann. Epidemiol.* 1990; **1**: 187–94.

13. Taylor, P.R., Dawsey, S. & Albanes, D. Cancer prevention trials in China and Finland. *Ann. Epidemiol.* 1990; **1**: 195–203.

14. Bonita, R. & Beaglehole, R. Cardiovascular disease epidemiology in developing countries: ethics and etiquette. *Lancet* 1994; **344**: 1586–7.

15. Wall, S.G. Epidemiology in developing countries – some experiences from collaboration across disciplines and cultures. *Scand. J. Soc. Med.* 1990; Suppl. **46**: 25–32.

16. Pearce, N., Beasley, R., Crane, J., Burgess, C. & Jackson, R. End of the New Zealand asthma mortality epidemic. *Lancet* 1995; **345**: 41–4.

17. Mitchell, E.A., Brunt, J.M. & Everard, C. Reduction in mortality from SIDS in New Zealand, 1986–92. *Arch. Dis. Child.* 1994; **70**: 291–4.

18. Doll, R. Progress against cancer: an epidemiologic assessment. *Am. J. Epidemiol.* 1991; **134**: 675–88.

19. Berridge, V. Passive smoking and its pre-history in Britain: policy speaks to science? *Soc. Sci. Med.* 1999; **49**: 1183–95.

20. Beaglehole, R. Science, advocacy and public health: lessons from New Zealand's tobacco wars. *J. Pub. Hlth Policy* 1991; **12**: 175–83.

21. Jha, P. & Chaloupka, F. (eds.). *Tobacco Control in Developing Countries*. Oxford; Oxford University Press, 2000.

22. Wing, S. Limits of epidemiology. *Med. Global Survival* 1994; **1**: 74–86.

23. Beaglehole, R. & Yach, D. Globalization and the prevention and control of noncommunicable disease: the neglected chronic diseases of adults. *Lancet* 2003; **362**: 903–8.

24. World Health Organization. *Diet, Nutrition and the Prevention of Chronic Diseases.* Report of a Joint WHO/FAO Expert Consultation. Geneva: WHO Technical Report 916, 2003.

25. Cochrane, A. *Effectiveness and Efficiency*. London: Nuffield Provincial Hospitals Trust, 1972.

26. Godlee, F. The Cochrane Collaboration. *Br. Med. J.* 1994; **309**: 969–70.

27. Cochrane Health Promotion and Public Health Field. http://www.vichealth.viv.gov.au.cochrane/overview/.

28. The Campbell Collaboration. http://www.campbellcollaboration.org/.

29. Liggins, G.C. & Howie, R.N. A controlled trial of antepartum glucocorticoid treatment for prevention of the respiratory distress syndrome in premature infants. *Pediatrics* 1972; **50**: 515–25.

30. The Cochrane Collaboration. *Introductory Brochure*. Oxford, 1993.

31. Yusuf, S. Two decades of progress in preventing vascular disease. *Lancet* 2002; **360**: 2–3.

32. Whincup, P.H., Emberson, J.R., Lennon, L., *et al.* Low prevalence of lipid lowering drug use in older men with established coronary heart disease. *Heart* 2002; **88**: 25–9.
33. Reddy, K.S. & Yusuf, S. Emerging epidemic of cardiovascular disease in developing countries. *Circulation* 1998; **97**: 596–601.
34. Last, J.M. What is clinical epidemiology? *J. Pub. Hlth Policy* 1988; **9**: 159–63.
35. Holland, W. Inappropriate terminology. *Int. J. Epidemiol.* 1983; **12**: 5–7.
36. Terris, M. In: Buck, C., Llopis, A., Napra, E. & Terris, M. (eds.). *The Challenge of Epidemiology: Issues and Selected Readings.* Washington DC: Pan American Health Organization, 1988.
37. Chalmers, I. & Haynes, B. Reporting, updating, and correcting systematic reviews of the effects of health care. *Br. Med. J.* 1994; **309**: 862–5.
38. Navarro, V. The future of public health in health care reform. *Am. J. Pub. Hlth.* 1994; **84**: 729–30.
39. Nijhuis, H.G.J. & Van Der Maesen, L.J.G. The philosophical foundations of public health: an invitation to debate. *J. Epidemiol. Commun. Hlth* 1994; **48**: 1–3.
40. Susser, M. Epidemiology today: 'a thought-tormented world'. *Int. J. Epidemiol.* 1989; **18**: 481–8.
41. McKinlay, J.B. The promotion of health through planned socio-political change: challenges for research and policy. *Soc. Sci. Med.* 1993; **36**: 109–17.
42. Skrabanek, P. Risk-factor epidemiology: science or non-science? In: Berger, P., Browning, R., Anderson, D., Skrabanek, P. & Johnstone, J.R. (eds.). *Health, Lifestyle and Environment: Countering the Panic.* London: Social Affairs Unit, Manhattan Institute, 1991.
43. Skrabanek, P. Has risk-factor epidemiology outlived its usefulness? *Am. J. Epidemiol.* 1993; **138**: 1016.
44. Savitz, D.A. In defense of black box epidemiology. *Epidemiology* 1994; **5**: 550–2.
45. Magnus, P. & Beaglehole, R. The real contribution of the major risk factors to the coronary epidemic: time to end the 50% myth. *Arch. Int. Med.* 2001; **161**: 2657–60.
46. Beaglehole, R. & Magnus, P. The search for new risk factors for coronary heart disease: occupational therapy for epidemiologists? *Int. J. Epidemiol.* 2002; **31**: 1117–21 and 1134–5.
47. McCormick, J. & Skrabanek, P. Coronary heart disease is not preventable by population interventions. *Lancet* 1988; **ii**: 839–41.
48. Pearce, N. The ecological study strikes back. *J. Epidemiol. Commun. Hlth* 2000; **54**: 326–7.
49. Skrabanek, P. The poverty of epidemiology. *Perspect. Biol. Med.* 1992; **35**: 182–5.
50. Skrabanek, P. The epidemiology of errors. *Lancet* 1993; **342**: 1502.
51. Skrabanek, P. The emptiness of the Black Box. *Epidemiology* 1994; **5**: 553–5.
52. Vandenbroucke, J.P. & Pardoel, V.P.A.M. An autopsy of epidemiologic methods: the case of 'poppers' in the early epidemic of the acquired immunodeficiency syndrome (AIDS). *Am. J. Epidemiol.* 1989; **129**: 455–7.
53. Bailar, J.C. When research results are in conflict. *New Engl. J. Med.* 1985; **313**: 1080–1.
54. Writing Group from the Women's Health Initiative Randomized Controlled Trial. Risks and benefits of estrogen plus progestin in healthy postmenopausal women. *J. Am. Med. Assoc.* 2002; **288**: 321–33.

55. Stehbens, W.E. The quality of epidemiological data in coronary heart disease and atherosclerosis. *J. Clin. Epidemiol.* 1993; **46**: 1337–46.
56. Feinstein, A.R. Scientific standards in epidemiologic studies of the menace of daily life. *Science* 1988; **242**: 1257–63.
57. Stebhens, W.E. An appraisal of the epidemic rise of coronary heart disease and its decline. *Lancet* 1987; **i**: 606–11.
58. Gordis, L. Challenges to epidemiology in the next decade. *Am. J. Epidemiol.* 1988; **128**: 1–9.
59. Rothman, K.J. & Greenland, S. Modern Epidemiology. 2nd edn. Philadelphia: Lippincott-Raven, 1998.
60. Krieger, N. Epidemiology and the web of causation: has anyone seen the spider? *Soc. Sci. Med.* 1994; **39**: 887–902.
61. Tesh, S.N. Miasma and 'social factors' in disease causality: lessons from the nineteenth century. *J. Hlth Policy, Policy Law* 1995; **20**: 1001–24.
62. McKinlay, J.B. & Marceau, L.D. A tale of two tails. *Am. J. Pub. Hlth* 1999; **89**: 295.
63. Arnoux, L. & Grace, V. Method and practice of critical epidemiology. In: Spicer, J., Trlin, A. & Walton, J.A. (eds.). *Social Dimensions of Health and Disease: New Zealand Perspectives.* Palmerston North: Dunmore Press, 1994.
64. McKinlay, J.B. & Marceau, L.D. To boldly go . . . . *Am. J. Pub. Hlth* 2000; **90**: 25–33.
65. McMichael, A.J. Prisoners of the proximate: loosening the constraints on epidemiology in an age of change. *Amer. J. Epidemiol.* 1999; **149**: 887–97.
66. Pearce, N. Traditional epidemiology, modern epidemiology, and public health. *Am. J. Pub. Hlth* 1996; **86**: 678–83.
67. Nijhuis, H.G.J. & Van Der Maesen, L.J.G. The philosophical foundations of public health: an invitation to debate. *J. Epidemiol. Commun. Hlth.* ss 1994; **48**: 1–3.
68. Baum, F. Social capital: is it good for your health? Issues for a public health agenda. *J. Epidemiol, Commun. Hlth* 1999; **53**: 195–6.
69. Pearce, N. & Davey Smith, G. Is social capital the key to inequalities in health? *Am. J. Pub. Hlth* 2003; **93**: 122–9.
70. Reich M. Applied policy analysis for health policy reform. *Curr. Iss. Pub. Hlth* 1996; **2**. 186–91.

6

Challenges for epidemiology: historical and contemporary

6.1 Introduction

The central purpose of epidemiology is the study of epidemics so that they might be prevented and controlled. The main challenges facing epidemiology stem from its two concerns: the scale and nature of human health problems and the desire to improve health. In this chapter we identify several challenges which, if met, will allow epidemiology to flourish, and will ensure that worldwide the public's health will receive the full benefit of what epidemiology can offer. This chapter outlines five priority challenges facing epidemiologists.

6.2 Improving basic epidemiological information

As discussed in Chapter 3, there are still major gaps in what is known about the global burden of disease and even less about the global distribution of health. Even the most rudimentary data on the number of deaths are missing for much of the world; for the two most populous nations, China and India, the best data comes from sentinel surveillance sites and this is used to estimate national data[1]. Methods that estimate the total number of deaths occurring globally each year provide an indication of the huge global burden of preventable premature death, as we have seen in Chapter 2. The information on cause of death is even more scanty and, where it does exist, its validity often is not known. Collecting even the most basic data leads to the recognition of shortcomings which, in turn, prompts the need for improved information. At a more general level, methods for measuring health status at a population level are seriously deficient. Recent concern about Creutzfeldt–Jakob disease in Europe has highlighted the failure of epidemiology to monitor the occurrence of bovine spongioform encephalopathy[2]. Addressing these gaps is a central challenge facing epidemiologists.

The only readily available information for monitoring international trends in death and disease is the death data provided to the WHO from comprehensive national vital registration systems, covering about one-third of the world's population. Data on disease incidence and case fatality, which are necessary to understand the reason for mortality trends, are not available routinely. The exceptions are data from cancer registries, which are available from 48 cancer registries for approximately 60 populations in 28 countries[3]. These registries require long-term commitment from official agencies and permissive privacy laws.

Information is lacking for the major cause of death worldwide[4], although a WHO project which *moni*tored the trends and determinants of *ca*rdiovascular disease (WHO MONICA Project) filled the gap for some, mostly European, countries[5–7]. This project under WHO leadership was facilitated by the relative strength of CVD epidemiology; in turn, it has strengthened further the practice of CVD epidemiology and prevention. The Global Burden of Disease (GBD) Project has also highlighted the lack of reliable information on the impact of disease on disability[8]; the basic data necessary for assessing this burden are, for the most part, simply not available although there have been major improvements over the last decade, stimulated by the GBD project[9]. In time, this project may produce reliable trend data in a small number of countries. New international collaborations have recently developed to fill gaps in our understanding of the occurrence of diabetes and asthma.

Measuring the burden of disease has not been a priority for epidemiologists, despite the central importance of this task. It is not a glamorous activity and not likely to result in major peer-reviewed publications. It is tedious and time consuming and many agencies decline responsibility for its funding. Health research institutions believe it to be a governmental responsibility, and governments in turn accord it a low priority. Furthermore, epidemiologists have not developed methods suitable for the widespread assessment of morbidity. Reliance has been placed on laborious and expensive methods that are barely suitable for ongoing use even in wealthy countries, let alone for countries with limited expertise, fewer resources and almost no appropriately trained workforce. The WHO Global Burden of Diseases Project has refocused attention on the importance of this activity and has stimulated many national GBD projects, for example, in New Zealand and Australia[10]. Globally, and in some countries, this has had a beneficial impact on health policy by underscoring the importance of neglected major diseases.

The challenge is to develop and implement cost-effective methods of monitoring the global burden of disease and the major risk factors. Traditional methods, involving disease registers and community surveys, are too expensive and cumbersome to be generally applicable. New methods, such as the capture–recapture method offer more promise[11], but require evaluation and testing, especially in poor countries. Information from sentinel sites could be aggregated easily using modern telecommunication networks. WHO has developed and implemented a simple standardised and step-wise approach to the collection of data on the major risk factors for chronic disease and this approach is providing useful information already for policy purposes by drawing attention to the high levels of risk factors in many poorer countries[12]. There is also scope for low-cost, but high-powered, modern information technologies for monitoring purposes[13]. This type of epidemiological action is not glamorous but should be supported more actively and encouraged by international health agencies and donors, even though it requires long-term funding.

6.3 Causal inference

There are two aspects to the challenge of determining whether an observed association is likely to be a causal relationship. The first is the need to increase knowledge of causal mechanisms and pathways, focusing especially on the social origins of disease. Much of contemporary epidemiology is guided by the principle that the origins of disease are due to gene–environmental interactions. This 'black box' approach to epidemiology emphasises exposure–disease associations and the idea that disease can be prevented by altering the environment without detailed knowledge of mechanisms[14]. The contributions of this approach have been enormous; one of the best examples is the way smoking was identified as a cause of cancer in the absence of knowledge of mechanisms. Advocates of this approach suggest that a commitment to the search for mechanisms will divert attention from the search for causes. Some commentators encourage an exploration of the 'black box' of mechanisms so as to avoid epidemiology being swept away, like the miasmists in the twentieth century[15]. This approach fails to acknowledge the history of epidemiology. Indeed, the miasma and the contagion theories are still with us, although neither is in its nineteenth-century form. Although the contagious and the environmental approaches are converging, neither approach adequately describes the origin of disease.

A more comprehensive understanding of causal pathways is necessary. For example, although much is known about the causes of coronary heart disease from the level of individual risk factors to the cellular mechanisms in the arterial wall, the huge population differences in risk factor levels are not well understood[6]. The process of causal inference runs the danger of adopting a

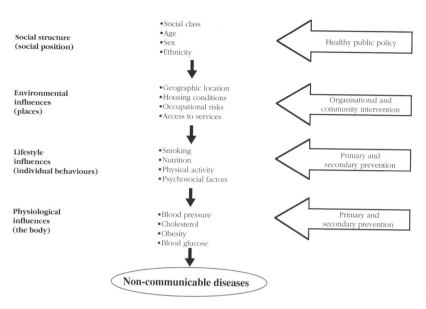

Fig. 6.1. Levels of causation.

narrow individualistic focus, and ignoring the social, economic and political contributions to the cardiovascular disease epidemic, the so-called upstream determinants which are outside the control of individuals (Fig. 6.1)[16].

The challenge for epidemiology is to develop sophisticated theories of disease causation that acknowledge the complex social, environmental and economic systems in which the health–disease process is embedded. Various attempts have been made to outline these relationships[17–20], but they are all largely schematic and, as yet, of unproven utility. These multi-level models – or Chinese boxes[20] – emphasise the importance of research, which places individuals firmly in the context of their social, economic and physical environment. This broad perspective is essential for a fuller understanding of the pathways to health and disease and thus an optimal approach to health improvement.

The second aspect of this challenge is to deepen understanding of the health transition and the reasons for changing mortality patterns. Although this transition has been known to epidemiologists and demographers for a long time, efforts to understand the relative roles of contributory factors are rudimentary, as discussed in Chapter 1. Three components of the health transition are described but their relative importance is only guessed at, and our ability to predict the evolution of the ongoing transition is limited. We cannot, for example, be sure as to what will happen to the major non-communicable diseases in poor countries if the transition progresses. The relative contribution of public health and individual medical care to the health transition requires further research.

6.4 Global problems require global solutions

Observers of epidemiology could be excused for thinking that epidemiologists are concerned increasingly with rediscovering and reinforcing the known. The availability of large public domain data sets, the career importance of publications, and the time pressure for producing dissertations, have all encouraged the repetition of safe (and sometimes boring) epidemiological studies[21] . By contrast, the big public health problems have been neglected; the health effects of war, poverty, and global environmental change, have not received the attention they, and the public, deserve.

The potential problems posed by a changing environment have reached the epidemiological agenda now[22–24]. The problems of war and poverty, although long on the public health agenda, are not a major concern of epidemiologists, most of whom are based in urban centres in wealthy countries (World Violence Report)[25]. The impact of urbanisation and development on the health transition in poor countries is of critical importance for determining the future global burden of disease. Yet, this topic also remains neglected. It is easier to receive research funds to investigate the role of lipoprotein fractions in heart disease, than to explore the burden of disease in poor countries. Epidemiologists must overcome their parochialism and recognise the importance to global health of the disease problems of the poor world[26].

In part, progress has been slow because of the difficulties in studying the health effects of widespread changes at a global level, for example the effect of World Trade Organization Multilateral Trade Agreements on health and health services in poor countries[27]. New methods and techniques are required as well as new approaches to causal inference, given the complete lack of experimental data, the complex relationships involved and the long time delay between cause and effect. This is a qualitatively different research challenge from ones faced in the past[28]. The emphasis will need to be on prediction rather than estimation and on model building that incorporates other biological data as well as extrapolation from limited empirical data.

More general factors have operated to discourage epidemiologists from dealing with the new global big health problems, most of which are social and economic in origin. The main sources of funding for epidemiological studies are governmental or voluntary agencies, which are most supportive of safe and uncontroversial studies of individual risk factors. In turn, this has led to epidemiologists concentrating on research areas that are likely to be funded and which avoid 'political' issues. Furthermore, the study of the big health problems presents enormous difficulties which are outside the traditional skills and techniques of traditional epidemiology and require close collaboration with a range of other disciplines. Most of the new funds for global health have been established to respond to priority health problems, for example, HIV/AIDS, malaria and vaccine preventable diseases of childhood[29]. This is an understandable approach and is attractive to donors and it may produce short-term gains. It is also important to respond to the other complex social, economic and civil causes of immediate health problems and to the long-term – and potentially even more devastating – problems.

The long-term solution to the neglect of the global public health problems is a re-orientation of epidemiology. The big problems will begin to receive the necessary attention when epidemiology returns to being a problem-solving discipline, as it was 150 years ago. Noteworthy attempts have been made to deal with the broad health effects of underdevelopment at a population level, not through public health programmes, but by changing the dominant social, economic and political systems, for example, in Nicaragua and Chile[30, 31].

The global problems in turn will require the development of new theories, methods and techniques, and not just data; existing study designs are unhelpful when studying, for example, the effects of global warming. Epidemiologists will need to become familiar with, and skilled in, the creative use of new information technologies in the context of a collaborative and inclusive vision of public health in an electronic world[32]. There are useful lessons from the recent development of epidemiology in Latin America, where it has become closely integrated with public health practice and has responded to the need to research the socio-economic determinants of health[33]. A global agenda for research in epidemiology and public health might help refocus the attention of epidemiologists[34].

6.5 Linking epidemiology and public policy

There are several aspects to the challenge of forging closer links between epidemiology and policy formation.

6.5.1 Building links with policy makers

A most important challenge facing epidemiologists is to develop and strengthen the tenuous link between epidemiological findings and their application. For the last 150 years the justification for epidemiology has been its close connection with public health policy. Epidemiological findings on the causes and prevention of disease always have implications for health policy and public policy more generally. Unfortunately, these implications are not always acted upon, with the majority of research attention being at the individual level to the neglect of the policy and programmatic requirements of research findings[35].

There are many fine examples of epidemiological results having policy impact, from fluoridation of water supplies – despite the weakness of the evidence[36] and seat belt legislation, to the withdrawal of potentially dangerous pharmaceuticals. There is a vast amount of sound epidemiological information, however, which has not been translated into appropriate policy, and neglected or misinterpreted data abound. Many of the issues studied by epidemiologists are also of great importance to a range of powerful vested interest groups, for example, the tobacco and food and alcohol industries[37]. Perhaps the most striking indictment of the failure to implement epidemiological data is the continuing inaction to prevent the global spread of the tobacco epidemic; the projections of the burden of disease caused by tobacco have done little to halt the spread of this epidemic[38, 39]. Other examples include encouragement of mammographic screening for women under the age of 50 years, despite the evidence showing that it is probably ineffective in reducing the death rate from breast cancer in younger women[40]; the failure to prevent the global spread of HIV infection despite a decade's knowledge of the means by which the infection is spread; the almost total reliance on the high risk strategy, for example for cardiovascular disease prevention; and the general failure to capitalise on the power of the population strategy for prevention[35].

There are many reasons for the lack of influence of epidemiology on policy. Many epidemiologists, especially those based in academic institutions, are remote from policy decisions and are not equipped to analyse the policy making process. Some epidemiologists believe in 'pure science'; others believe that their work is 'value free' and should be kept separate from the explicit values of policy. The epidemiological time frame for action is slow and epidemiologists tend to be cautious and pedantic. Yet policy makers often require information at short notice. Epidemiological results are often couched in careful, but ambiguous, terms and sometimes conflicting results emerge which generate debate and confusion and often the media trivialises the epidemiological debates. If epidemiologists cannot agree on the meaning of conflicting results, it is easy to see why policy makers will ignore calls for action.

For some epidemiologists remoteness from policy is not an accident, but a conscious choice. There is a view that the science and its policy application should be kept separate, in the interests of maintaining scientific integrity.

The editor of the journal *Epidemiology*, for example, discourages authors from linking policy implications with their research finding on the basis that brief discussions of policy, usually at the end of the discussion section of articles, are likely to be facile[41]. This editorial approach which distances epidemiology from its social and policy context is particularly strong in the United States of America and encourages the separation of science from policy . In this view, the only policy role of epidemiologists is as private citizens[42,43]. If epidemiology serves only to study the occurrence of disease and is not involved in prevention and control, this position is understandable. In our view, epidemiologists have an obligation to discuss policy implications which are, after all, the main justification for epidemiology.

The process of influencing health policy and, more generally, public policy, is extraordinarily complex. Epidemiologists are only one rather small group of actors in the process of policy making which balances competing risks and benefits. By informing policy decisions, epidemiology can contribute directly to provide the necessary information to assist in this process, thereby ensuring an improvement in the public's health. Also involved in the policy making process are other scientists, bureaucrats, various professional groups, politicians, and powerful commercial vested interest groups. For many issues, it is only recently that the process of causal inference has become sufficiently developed by epidemiologists for a hypothesis to be supported with enough strength to justify action. Additional reasons for policy ineffectiveness are related closely to several of the other challenges including the isolation of epidemiology from communities, and our inability to develop a comprehensive understanding of the causes of disease and of the importance of the political process in policy making.

As with all the challenges to epidemiology, the solution is neither simple nor straightforward. In the first instance, it is necessary for epidemiology to affirm its connection with policy and to reject scientific isolation and value free objectivity[16]. More coherent policy advice will arise if epidemiologists work more closely with other social scientists. The policy-making process itself requires greater scientific scrutiny. Secondly, epidemiologists and policy makers, irrespective of their background, institutional location or political affiliation, need to establish close links. These links can be based on formal contractual relations or on informal networks. Thirdly, epidemiologists must be exposed in training and in practice to the complexity of policy making. Fourthly, the editorial and peer-review process must focus not only on the scientific merit of a paper, but should also encourage discussion of policy implications as is now undertaken, for example, in the *British Medical Journal*. Epidemiological data inevitably illuminates policy options and these should be discussed. Fifthly, grant funding agencies should consider, as one of their criteria, evidence of prior discussions with potential users of the results of the proposed study.

6.5.2 Communicating risk

The process of communicating quantitative estimates of disease risks to the public and policy makers is a serious challenge facing epidemiologists[44] and is closely related to the more general challenge of linking epidemiology to public health[9]. A central task of epidemiologists is the measurement of the strength of observed associations. Various measures of risk are used: relative risk to assess the strength of a relationship; risk differences to measure the impact of the risk factor; and measures of attributable risk to assess the importance of the risk factor from a population perspective.

Almost daily new risks, or 'menaces to daily life', based on epidemiological studies are presented to the public by the media. The proliferation of so-called 'health information' allows fatalists to shrug their shoulders and say 'well, what's the point, everything is dangerous', and epidemiology is mocked. Recent examples of small increased relative risks which received media publicity include: passive smoking and heart disease; margarine (*trans*-fatty acids) and heart disease; iron and heart disease; abortion and breast cancer; smoking and breast cancer; hormone replacement therapy and prevention of heart disease; low dose oral contraceptives and pulmonary embolism; and beef eating and the risk of Creutzfeldt–Jakob disease.

Epidemiological findings can be powerful enough to cause epidemics[45]. For example, in 1986, a cancer agency conducted a study of cancer incidence in two suburbs of Edmonton, Alberta, and reported publicly an increase of about 25% over the expected occurrence for most sites of cancer[46]. Residents in these communities had been concerned for several years about an apparently elevated rate of cancer among adults because of the presence nearby of oil refineries and petrochemical factories. Re-analysis of the data several months later revealed an error and correction brought the rates into line with Alberta as a whole. A survey of residents, after realisation of the mistake and before its public correction, studied the response of the communities. The perception of any elevated cancer risk, in the absence of a true risk, had negative effect on the communities, both psychologically and economically.

Another example demonstrates that the way in which data from randomised trials are presented significantly influences health policy decisions[47]. For example, the willingness to fund a mammography screening programme (see Box 6.1) was far greater when results of a trial were presented as a relative risk reduction (A) compared with other methods: absolute risk reduction (B), proportion of event free patients (C), or as the number of patients needed to be treated to prevent an adverse event (D).

Box 6.1   Different, but equal, ways of communicating risk[47].

The following four statements based on the results of a randomised controlled trial of mammographic screening [48] are equivalent. Over a 7-year follow-up period:

- the **rate** of deaths from breast cancer was reduced by 34%
- the **absolute reduction** in deaths from breast cancer was 0.06%
- the **survival rate** of patients with breast cancer was increased from 99.82 to 99.88%
- 1592 women **needed to be screened** over 7 years **to prevent one death** from breast cancer.

When relative risk estimates are high, communication is easier, but still not necessarily effective. For example, the relative risk of lung cancer for a cigarette smoker after 20 years of heavy smoking compared with a non-smoker is about 20; that is, the heavy smoker has a 20-fold increased risk of developing lung cancer. In epidemiological terms, this is a very strong relative risk and most people are aware of this risk, even smokers. Of course, not every heavy smoker develops lung cancer and the risk is not instantaneous. Young people, in particular, are more concerned with immediate social and peer pressures than with long-term risks; and all smokers can point to a healthy heavily smoking octogenarian. Other high relative risks are found with exposure to asbestos in association with smoking, and with some drugs, for example thalidomide in pregnancy.

Most relative risks are an order of magnitude lower, around two, and increasingly, epidemiologists struggle with the meaning of relative risks in the range 1.1 to 1.5. The lower the estimate of risk, the more likely it is due to bias in the design or conduct of the study, especially if it has been found in only a single study. Although epidemiologists may order their lives on the basis of quantitative results (less animal fat, more or less alcohol, more exercise), most people are more fatalistic, especially young people with limited social and economic prospects.

The challenge of communicating notions of risk to policy makers and, even more importantly, to the public, has yet to be contemplated seriously[9]. The old messages of gloom and doom, so beloved by health educationalists, which might be effective for small segments of the population, do not impact on the great majority of the population. In fact, this type of message contributes to the growing social inequalities in health status within populations. All epidemiological studies require independent scientific scrutiny and the journal peer-review process is not always adequate for this purpose. It is imperative that epidemiologists, peer reviewers and journal editors appreciate the limitations of the data and ensure that the results are presented in a balanced manner, even at the risk of missing media attention. Doll and Hill, in their pioneering studies of smoking and lung cancer, set a fine example. When their first study produced an unexpected result (after all, they were also interested in the health effects of pollution), further studies were planned which confirmed their original findings. In general, less rush to publication and more discussion and thought will improve communication with the public.

Much more work is required to ensure that epidemiological risks are translated into terms and images that can be readily understood. This is one prerequisite for influencing behaviour. Simple quantitative and probabilistic statements mean little; for example, 'passive smokers have an increased risk of cancer of 30%', oversimplifies a complex epidemiological issue. Statements such as 'each cigarette smoked reduces life expectancy by 5 minutes' may carry more weight, but this type of message requires testing with smokers of different ages and sex. From a public health perspective, population attributable risk is more important than relative risk; and from a clinical perspective, absolute risk is more important for treatment guidelines[49,50]. Once the epidemiological data are firm, creativity is required in communicating the appropriate messages in a meaningful manner so that all segments of society benefit.

6.5.3 Overcoming isolation

The isolation of epidemiology from other sciences, public health practitioners, policy makers and the public, limits the ability of epidemiologists to influence policy. There are several aspects to the isolation of epidemiology. Although epidemiologists have usually worked closely with biostatisticians (often out of necessity), collaboration with other public health disciplines such as social scientists, health economists, laboratory-based scientists and clinicians has been less obvious. Partnership and collaboration with the public is critical – putting the public back into public health.

Part of the problem arises from the separation (or 'schism') between epidemiology and clinical medicine, as in the United States of America, where separate schools of public health were developed in the first half of the last century, often with the support of the Rockefeller Foundation[51]. This separation is also important in countries that have not developed separate public health institutions. For example, even where epidemiology has been located primarily within schools of medicine, as in the United Kingdom, there has been a separation of epidemiology from clinical and laboratory-based disciplines.

There is much to be gained from collaboration between epidemiologists with other biological scientists. Findings which may not make biological sense initially may lead to real advances in knowledge. Biological implausibility, however, should alert us to the possibility that epidemiological results have other, more mundane, explanations related to insufficient adherence to basic scientific principles. The distance from biology may be one explanation why distinguished statisticians such as Fisher took a negative position, from a purely statistical viewpoint, on the relationship of smoking to lung cancer[52]. Equally important is the isolation of epidemiology from the full range of social science methods including the political sciences. As a consequence, much of the policy recommendations coming from epidemiology have been one dimensional.

It will not be easy to overcome the isolation of epidemiology from other scientific disciplines. A reorientation and integration of epidemiology teaching with other public health disciplines has enormous potential. Exposure to a broad range of public health disciplines should be mandatory for epidemiology students.

The remedy for the separation of epidemiology from clinical medicine was the development of clinical epidemiology. Clinical epidemiology has taken off in some institutions in wealthy countries, for example, at McMaster University in Canada and at the University of Newcastle in New South Wales, Australia. The International Clinical Epidemiology Network was relatively successful in strengthening clinical expertise in some clinical groups in several poor countries [53,54] but was much less successful in supporting the academic public health workforce. Clinical epidemiology, as its name implies, is more important for clinical medicine than for public health and has yet to make major contributions to the development of public health or health policy.

Another aspect of isolation is the separation of academic epidemiology from public health practitioners, especially from members of local and central departments of health. A special manifestation of epidemiological isolation, all too common in the United States of America, is the analysis, often by graduate students, of data gathered by someone else. The epidemiological analysis often proceeds in ignorance of the true nature of the data and with a lack of

understanding of its strengths and weaknesses. Making connections with public health practitioners to ensure an involvement with public health policy is
essential for all graduate students.

An important and fundamental aspect of the isolation of epidemiologists
is that epidemiology is all too often divorced from the public it serves[55,56].
Only rarely are epidemiological studies designed in close collaboration with
representatives of the public. The word 'epidemiology' gives full weight to
'the people' (*demos*). The involvement of the public in epidemiological studies
encourages a greater understanding of disease occurrence and is important for
a well-rounded approach. This involvement is essential, given the paramount
importance of social factors in disease. In addition, this approach will facilitate
disease prevention because it is based on the experience of people in their own
social and economic environments. For example, participatory epidemiology
(or 'popular' epidemiology) has developed around the work of toxic waste activists[57]. These activists have created a social movement and have helped to
broaden the overall environmental movement. Most often, however, epidemiologists consider the people they study as their 'subjects' or 'patients', though
there is now a move to relabel them as 'participants'. Although the labels may
have changed, the nature of the relationship is unchanged.

The participation of lay people in popular epidemiology, and public health
programmes generally, is difficult because of differing conceptions of risk, lack
of resources, poor access to information, and unresponsive public health bureaucrats and scientists[58]. Slowly environmental epidemiologists and other public
health professionals are recognising and responding to the special challenges of
working closely with lay people and their communities[59]. The great attraction of
such participation is that it may expand traditional epidemiological approaches
to include social and economic factors as part of the causal pathways as well
as facilitating the use of the data.

6.5.4 Achieving breadth and depth

Modern epidemiology is becoming concerned increasingly with technique[26].
This trend runs the risk of divorcing epidemiology from biology and society,
giving rise to criticism that it lacks depth and breadth thereby limiting its relevance to public health[60].

The challenge of increasing the breadth and depth of epidemiology is related
to the need to overcome isolation, and it goes beyond the breaking down of
barriers. The value of an epidemiological study depends on the hypothesis
under investigation which, in turn, requires well-developed epidemiological
theories of the social dynamics of health and disease. Epidemiology, however,

is much more than a set of designs and methods. Unfortunately, undue attention in epidemiological teaching is focused on hypothesis testing to the neglect of explicit theories.

The implicit theory underlying most epidemiology is 'biomedical individualism'[61]. While in practice this involves the exploration of the biological determinants of disease amenable to medical care, it too often ignores the social determinants of disease, and treats populations as the sum of individuals. More attention needs to be directed to the creation of productive and illuminating hypotheses. Much can be learnt from historical examples, such as the hypotheses concerning scurvy, pellagra, retrolental fibroplasia, the nineteenth-century debate on the relationship of poverty and disease, and more recently from HIV/AIDS[62].

A good example of the limitation of a narrowly focused epidemiology is the continuing neglect of the striking impact of social class on the incidence of disease[63]. Another example is the ongoing concern for identifying the causes of disease in individuals to the neglect of the causes of a population's health status. Stressing public health as a prime value will ensure that research is placed in its social context[64]. Multi-disciplinary collaboration, firmly grounded in biology, will help develop a creative epidemiology that is purposeful and focused on the need to prevent and control epidemics. This will also involve greater concentration on the multiple health outcomes of environmental determinants, rather than working backwards from a single disease to its multiple causes. From this perspective, cohort studies are the preferred study design as each case control study can investigate only one outcome.

Creative approaches are also required to ensure that new diseases are investigated efficiently, irrespective of their origin, utilising a full range of techniques. Although not the focus of this book, much more creative epidemiology is also required in measuring the effectiveness and efficiency of health services. Without this creativity, epidemiology will surely become a 'lost cause'.

6.6 The ethical challenge

The final challenge is to ensure that epidemiology reaches and maintains a high ethical standard[65]. The Helsinki Declaration requires that biomedical research with humans must conform to accepted scientific principles; it must be truthful, honest, impartial and objective[66]. Only in the last few years have epidemiologists seriously considered the ethical implications of their work[67]. Epidemiologists, along with all other biomedical scientists, must strive to up hold the four basic principles of biomedical ethics: autonomy, the respect for human rights,

dignity and freedom; non-maleficence, the principle of not harming; beneficence, the principle of doing good; and justice, the principle concerned with
equity, fairness and truth telling.

Epidemiologists come into conflict with the principles of autonomy and
non-maleficence when dealing with the privacy of personal information stored
in health records. The protection of personal privacy is, of course, a laudable
aim. There is a conflict between this right and the need for research which
is in the interest of the 'public good'. Epidemiologists require access to this
type of information because, ultimately, it is in the public interest to use this
information to identify new knowledge about the causes of many diseases; strict
confidentiality rules must be observed.

By contrast with the potential restriction on epidemiological data, is the
much greater freedom allowed journalists[68]. It is a poor reflection on societal
values that we are willing to accept journalists' right to invade privacy, but not
prepared to protect epidemiological research, which is much more in the public
interest and less likely to do harm to individuals[69]. There are, in addition, other
national threats to epidemiological research. In Germany, for instance, access
to death certificates and post-mortem reports for research purposes has long
been prohibited and psychiatric registers have been closed in both Norway and
Germany[68].

A European Union directive on the confidentiality of data balances the rights
to privacy with the needs of epidemiological research[70]. This emerged only
after an extensive exchange of view points and facts between epidemiologists
and legislators. In its original proposal it would have prohibited record linkage
studies using existing data sets on the basis that they were unethical[71]; stipulated
how long data could be kept; required written consent before data could be
processed; required that the subject of the data should be told about disclosure
of data to a third party; and made provision for the subject's right of access to
the data. These requirements would have prohibited observational studies using
historical data, for example the studies of Barker and colleagues on the prenatal
origins of non-communicable diseases[72]. The original European proposal was
potentially so restrictive because it aimed to ensure high and uniform levels of
protection.

So far epidemiology has not had to contend with large-scale fraudulent
investigations, although questions have been raised about some data contributed
to multi-centre studies of the management of breast cancer in North America[73].
There is an increasing tendency for epidemiological studies to be sponsored
by agencies with a direct interest in the association under study. The tobacco
industry is notorious in this regard, although it now channels research funds
through 'independent' trusts. The pharmaceutical industry is now one of the

major funders of drug evaluation trials. This type of funding poses enormous ethical problems for epidemiology.

Epidemiological studies in poor countries present particular ethical problems[65]. Western models of science are not accepted universally and epidemiologists working in poor countries may be alienated from the populations studied[74]. Poverty and helplessness is a striking feature of many communities, and not just in the poor world. If communities do not perceive the benefits of epidemiological studies, participation will be low and the community may feel exploited. Randomised controlled trials in poor communities entail additional ethical problems if local health services are poorly organised and health budgets are inadequate to ensure that the local population receives the benefits of the intervention, assuming that it was shown to be effective. Difficult ethical issues arise when trials do not use the best available regimes in the control arm, even if this best therapy is unlikely to be available in the host country[65]. Recently attention has also been given to the particular ethics of epidemiology of women's health[75]. For example, the United States Food and Drug Administration in 1993 lifted its ban on including women of child-bearing age in early drug trials because of the scientific benefits of their inclusion[76].

The solution to this ethical challenge will depend on how epidemiologists meet the previous challenges. If epidemiology can establish a sound and socially responsible theoretical base and communicate more easily with the public and policy makers, it will be in a more secure position. If, at the same time, epidemiologists accept and adhere to the guidelines proposed by the Council of International Organisations of Medical Sciences (CIOMS), the discipline will rest on a firmer ethical base[77]. Specific guidelines are also required on funding, especially of consultancies, to avoid conflicts of interest. Epidemiologists must not become beholden to vested interests. Researchers sponsored by industry should insist that they retain the right of unrestricted publication. It is likely that many such studies have been censored by the sponsoring industry, although the extent of this problem is unknown[78]. There is a pressing need for more formal ethics curricula in epidemiological teaching programmes especially in poor countries[65,79].

The issue of advocacy in epidemiology raises important ethical issues. Various ethical guidelines endorse the role of advocate, although the recommendations differ[80]. The guidelines of the International Epidemiological Association recommend separating the roles of scientists and advocates. The CIOMS guidelines recommend advocacy dependent on the quality of epidemiological research and on causal interpretations of the data. The ethical principle of beneficence supports the advocacy role. Advocacy becomes a central obligation when epidemiologists accept a commitment to disease prevention and control; unfortunately, this commitment is not universal[81].

6.7 Conclusions

If epidemiology rises to these five key challenges, its healthy development will be assured. If, on the other hand, it ignores the challenges, its future will be bleak, with epidemiologists increasingly confined to clinical epidemiology and health services research.

A flourishing discipline of epidemiology will conform to the following principles: it will be interconnected closely with the population being studied; it will be informed and guided by a theory which integrates the historical, social and economic determinants of health and disease in populations; and it will address the health problems of all groups in both the rich and poor worlds. A socially responsible epidemiology will be closely connected with public health practice at local, national and global levels. If these conditions are met, comprehensive solutions will emerge and be implemented to respond to the major health problems.

Chapter 6   Key points

The major challenges facing epidemiology are:

- to improve basic epidemiological information;
- to refine causal mechanisms and pathways and clarify the process of causal inference, focusing especially on the social origins of disease;
- to study and confront the health effects of war, poverty and global environmental change;
- to develop and strengthen the links between epidemiological findings and their application in public policy; and
- to ensure that epidemiology reaches and maintains a high ethical standard.

References

1. Lopez, A.D. Counting the dead in China: measuring tobacco's impact in the developing world. *Br. Med. J.* 1998; **317**: 1399–40.
2. Gore, S.M. Bovine Creutzfeldt–Jakob disease? Failures of epidemiology must be remedied. *Br. Med. J.* 1996; **312**: 791–3.

3. Coleman, M.P., Esteve, J., Damiecki, P., Arslan, A. & Renard, H. *Trends in Cancer Incidence and Mortality.* Lyon: World Health Organization International Agency for Research on Cancer, 1993.

4. Reddy, K.S. & Yusuf, S. Emerging epidemic cardiovascular disease in developing countries. *Circulation* 1998; **97**: 596–601.

5. Kuulasmaa, K., Dobson, A., Tunstall-Pedoe, H. *et al.* Estimation of the contribution of changes in risk factors to trends in coronary event rates across the WHO MONICA Project populations. *Lancet* 2000; **355**: 675–87.

6. Tunstall-Pedoe, H., Vanuzzo, D., Hobbs, M. *et al.* Estimation of contribution of changes in coronary care and coronary heart disease mortality across the WHO Monica Project populations. *Lancet* 2000; **355**: 688–700.

7. *WHO MONICA Monograph and Multimedia Sourcebook.* World's largest study of heart disease, stroke, risk factors, and population trends 1979–2002. Edited by Hugh Tunstall-Pedoe for the WHO MONICA Project.

8. Murray, C.J.L., Lopez, A.L. & Jamison, D. The global burden of disease in 1990: summary results, sensitivity analysis and future directions. *Bull. WHO* 1994; **72**: 495–509.

9. World Health Organization. *World Health Report 2002. Reducing Risks, Promoting Healthy Life.* Geneva: World Health Organization, 2002.

10. Mathers, C.D., Vos, T. & Stevenson, C. *The Burden of Disease and Injury in Australia.* Canberra: Australian Institute of Health and Welfare, 1999.

11. Laporte, R.E. How to improve monitoring and forecasting of disease patterns. *Br. Med. J.* 1993; **307**: 1573–4.

12. Armstrong, T. & Bonita, R. Capacity building for an integrated noncommunicable disease risk factor surveillance system in developing countries. *Ethnicity Dis.* 2003; **13**: (S2–S13).

13. LaPorte, R.E., Akazawa, S., Hellmonds, P. *et al.* Global public health and the information superhighway. *Br. Med. J.* 1994; **308**: 1651–2.

14. Loomis, D. & Wing, S. Is molecular epidemiology a germ theory for the end of the twentieth century? *Int. J. Epidemiol.* 1990; **19**: 1–3.

15. Vandenbroucke, J.P. Epidemiology in transition: a historical hypothesis. *Epidemiology* 1990; **1**: 164–7.

16. McKinlay, J.B. & Marceau, L.D. A tale of two tails. *Am. J. Pub. Hlth* 1999; **89**: 295.

17. Mosley, W.H. & Chen, L.C. An analytical framework for the study of child survival in developing countries. *Pop. Dev. Rev.* 1984; **10** (Suppl.):25–45.

18. Evans, R.G. & Stoddart, G.L. Producing health, consuming health care. *Soc. Sci. Med.* 1990; **31**: 1347–63.

19. Beaglehole, R. Conceptual frameworks for the investigation of mortality from major cardiovascular diseases. In: Lopez, A., Caselli, G. & Valkonen, T. (eds.). *Adult Mortality in Developed Countries: From Description to Explanation.* Oxford: Oxford University Press, 1995.

20. Susser, M. & Susser, E. Choosing a future for epidemiology: II. From black box to chinese boxes and eco-epidemiology. *Am. J. Pub. Hlth* 1996; **86**: 674–77.

21. Beaglehole, R. & Magnus, P. The search for new risk factors for coronary heart disease: occupational therapy for epidemiologists? *Int. J. Epidemiol.* 2002; **31**: 1117–21 and 1134–5.

22. Haines, A., Epstein, P.R. & McMichael, A.J. On behalf of an international panel. Global health watch: monitoring impacts of environmental change. *Lancet* 1993; **342**: 1464–9.

23. McMichael, A.J. *Human Frontiers, Environments and Disease*. Cambridge: Cambridge University Press, 2001.

24. McMichael, A.J. Population, environment, disease, and survival: past patterns, uncertain futures. *Lancet* 2002; **359**: 114.

25. World Health Organization. *World Violence Report*. Geneva: World Health Organization, 2002.

26. Pearce, N. The globalization of epidemiology. *Int. J. Epidemiol.* in press.

27. World Health Organization/World Trade Organization. *WTO Agreements and Public Health. A joint study by the WHO and the WTO Secretariat*. Geneva: World Health Organization/World Trade Organization, 2002.

28. McMichael, A.J. *Planetary Overload. Global Environmental Change and the Health of Human Species*. Cambridge: Cambridge University Press, 1993.

29. Brugha, R., Starling, M. & Walt, G. GAVI, the first steps: lessons for the Global Fund. *Lancet* 2002; **359**: 435–8.

30. Waitzkin, H., Iriart, C., Estrada, A. & Lamadrid, S. Social medicine in Latin America: productivity and dangers facing the major national groups. *Lancet* 2001; **358**: 315–23.

31. Wing, S. Limits of epidemiology. *Med. Global Survival* 1994; **1**: 74–86.

32. Milio, N. Beyond informatics: an electronic community infrastructure for public health. *J. Pub. Hlth Man. Pract.* 1995; **1**: 84–94.

33. World Health Organization. Ad Hoc Committee on Health Research Relating to Future Intervention Options. *Investing in Health Research and Development* Geneva: WHO, 1996.

34. Baretto, M. The globalization of epidemiology: critical thoughts from Latin America. *Int. J. Epidemiol.* in press.

35. Beaglehole, R. Global cardiovascular disease prevention: time to get serious. *Lancet* 2001; **358**: 661–3.

36. McDonagh, M., Whiting, P.F., Wilson, P.M. *et al.* Systematic review of water fluoridation. *Br. Med. J.* 2000; **321**: 855–9.

37. Beaglehole, R. & Yach, D. Globalization and the prevention and control of noncommunicable disease: the neglected chronic diseases of adults. *Lancet* 2003; **362**: 903–8.

38. Jha, P. & Chaloupka, F. (eds.). *Tobacco Control in Developing Countries*. Oxford: Oxford University Press, 2000.

39. Peto, R., Lopez, A.D., Boreham, J. & Thun, M. *Mortality from Smoking in Developed Countries 1950–2000*, 2nd Edn. Data updated 15 July 2003. www.ctsu.ox.ac.uk.

40. Horton, R. Screening mammography – an overview revisited. *Lancet* 2001; **358**: 1284–5.

41. Rothman, K.J. Policy recommendations in epidemiology research papers. *Epidemiology* 1993; **4**: 94–5.

42. Macdonald, S.C. Authors should be expected to elucidate policy implications of empirical data. *Epidemiology* 1993; **4**: 557–8.

43. Rothman, K.J. & Poole, C. Science and policy making. *Am. J. Pub. Hlth* 1985; **75**: 340–1.

44. Bennett, P. & Calman, K. (eds.). *Risk Communication and Public Health*. Oxford: Oxford University Press, 1999.

45. Anon. Do epidemiologists cause epidemics? *Lancet* 1993; **341**: 993–4.

46. Guidotti, T.L. & Jacobs, P. The implications of an epidemiological mistake: a community's response to a perceived excess cancer risk. *Am. J. Pub. Hlth* 1993; **83**: 233–9.

47. Fahey, T., Griffiths, S. & Peters, T.J. Evidence based purchasing: understanding results of clinical trials and systematic reviews. *Br. Med. J.* 1995; **311**: 1056–60.

48. Tabar, L., Fagerberg, G., Gad, A. *et al.* Reductions in mortality from breast cancer after mass screening with mammography. *Lancet* 1985; **i**: 829–32.

49. Jackson, R. Updated New Zealand cardiovascular disease risk–benefit prediction guide. *Br. Med. J.* 2000; **320**: 709–10.

50. Jackson, R. Guidelines on preventing cardiovascular disease in clinical practice. *Br. Med. J.* 2000; **320**: 659–61.

51. White, K.L. *Healing the Schism. Epidemiology, Medicine, and the Public's Health*. New York: Springer, 1991.

52. Stolley, P.D. When genius errs: RA Fisher and the lung cancer controversy. *Am. J. Epidemiol.* 1991; **133**: 16–25.

53. Editorial. The hidden epidemic of cardiovascular disease. *Lancet* 1998; **352**: 1795.

54. Macfarlane, S.B.J., Evans, T., Muli-Musiime, F. *et al.* Global health research and INCLEN. *Lancet* 1999; **353**: 502.

55. Macfarlane, S., Racelis, M. & Muli-Musiime, F. Public health in developing countries. *Lancet* 2000; **356**: 841–6.

56. Raeburn, J. & Macfarlane, S. Putting the public into public health: towards a more people-centred approach. In: Beaglehole, R. (ed.). *Global Public Health: A New Era*. Oxford: Oxford University Press, 2003.

57. Brown, P. Popular epidemiology challenges the system. *Environment* 1993; **35**: 16–41.

58. Lawlor, D.A., Frankel, S., Shaw, M. *et al.* Smoking and ill health: does lay epidemiology explain the failure of smoking cessation programs among deprived populations. *Am. J. Pub. Hlth* 2003; **93**: 266–70.

59. Pearce, N. Traditional epidemiology, modern epidemiology, and public health. *Am. J. Pub. Hlth* 1996; **86**: 678–83.

60. Susser, M. & Susser, E. Choosing a future for epidemiology: I. Eras and paradigms. *Am. J. Pub. Hlth* 1996; **86**: 668–73.

61. Nijhuis, H.G.J. & Van Der Maesen, L.J.G. The philosophical foundations of public health: an invitation to debate. *J. Epidemiol. Commun. Hlth* 1994; **48**: 1–3.

62. Fee, E. & Fox, D.M. *AIDS: The Burdens of History*. Berkeley: University of California Press, 1988.

63. Marmot, M. & Wilkinson, R.G. (eds.). *Social Determinants of Health*. Oxford: Oxford University Press, 1999.

64. Susser, M. & Susser, E. Choosing a future for epidemiology: II. From black box to Chinese boxes and eco-epidemiology. *Am. J. Pub. Hlth* 1996; **86**: 674–7.

65. Wikler, D. & Cash, R. Ethical issues in global public health. In: Beaglehole, R. (ed.). *Global Public Health: A New Era*. Oxford: Oxford University Press, 2003.

66. World Medical Association. *Declaration of Helsinki*. Adopted by the 18th World Medical Assembly, Helsinki, Finland, June 1964, and amended by the 29th

World Medical Assembly, Tokyo, Japan, October 1975; the 35th World Medical Assembly, Venice, Italy, October 1983; and the 41st World Medical Assembly, Hong Kong, September 1989.

67. Last, J.M. Guidelines on ethics for epidemiologists. *Int. J. Epidemiol.* 1990; **19**: 226–9.

68. Westrin, C.-G. & Nilstun, T. The ethics of data utilisation: a comparison between epidemiology and journalism. *Br. Med. J.* 1994; **308**: 522–3.

69. Anon. Protecting individuals; preserving data. *Lancet* 1992; **339**: 784.

70. Lynge, E. New draft on European directive on confidential data. At last, a step forward for epidemiological research. *Br. Med. J.* 1995; **310**: 1024.

71. Lynge, E. European directive on confidential data: a threat to epidemiology. *Br. Med. J.* 1994; **308**: 490.

72. Barker, D.J.P. *Fetal and Infant Origins of Adult Disease*. London: British Medical Journal, 1992.

73. Bailar, J.C. Surgery for early breast cancer – can less be more? *New Engl. J. Med.* 1995; **333**: 1496–8.

74. Khan, K.S. Epidemiology and ethics: the perspective of the Third World. *J. Pub. Hlth Pol.* 1994; **15**: 218–25.

75. Levine, C. Ethics, epidemiology, and women's health. *Ann. Epidemiol.* 1994; **4**: 159–65.

76. Merkatz, R.B., Temple, R., Sobel, S., Feiden, K. & Kessler, D.A. Women in clinical trials of new drugs: a change in Food and Drug Administration Policy. *New Engl. J. Med.* 1993; **329**: 292–6.

77. Bankowski, Z., Bryant, J.H. & Last, J.M. (eds.). *Ethics and Epidemiology: International Guidelines*. Geneva: CIOOMS, 1991.

78. Godlee, F. The Cochrane Collaboration. *Br. Med. J.* 1994; **309**: 969–70.

79. Coughlin, S.S. & Etheredge, G.D. On the need for ethics curricula in epidemiology. *Epidemiology* 1995; **6**: 566–7.

80. Weed, D.L. Science, ethics guidelines, and advocacy in epidemiology. *Ann. Epidemiol.* 1994; **4**: 166–71.

81. Chapman, S. & Lupton, D. *The Fight for Public Health. Principles and Practice of Media Advocacy*. London: BMJ Publishing Group, 1994.

PART III

Public health

The final part of this book considers the state of public health from both historical and contemporary perspectives. The underlying themes are the global threats to public health and the marginalisation of public health services. The prospects for major reform of public health services are assessed.

- Chapter 7 identifies recurrent themes in the history of public health which continue to influence public health practice and debates about the future of public health.
- Chapter 8 reviews the organisation and practice of public health in several wealthy countries.
- Chapter 9 examines the state of public health in selected poor countries.
- Chapter 10 assesses the prospects for public health in the twenty-first century.

public health and a sombre focus on the social and economic costs of drink

7

Public health themes: historical and contemporary

7.1 Introduction

This chapter outlines recurrent themes in the history of public health that continue to influence public health practice and debates about the future of public health. Of central importance is the realisation that public health is not proceeding along a linear and triumphant march[1]. Although the chapter focuses on these themes, it is not a systematic history of public health, which has been covered in numerous books and articles[1-7].

7.2 The nature and scope of public health

A recurrent and critical theme concerns the nature and scope of public health:

- What are the boundaries of public health?
- How does public health relate to medical care, social welfare, environmental and occupational health?
- Should public health be centrally and explicitly concerned with the social and economic determinants of health, such as income, housing and poverty?

The prevailing social and economic ideology has a great bearing on the answers to these questions and the emphasis given to various public health strategies. These questions are not new; the tension between a narrow medical view of public health and a broader focus on the social and economic causes of health and disease was a feature of nineteenth-century public health in England[8].

Public health has been defined in many different ways[9]. All definitions of public health have in common the idea that public health is defined in terms of its aims – to reduce disease and maintain and promote the health of the whole population – rather than by a theoretical framework or a specific body of knowledge.

In 1923 Winslow, a leading theoretician of the American public health movement during the first half of the twentieth century, proposed the following definition:

> the science and art of preventing disease, prolonging life, and promoting physical health and efficiency through organised community efforts for the sanitation of the environment, the control of community infections, the education of the individual in principles of personal hygiene, the organisation of medical and nursing service for the early diagnosis and preventive treatment of disease, and the development of the social machinery which will ensure to every individual in the community a standard of living adequate for the maintenance of health[10].

The scope of this definition is broad, includes early diagnosis and treatment, and incorporates the underlying economic determinants of health. Despite his broad definition, Winslow advocated the individual approach to public health and believed, for example, that the 'discovery of popular education as an instrument in preventive medicine, made by the pioneers in the tuberculosis movement, has proved almost as far reaching in its results as the discovery of the germ theory of disease thirty years before'. Winslow also noted, with approval, the increasing use of physicians for the examination of well people suggesting that control of the 'degenerative diseases requires nothing less than the systematic medical examination of presumably normal individuals'. More recently, the US Institute of Medicine defined public health as 'what we, as a society, do collectively to assure the conditions in which people can be healthy'[11]. This definition, as the Committee recognised, places a huge responsibility on America's public health agencies, as it includes the provision of personal health care to the millions of people rejected by the rest of the health system. The favoured definition in the United Kingdom, and in many other countries, was proposed by the Acheson Report in 1987 as:

> *'the art and science of preventing disease, promoting health, and prolonging life through organised efforts of society'*[12].

Our preferred definition is 'collective action for sustained population-wide health improvement', which emphasises the hallmarks of public health practice: the focus on actions and interventions which require collective (or collaborative or organised) actions; sustainability, that is, the need to embed policies within supportive systems; and the goals of public health: population-wide health improvement implying a concern to reduce health inequalities. A fundamental characteristic of public health action is that it acts primarily on the determinants of health that lie outside the control of individuals and are not responsive to market forces.

Resolution of the dilemma posed by varying interpretations of the scope of public health remains a priority. The continuing failure to agree on the scope of public health and, most importantly, on an appropriate set of strategies is confusing and debilitating. The main themes of modern public health practice are summarised in Box 7.1. Public health should remain inclusive and broad in scope and strategies should be developed to achieve the broad aims. It is counter-productive to espouse a broad definition and apply minimalist strategies, as has been the case for much of the last 150 years. We return to this theme in Chapter 10.

Box 7.1 The essential elements of modern public health theory and practice are:

- the emphasis on collective responsibility for health and the prime role of the state in protecting and promoting the public's health;
- a focus on whole populations;
- an emphasis on prevention, especially the population strategy for primary prevention;
- a concern for the underlying socioeconomic determinants of health and disease, as well as the more proximal risk factors;
- a multi-disciplinary basis which incorporates quantitative and qualitative methods as appropriate; and
- partnership with the populations served.

7.3 A 'Golden Age' of public health?

One of the enduring themes in public health is the idea of a past 'golden age' of public health. The origins of modern public health are usually traced back to the Victorian age in Britain, and the response to the social and health problems generated by rapid industrialisation. As Rosen has shown, however, the history of public health stretches back at least as far as the ancient Greeks and the Hippocratic School; and Sweden instituted public health measures to monitor the population and promote population growth in the early eighteenth century, well before industrialisation[13].

The birth of a systematic approach to public health at the beginning of the nineteenth century can be attributed to the development of the scientific spirit, the humanitarian ideal and the sense of 'public virtue', as well as the presumed economic value of preventing premature mortality. In both Britain and the United States of America, the public health movement was created by social reformers and included, but was not led by, medical practitioners.

Two main nineteenth-century phases of public health are usually described: the environmental sanitation phase lasting from around 1840 to 1890, and the period of the scientific control of communicable disease, based on bacteriological discoveries and the germ theory, from 1890 to 1910. Winslow regarded this later phase as the 'Golden Age'. Most historians, however, date the beginning of the 'golden' age to the middle of the nineteenth century with the publication in 1842 of Chadwick's report on the sanitary conditions of the labouring class and the subsequent Public Health Act of 1848. Another suggestion is that the 'golden age' included both the second half of the nineteenth century and the first half of the twentieth century[14].

The late nineteenth-century public health movement, and especially the locally administered preventive health measures, which led to the reduction of the major adverse health effects of industrialisation, made an important contribution to the development of public health[15]. The importance of the mid-nineteenth century 'golden age' of public health has been exaggerated as there was little real concern with the underlying social and economic determinants of disease[16]. As both professional and lay people saw disease causality in terms of precise invisible entities (disease agents), prevention policies were often narrow and reductionist.

Chadwick, an ardent disciple of Bentham, the utilitarian political philosopher, was appointed as Assistant to the Royal Commission to inquire into the operation and administration of the Poor Laws, and his report revealed the ugly and dangerous conditions in which the working class lived. He believed the people's health was a matter of public concern and supported the principle that the state has responsibility for the health of the public but primarily because of the desire to reduce the economic burden on the state[8]. As a result, public health was seen as a political activity with social and economic changes as its goal, and with local government having a major role to play[17]. Chadwick was not interested primarily in reducing disease. His major concern was tax reduction[16]. Chadwick and his colleagues were interested primarily in the miasmas or odours thought to be the cause of disease that arose from decaying organic matter, not the underlying poverty and general squalor. Filth became an important 'public enemy of community health'. Garbage removal was seen as the solution rather than alleviation of poverty.

The focus on miasma was a reflection of scientific orthodoxy, although a complex range of theories of disease causation coexisted[18]. Chadwick minimised the influence of poverty, believing that '. . . high prosperity in respect to employment and wages and abundant food have afforded to the labouring classes no exemptions from attacks of epidemic disease, which have been as frequent and as fatal in periods of commercial and manufacturing prosperity as in any others'[18]. This conclusion is understandable more readily in the context of Chadwick's starting point, which was the concern with the cost of charitable aid and the widespread Victorian belief that disease caused poverty; an extension of this idea – that responding to the disease burden will stimulate economic growth – has recently gained credibility[19]. Environmental reforms, especially sanitary engineering, were supported in the belief that they would reduce disease and mortality and thus address the problem of poverty indirectly, without compromising individual responsibility or challenging personal liberty. The problems of commercial profit, disease prevention, environmental conditions and government action were intertwined but there was no serious attempt to challenge the social and political fabric of society[20,21].

The Board of Health, established by the Act of 1848, was both unpopular and short-lived because of the power of the vested interests it challenged. This situation has a parallel with the fate of the New Zealand Public Health Commission 150 years later, as discussed in Chapter 8. Following its demise, public health work passed from the Board of Health to a newly established committee of the Privy Council, where, under the direction of the Medical Officer, John Simon, the foundations of a modern public health service were laid. Simon repudiated the Chadwick equation of public health with sanitary engineering and brought both medicine and science back into public health[8]. By 1870 the medical profession dominated public health in Britain and the focus had shifted from legislative action to administrative implementation[17]; this dominance continues in the United Kingdom[22].

From the 1870s a new profession emerged with the establishment of a national network of medical officers of health; social reformers were replaced by professional public health administrators[20]. The history of this professional group is central to the development of public health in Britain in the late nineteenth century. The failure to clarify the goals and practice of this profession ultimately undermined its influence over the political and economic development of the public health system. With the development of a national civil service, public health as a process of social reform, became diffused and the role of public health practitioners as engaged citizens was reduced.

Despite their limited focus, the achievements of the sanitary reformers were impressive[15]; cholera, for example, was controlled basically by impressive feats of engineering. Chadwick was a powerful and influential person and, even by modern standards, his Report is an outstanding example of the use of quantitative and qualitative data to improve the public's health. By stimulating and initiating the legislative basis of public health, Chadwick did much to promote public health. Chadwick was a combination of social investigator, coalition builder, ideologue and administrator[6]. His legacy did not, in the long term, lead to a strong and vigorous public health movement; his ideas merged easily with the reductionist pressure stemming from the germ theory at the end of the nineteenth century. Chadwick and many of his colleagues were not able, or willing, to distinguish the agent of disease from the underlying causes, and when social and economic factors were identified, such as overcrowding and poor housing, the appropriate remedy (preventing poverty) was not recommended. Instead, the focus was on sanitation and water supply, which although great advances in themselves, did not deal with the impact of the underlying poverty.

An important exception to the narrow view expressed by the majority of the English sanitary reformers was provided by Virchow who identified the fundamental importance of the social origins of disease and urged doctors to become advocates for the poor[23]. Virchow's views on the importance of social medicine are summarised in his report on an 1848 typhus epidemic in Upper Silesia. His analysis, based on only a 3-week visit to the region at the request of the Prussian Government, emphasised the underlying social, economic and cultural factors responsible for the epidemic. Instead of recommending a medical response, and in contrast to Chadwick, Virchow outlined a radical programme including full employment and universal education. The impact of these recommendations on the health of the people of Upper Silesia was limited because Virchow's ideas were not welcomed by the Government. Shortly after the publication of the report, he was suspended from his hospital post.

With the liberalisation of Prussian politics, Virchow entered politics in 1861 and actively promoted the concept of the social origins of disease. Virchow firmly believed that a central concern of government should be the health of the people: 'a . . . sound constitution must affirm beyond any doubt the right of the individual to a healthy life'[23]; Virchow supported the formation of a national ministry of health with a physician as minister[24]. At a practical level he planned and implemented a sewerage disposal system for Berlin. Throughout his life he promoted public health against those who wanted to leave the field to private endeavour. He believed passionately that the state had to practise public health, although he was also a strong advocate for local government and decentralised interventions. Unfortunately, Virchow's ideas have not prevailed in the last 150 years.

From a historical perspective, the second half of the nineteenth century was important for public health, even if the period does not warrant the 'golden age' label. Progress was made in improving the health of the public by the sanitary reformers and their engineers. Unfortunately, the critical public health issue of poverty did not receive the attention it deserved and the sanitary reformers directed attention away from the other fundamentally important social factors. From the contemporary perspective, it is still necessary for public health practitioners to focus attention on the underlying social and economic causes of health and disease. We are still awaiting the 'golden age' of public health.

7.4 Role of the state

The state has always had a major influence on public health. Ideally, the state acts proactively and positively to promote health. Unfortunately, examples abound of actions taken by states that have been detrimental to health; for example, war, now more often civil than international, is one of the most harmful public health actions a state can become involved in.

Since antiquity, the state has responded to public health problems by enacting laws, promulgating regulations and establishing organisations. Some of the earliest and most impressive responses were the engineering achievements of the Peruvians, Etruscans and Romans. Medieval citizen governments, like their Roman predecessors, hired labourers to clean streets, cisterns, and sewers, and remove garbage. Furthermore, they attempted to enforce the laws[25]. From the thirteenth century, Italian city states were at the forefront of sanitary endeavours, although progress was slow and public hygiene laws in 1700 strongly resembled those of 1300. Creation of public boards of health by Italian cities from about 1500 represented a major advance in public health practice. Quarantine was used first by Ragusa, the tiny Dalmatian colony of Venice, in 1377 but did not become widespread until the sixteenth century[25].

During the eighteenth century, the impetus for reform in public health moved northwards from Italian cities. Northern Europeans rejected the political basis for protecting public health and, instead, turned their attention to cleanliness, hospital building and information gathering. With the political assertion of health as a right of citizenship, which became common after 1800, the state was obliged to take a more active interest in public health[1]. Until the mid-nineteenth century, however, public health efforts were largely the work of voluntary groups or of local or regional governments, especially in Great Britain where there was a great distrust of the central government which, in general, had little interest in public health. The public health actions of the early nineteenth-century governments were usually in response to specific epidemic threats and were piecemeal and tentative actions motivated by fear, civic pride and religious zeal[20]. The first major national health law was the British Public Health Act of 1848. This Act was a landmark and foreshadowed the public health role of central governments even though it was strongly opposed by the medical profession and local government officials reluctant to surrender authority to a central agency.

In France, a system of weak local advisory health councils was established following the Revolution of 1848 and remained in effect until the end of the nineteenth century. Despite the work of the French hygienists, public health in France lagged far behind that of Britain, largely because of the lack of central government action[26]. The public health regulations in Russia, although advanced, were not enforced systematically, even in response to cholera epidemics; the state completely dominated public health practice in the Soviet Union, ultimately with adverse effects on the health of the public.[27] In Germany there has been a great array of systems with considerable local and regional diversity[24]. In the United States of America there was a greater exertion of local control and delayed action by the federal Government.

In the twentieth century, the state became increasingly involved in public health. For example, the United States Federal Children's Bureau was established in 1912 to protect the health of children. Federal activities in public health in the United States of America gradually expanded and the Marine Hospital Service was renamed the Public Health Service in 1912. Increasing federal support was stimulated by the poor state of recruits for World Wars I and II, and in response to the economic depression of the 1930s. The federal funds were directed toward specific diseases, especially tuberculosis, and specific population groups, especially children[28]. Following the Second World War, debate occurred in the United States of America on the relationship between public health and medical care, but the federal programme for building hospitals set the agenda and diverted the bulk of federal resources into hospitals. The postwar boom in expenditure for laboratory research and hospitals was associated with the relative neglect of public health services and a failure to adopt and implement a broad view of public health[29]. By the 1970s, the financial impact of the expansion in public health activities from the 1930s, particularly the costs of medical care, began to be felt in the United States of America. As new public health issues surfaced, separate agencies were established, for example, the Environmental Protection Agency. In the process, public health lost a clear institutional base and an associated loss of visibility and credibility. In the 1980s federal funding for public health programmes was cut and responsibilities shifted to the states which had the unenviable aim of tailoring limited funds to a vast array of problems. It remains to be seen whether the recent injection of funds into the public health services in response to the threats of bioterrorism will contribute to a long-term strengthening of the public health infrastructure[30].

The United States of America, along with most other countries, continues to grapple with the problems of cost escalation in health services, the emergence of new health problems, such as AIDS, and the large segment of the population without organised medical care coverage[31]. Central to this dilemma is the argument about the scope of public health and the extent of public sector responsibility for medical care. In many countries this dilemma has been resolved by the state taking as much responsibility for individual medical care as it does for public health.

Although the state has ultimate responsibility for public health, it is often unwilling to exercise this responsibility in a planned and coordinated manner. Throughout history the state has been confronted by a combination of strong vested interests and a weak public health constituency and this contributes to the neglect of public health in the face of other pressing priorities. In all countries, the resources devoted by the state to public health are only a tiny fraction of those spent on medical care. The changing nature of the state in recent decades has added complexity to the process of strengthening the role of the state in the practice of public health; for example, external pressures to 'downsize' the role of the state are a direct threat to many public health functions[32].

7.5 Individual liberty and collective responsibility

By definition, public health involves collective action to protect and promote health. The degree of emphasis, however, placed on collective as opposed to individual actions, has varied, often quite markedly[33]. As a result, surprisingly rapid changes have occurred in the balance of responsibilities. Collective actions have been easier to initiate, organise and implement in response to public health crises and public panic. These crises have usually involved epidemics of infectious disease, although the general and severe health problems caused by rapid industrialisation in the eighteenth and nineteenth centuries were seen as a major threat to social order.

In the United States of America, organised public health activities began in the eighteenth century with the initiation of laws for the isolation of smallpox patients and for ship quarantine. The need for quarantine was balanced against the need to maintain trade; quarantine regulations were vigorously opposed by those whose economic investments were threatened. Prior to the twentieth century, there were few formal institutional bases for public health officials in the United States of America and, at least until the mid-nineteenth century, public health was usually the responsibility of the social elite with public health programmes being organised locally. This pattern was also common in other countries, for example Russia, where the gentry took responsibility, albeit limited, for the health of their serfs.

The recurring threat of cholera from the 1830s provided the stimulus to create boards of health in many eastern cities of the United States of America. Quarantine regulations fluctuated depending on the balance of threats from epidemics and merchants. The Civil War, in which more casualties were the result of disease than battle, emphasised the importance of infectious diseases. The industrial transformation of the north, which followed the war, exacerbated public health problems. An increasing number of reform groups took an interest in these problems and supported the need for sanitary reform. Public health reform offered a safe response to pressing social problems. In the United States of America, as elsewhere, little effort was made to tackle the underlying issue of poverty. The nineteenth-century sanitarians were not afraid to tackle vested interests (water companies, landlords) but they did not oppose the underlying social and political framework. Public health had little impact on the social and economic factors crucial to the prevention of disease and the promotion of health for a number of reasons (see Box 7.2).

Box 7.2   There are several reasons why public health has taken a narrow path:

- The domination of the narrow engineering view of public health, stemming from Chadwick and other nineteenth-century reformers, is of critical importance.
- The difficulty in converting a broad view of public health into appropriate strategies. All too often, minimalist strategies have been advocated by public health practitioners as a way of avoiding political conflict.
- The enormous success and popularity of the germ theory of disease undermined a broader public health approach at the end of the nineteenth century.
- The continuing lack of a public health constituency; public support for public health is, at best, limited. Even the limited public support is easily overcome by vested interests and the pressing need for governments to respond to immediate crises.

The main contemporary 'health crisis' in all countries is the cost of medical care stimulated by technological developments, ageing of the population, epidemics of infectious and non-communicable diseases, and by the need for the medical profession to maintain its status and income[34]. Cost containment and ideological pressures are the main motivation for health reforms in all countries, and a focus on individual responsibility has become the main strategy for the control and prevention of non-communicable diseases. 'Blaming the victim' (from the 'unworthy poor' to the 'irresponsible smoker') becomes a powerful excuse for limiting government action, a theme that has been recurrent in public health for centuries. This tendency has been exacerbated by top down pressure from external donors and global policy networks under the guise of improving health service efficiency[35]. Accountability for the health of populations is still low on the priorities of most governments.

The basis of effective public health strategies is sustainable collective action. Regrettably, most government actions are a result of strong and persistent lobbying pressure from health advocacy groups and other vested interest groups and do not stem from a coherent approach to disease prevention and health promotion.

7.6 The role of scientific knowledge

The prevailing scientific paradigm has a strong influence on public health practice. For centuries, the miasma theory competed with the contagion theory of disease transmission, although these and other theories often coexisted. The most striking impact of medical knowledge on public health was the explosion of interest in bacteriology in the half century from 1870. The bacteriological era overshadowed the environmental approach to public health which had been the major strategy in the earlier decades of the nineteenth century. By the early 1900s, bacteriology dominated the public health agenda in both the United States of America and Europe. Once it was believed widely that it was not dirt itself that caused disease, the public health focus narrowed and attention was deflected from the primary role of the environment in disease causation.

Public health agencies began to expand their activities into laboratory science and infectious disease epidemiology. More generally, specific control measures based on laboratory sciences came to replace social and sanitary reform measures to combat disease. The focus was now on specific routes of transmission, rather than on cleaning up cities. Bacteriology became the foundation of the new scientific public health and drew attention away from the larger and more difficult problems created by poverty[36].

The role of public health science in health improvement has been critical. For example, the decline of lung cancer in men in the last third of the twentieth century in many wealthy countries was a reflection of the dissemination of epidemiological research results[37]. At the end of the twentieth century another paradigmatic shift occurred with an increasing emphasis on the molecular and genetic basis of disease. The implications for public health of this shift could be profound because molecular epidemiology emphasises the technical, rather than the social and environmental, approach to disease control. Health economics has also become an important influence on public health because of the worldwide economic constraints on health spending. The World Bank took the initiative by identifying cost effective public health initiatives which may yield large benefits at low cost. An 'essential public health package' includes:

- childhood immunisation and micronutrient supplementation;
- school health programmes;
- public information programmes;
- programmes to reduce tobacco and alcohol consumption; and
- AIDS prevention programmes[38].

While it is, of course, important to ensure that resources are used effectively, the World Bank's approach reduces public health practice to a series of specific interventions far removed from the broad social movements which, historically, have had a greater impact on the public's health. A challenging research issue concerns the nature and origins of social movements for health and their relationship with democratic traditions. Some insights into this issue can be gained from countries that have achieved an exceptional health status at relatively low cost, as will be discussed in Chapter 9.

7.7 The professionalisation of public health

The professionalisation of public health is linked to the development of specialised knowledge in medicine. The history of public health in early nineteenth-century Europe and the United States of America is replete with reformers, many of whom were not health professionals; the role of doctors was limited in the Victorian public health efforts. All reforms were motivated by the notion that ill health caused poverty which, in turn, led to unproductive expenditure on poor relief and further demoralisation of the poor.

Public health programmes in the nineteenth century were promoted by a variety of interest groups for many different reasons. Some were directly concerned about health on humanitarian or religious grounds. Others saw health as a social issue central to the stability of the state. Nineteenth-century public health adopted a healthy public policy approach only in so far as central and local governments were involved in episodic attempts to regulate against public health dangers and to implement sanitary reform. The early public health reformers, often described as 'zealots', were strong-minded and dedicated people[20]. Unfortunately, the concept of public health remained indistinct and was characterised by the absence of a coherent philosophy. Despite the professionalisation of public health, this criticism remains valid today.

The public health movement in the United Kingdom embraced medical practitioners only towards the end of the nineteenth century. The first medical officer of health was appointed in Liverpool in 1847[39]. The professionalisation of public health in Great Britain continued with the Public Health Act of 1872, which made the appointment of a medical officer of health obligatory for local sanitary authorities. Medical officers of health were responsible for enforcing public health acts in their communities, for inspecting food, sanitation and housing, and for publishing an annual report on their activities and the state of public health in their communities.

In the early years of the twentieth century there was a narrowing of focus towards the responsibility of the individual for 'personal prevention', with health education as the main strategy. Medical officers of health in the United Kingdom also became involved in hospital administration, although this responsibility was removed with the formation of the National Health Service in 1948[4] . At the same time, public health moved closer to clinical medicine despite the desire of some academic social medicine advocates and political lobby groups to broaden the focus of public health. As public health became a 'special kind of clinical medicine', practical public health was neglected, especially in the 1930s when medical officers of health became responsible for administering clinical services and hospitals. Social medicine, which espoused a broad view of public health, remained confined to universities. Social medicine was quite separate from health policy and practical public health[40] and, because it assumed intellectual authority as a new academic discipline, it contributed to the rift between public health teaching and practice[41].

In the United States of America the medicalisation of public health occurred later, beginning in the 1920s. Until this time it was largely the field of engineers, biologists and a few social scientists[42]. The key event in this process was the establishment in 1916 of the Johns Hopkins School of Hygiene and Public Health with the financial support of the Rockefeller Foundation. The Foundation supported the development of the early schools of public health in many countries[43].

In the United Kingdom, the speciality of Community Medicine was established in the early 1970s as the 'speciality practised by epidemiologists and administrators of medical services'[20]. The role of the community physician was as a specialist health strategist in the integration of services but it was an unsatisfactory role with limited authority. This speciality became embedded within the structure of the health service and was not able, or willing, to articulate a concern for a broad vision of public health. A few notable public health academics, such as Cochrane, were willing to question the value of medical care activities[44]. In general, the difficult task of addressing the underlying causes of ill health was not given priority by the public health professions. To its credit, the Community Medicine speciality has, at times, argued for a social view of public health, for example, in response to the Black Report on inequalities[45].

The speciality of public health has continued to evolve. In many countries, such as the United Kingdom, Australia and New Zealand, it is still strongly influenced by the medical profession. In the United States of America, public health has a much broader constituency and the medical profession is not so dominant. A broad and inclusive public health speciality is the only viable option in countries where public health specialists of all disciplinary backgrounds are rare. One possible outcome of a broad based disciplinary grouping is the lowering of status of public health professionals, in comparison with the medical profession. This is a small price to pay, however, as the medicalisation of public health has itself resulted in a narrowing of the focus of public health practice. The medical dominance of the profession was exemplified by the bar, until recently, of non-medically qualified individuals becoming full members of the United Kingdom Faculty of Public Health Medicine. This situation had two consequences. One was to constrain the development of a multidisciplinary profession; the other was to strengthen the role of health services research within public health. The Faculty of Public Health Medicine (the modern form of the speciality of Community Medicine) has now opened its membership to non-medically qualified public health practitioners. An unresolved issue for medically qualified public health practitioners is their relationship with clinical medicine[40]. In the United Kingdom, Australia and New Zealand, public health medicine has emerged as a distinct entity on the basis of clinical epidemiology and 'evidence-based medicine'. While this development is good for clinical medicine and increases the status of public health medicine, it is a diversion from the main challenges facing public health. It is unlikely that this development will, in itself, renew public health. In the medium term, it would be more productive for public health doctors to return to the mainstream of public health and to resist cooption and integration with clinical medicine[46].

7.8 Globalisation of public health

Victorian England influenced the development of public health in North America, although, largely because of the size of the continent, there was a greater tendency for decentralised activity at the state level. The impact of the

Victorian approach to health and welfare was felt most directly on the English colonies, especially in India[47], Africa and Australasia[48]. As we will see in Chapter 9, this influence continues today. Other colonial powers had a similar and longstanding impact on the practice of public health in their colonies. This influence is not new; the Hippocratic writings on the effects of the environment provided useful advice for the colonisation of ancient Greece[1].

The experience of the United States Army in the Spanish–American War in Cuba and the Philippines with yellow fever and malaria illustrates the importance of public health for successful colonisation[49]. These lessons were applied in the southern United States of America with the support of Rockefeller money. By 1915 the Public Health Service, the United States Army and the Rockefeller Foundation were the major agencies involved in public health in the United States and its colonies.

The modern form of 'colonialism' is less direct, but equally influential. Many international agencies, including the World Bank and the International Monetary Fund, play an important part in shaping economic, welfare and health policies in poor countries. Structural adjustment programmes in the 1980s, put in place to facilitate debt repayment, encouraged the move towards market-based approaches to medical care and public health policy. It appears that the health problems of many people in poor countries have been exacerbated by these programmes, especially in sub-Saharan Africa[50]. We return to this theme in Chapter 9.

A feature of international public health has been the attempts to eradicate selected diseases. This concept probably originated with the Rockefeller Foundation at its inception in 1913[51]. Eradication of hookworm was the major goal, although the technology was not, and is still not, available for this task. Yellow fever and malaria eradication programmes followed in 1955, both of which were only partially successful; there has been a massive resurgence in malaria since the successes of the 1950s and 1960s. It is now appreciated that the discipline of tropical medicine achieved more for the health of the colonialists than for tropical countries[52].

The eradication of smallpox was successful with the last naturally occurring case being found in Somalia in 1977 after a 10-year campaign led by WHO. Despite this success, there was some disillusionment with disease targeted approaches. The Alma Ata Declaration of 1978 encapsulated the comprehensive primary health care approach defined as 'essential health care made universally accessible to individuals and families in the community by means acceptable to them, through their full participation and at a cost that the community and country can afford'[53]. The overall goal endorsed by WHO was the 'attainment by all peoples of the world by the year 2000 of a level of health that will permit them to lead a socially and economically productive life'. Fine words, but the year 2000 has passed and the rhetoric has not matched the achievements. In part, the recession of the 1980s is to blame. The resources made available, however, did not match the policy goals and where resources were available, they were not directed necessarily to public health policy goals.

In the 1980s the international goal of comprehensive primary health care was replaced by 'selective primary health care' which targets, in the interim, the few most important diseases for which cost effective therapies are available (Box 7.3). Four key interventions were developed and implemented: immunisation, oral rehydration, breast feeding and antimalarial drugs. In 1983, UNICEF spearheaded this initiative with the goal of universal childhood immunisation[35]. The selective or vertical approach to disease control continues with many programmes directed at specific diseases, for example, HIV/AIDS, tuberculosis and malaria[54–57]. The eradication of polio, with major support from Rotary International, is close to achievement although problems remain in a few countries such as India and Nigeria[58].

Box 7.3   Differing approaches to health care

Comprehensive primary health care and selective primary health care are fundamentally different approaches[59].

- Primary health care is based on the broad definition of health; selective primary health care views health as the absence of disease.
- Primary health care stresses equity; selective primary health care consolidates the power of health professionals and promotes technological solutions to health problems. Selective primary health care has been particularly directed towards improving child health, although the 1993 World Development Report expanded this approach to adults.
- Comprehensive primary health care stresses the necessity of multisector approaches to health; selective primary health care focuses on the prevention and management of selected important disease problems.
- Primary health care is firmly rooted in community empowerment; with selective primary health care, community involvement is necessary only for compliance, not for decision making and control. Comprehensive primary health care is an essential component of broad and inclusive public health practice.

Chapter 7 Key points

The recurrent historical themes that continue to influence public health practice are:

- the lack of agreement on the scope of public health and the appropriate strategies;
- the belief in a 'golden age' of public health;
- the central but varying role of the state;
- the tension between individual liberty and collective responsibility;
- the influence of scientific knowledge on public health practice;
- the professionalisation of public health; and
- the globalisation of public health.

7.9 Conclusions

The challenges facing public health at the beginning of the twenty-first century are not new. All current challenges have historical antecedents and lessons abound for advancing public health practice. Unfortunately, the situation confronting public health practitioners is now especially difficult. The globalisation of finance and trade, the dependence of poor countries on a few wealthy countries for access to markets and even basic aid, the integration of labour markets in poor countries with the needs of multinational companies, all increase the difficulty of dealing with public health issues at a country level. A central challenge is to strengthen the global approach to public health: a challenge we return to in Chapter 10.

References

1. Porter, D. (ed.). *The History of Public Health and the Modern State*. Amsterdam: Editions Rodopi BV, 1994.
2. Rosen, G. *From Medical Police to Social Medicine: Essays on the History of Health Care*. New York: Science History Publications, 1974.
3. Duffy, J. *The Sanitarians. A History of American Public Health*. Chicago: University of Illinois Press, 1990.
4. Lewis, J. The origins and development of public health in the UK. In: Holland, W.W., Detels, R. & Knox, G. (eds.). *Oxford Textbook of Public Health: Influences of Public Health*. Oxford: Oxford University Press, 1991.
5. Lewis, J. The public's health: philosophy and practice in Britain in the twentieth century. In: Fee, E. & Acheson, R. (eds.). *A History of Education in Public Health. Health that Mocks the Doctors' Rules*. Oxford: Oxford University Press, 1991.

6. Hamlin, C. The history and development of public health in developed countries. In: Detels, R., McEwen, J., Beaglehole, R. & Tanaka, H. (eds.) *Oxford Textbook of Public Health*, 4th Edition. Oxford: Oxford University Press, 2002.

7. Porter, D. *Health, Civilization and the State. A History of Public Health from Ancient to Modern Times*. London: Routledge, 1999.

8. Hamlin, C. State medicine in Great Britain. In: Porter, D. (ed.) *The History of Public Health and the Modern State*. Amsterdam: Editions Rodopi B.V., 1994.

9. Beaglehole, R. (ed.). *Global Public Health: A New Era*. Oxford: Oxford University Press, 2003.

10. Winslow, C.E.A. *The Evolution and Significance of the Modern Public Health Campaign*. New York: Yale University Press, 1923.

11. Committee for the Study of the Future of Public Health. *The Future of Public Health*. Washington: National Academy Press, 1988.

12. Committee of Inquiry into the Future Development of the Public Health Function. *Public Health In England*. London: HMSO, Cmd 289, 1988.

13. Johannisson, K. The people's health: public health policies in Sweden. In: Porter, D. (ed.). *The History of Public Health and the Modern State*. Amsterdam: Editions Rodopi B.V., 1994.

14. Nijhuis, H.G.J. & Van Der Maesen, L.J.G. The philosophical foundations of public health: an invitation to debate. *J. Epidemiol. Commun. Hlth* 1994; **48**: 1–3.

15. Szreter, S. The importance of social intervention in Britain's mortality decline c.1850–1914: a re-interpretation of the role of public health. *Soc. Sci. Med.* 1988; **1**: 1–37.

16. Tesh, S.N. Miasma and 'social factors' in disease causality: lessons from the nineteenth century. *J. Hlth Pol. Pol. Law* 1996; **20**: 1001–31.

17. Fee, E. & Porter, D. Public health, preventive medicine and professionalization: England and America in the nineteenth century. In: Wear, A. (ed.). *Medicine in Society*. Cambridge: Cambridge University Press, 1992.

18. Pelling, M. *Cholera, Fever and English Medicine 1825–1865*. Oxford: Oxford University Press, 1978.

19. World Health Organization Report of the Commission on Macroeconomics and Health. *Macroeconomics and Health: Investing in Health for Economic Development*. Geneva: World Health Organization, 2001.

20. Lewis, J. *What Price Community Medicine? The Philosophy, Practice and Politics of Public Health since 1919*. Sussex: Wheatsheaf Books, 1986.

21. Ringen, K. Chadwick, the maket ideology, and sanitary reform: on the nature of the 19th-century public health movement. *Int. J. Hlth Serv.* 1979; **9**: 107–20.

22. Griffiths, S. Public Health in the United Kingdom. In: Beaglehole, R. (ed.) *Global Public Health: A New Era*. Oxford: Oxford University Press, 2003.

23. Taylor, R. & Rieger, A. Medicine as social science: Rudolf Virchow on the typhus epidemic in Upper Silesia. *Int. J. Hlth Serv.* 1985; **15**: 547–59.

24. Weindling, P. Public Health in Germany. In: Porter, D. (ed.). *The History of Public Health and the Modern State*. Amsterdam: Editions Rodopi B.V., 1994.

25. Carmichael, A.G. History of public health and sanitation in the west before 1700. In: Kiple, K.F. (ed.). *The Cambridge World History of Human Disease*. Cambridge: Cambridge University Press, 1993.

26. Ramsey, M. Public Health in France. In: Porter, D. (ed.). *The History of Public Health and the Modern State.* Amsterdam: Editions Rodopi B.V., 1994.

27. McKee, M. & Zatonski, W. Public health in eastern Europe and the former Soviet Union. In: Beaglehole, R. (ed.). *Global Public Health: A New Era.* Oxford: Oxford University Press, 2003.

28. Snyder, L.P. Passage and significance of the 1944 Public Health Service Act. *Pub. Hlth Rep.* 1994; **109**: 721–4.

29. Fox, D.M. The Public Health Service and the Nation's health care in the post-World War II era. *Pub. Hlth Rep.* 1994; **109**: 725–7.

30. Horton, R. Bioterrorism: the extreme in Public Health. In: Beaglehole, R. (ed.). *Global Public Health: A New Era.* Oxford: Oxford University Press, 2003.

31. Scutchfield, F.D. & Last, J.M. Public health in North America. In: Beaglehole, R. (ed.). *Global Public Health: A New Era.* Oxford: Oxford University Press, 2003.

32. Reich, M.R. Reshaping the state from above, from within, from below: implications for public health. *Soc. Sci. Med.* 2002; **54**: 1669–75.

33. Beaglehole, R., Bonita, R., Horton, R. *et al.* Public health for the new era. Improving health through collective action. *Lancet* 2003 in press.

34. Evans, R.G. & Stoddart, G.L. Producing health, consuming health care. *Soc. Sci. Med.* 1990; **31**: 1347–63.

35. Lee, K. & Goodman, H. In: Lee, K., Buse, K. & Fustukian, S. (eds.). *Health Policy in a Globalising World.* Cambridge: Cambridge University Press, 2002.

36. Hill, H.W. *The New Public Health.* New York: Macmillan, 1916.

37. Powles, J. & Comim, F. Public health infrastructure and knowledge. In: Smith, R., Beaglehole, R., Woodward, D. & Drager, N, (eds.). *Global Public Goods for Health.* Oxford: Oxford University Press, 2003.

38. World Development Report, 1993. *Investing in Health, World Development Indicators.* New York: Oxford University Press, 1993.

39. Porter, D. Stratification and its discontents: professionalization and conflict in the British Public Health Service, 1848–1914. In: Fee, E. & Acheson, R. (eds). *A History of Education in Public Health. Health that Mocks the Doctors' Rules.* Oxford: Oxford University Press, 1991.

40. Holland, W.W., Fitzsimons, B. & O'Brien, M. 'Back to the future' – public health research into the next century. *J. Pub. Hlth Med.* 1994; **16**: 4–10.

41. Porter, D. How soon is now? Public health and the BMJ. *Br. Med. J.* 1990: **301**: 738–40.

42. Acheson, R.M. The medicalization of public health; the United Kingdom and the United States contrasted. *J. Pub. Hlth Med.* 1990; **12**: 31–8.

43. Waitzkin, H., Iriart, C., Estrada, A. & Lamadrid, S. Social medicine in Latin America: productivity and dangers facing the major national groups. *Lancet* 2001; **358**: 315–23.

44. Cochrane, A. *Effectiveness and Efficiency.* London: Nuffield Provincial Hospitals Trust, 1972.

45. Smith, A. & Jacobson, B. *The Nation's Health: A Strategy for the 1990s.* London: King Edward's Hospital Fund, 1988.

46. Leeder, S.R. Improving our self-episteme. *Aust. J. Pub. Hlth* 1994; **18**: 355.

47. Harrison, M. *Public Health in British India: Anglo-Indian Preventive Medicine 1859–1914.* Cambridge: Cambridge University Press, 1994.

48. Maclean, F.S. *Challenge for Health. A History of Public Health in New Zealand.* Wellington: Government Printer, 1964.

49. Fee, E. Public health and the state: the United States. In: Porter, D. (ed.). *The History of Public Health and the Modern State.* Amsterdam: Editions Rodopi B.V., 1994.

50. Sanders, D., Dovlo, D., Meeus, W. & Lehmann, U. Public health in Africa. In: Beaglehole, R. (ed.). *Global Public Health: A New Era.* Oxford: Oxford University Press, 2003.

51. Warren, K.S. Tropical medicine or tropical health: the Heath Clark Lectures, 1988. *Rev. Infect. Dis.* 1990; **12**: 142–56.

52. Ramirez, V.D. Will tropical medicine move to the tropics? *Lancet* 1996; **347**: 629–31.

53. World Health Organization. *Alma-Ata. Primary Health Care (Health For All Series No.1).* Geneva: World Health Organization, 1978.

54. Brugha, R. & Walt, G. A global health fund: a leap of faith? *Br. Med. J.* 2001; **323**: 152–4.

55. Yamey, G. Global campaign to eradicate malaria. *Br. Med. J.* 2001; **322**: 1191–2.

56. Global Forum for Health Research. *The 10/90 Report on Health Research 2001–2002.* Geneva: Global Forum for Health Research.

57. World Health Organization. Final Report of the External Evaluation of Roll Back Malaria. August 2002. http://mosquito.who.int.

58. Aylward, R.B., Acharya, A., England, S. *et al.* Global health goals: lessons from the worldwide effort to eradicate poliomyelitis. *Lancet* 2003; **362**: 909–14.

59. Rifkin, S.B. & Walt, G. Why health improves: defining the issues concerning 'comprehensive primary health care' and 'selective primary health care'. *Soc. Sci. Med.* 1986; **6**: 559–66.

8

Public health organisation and practice in wealthy countries

8.1 Introduction

This chapter assesses the current state of public health in five wealthy countries: the United Kingdom, United States of America, Sweden, Japan and New Zealand. The United Kingdom is included because of its historical importance for the development of modern epidemiology and public health. The United States is important because of its wealth and the dominance of the private sector in the provision of health care. Sweden, by contrast, has a stronger commitment to public welfare and one of the best public health systems. Japan has undergone remarkable improvements in health standards over the last half century and it is of interest to see whether public health reforms have been a key to these changes. New Zealand, although a tiny country by world standards, has had a long commitment to public welfare, and recent major changes to the organisation and delivery of health care have had a major impact on the practice of public health.

An obvious gap is a country from Central and Eastern Europe. As the rate of change is so rapid in most of these countries and information scarce, it was not easy to include one of these countries[1]; the developing role of the European Union in health affairs is described. It is also apparent that some countries which have made major gains in public health recently, such as The Netherlands[2], have been omitted, as have states which have achieved more than the country as a whole, for example, Victoria in Australia[3]. The situation in selected poorer countries will be described in the next chapter.

There have been several international comparisons of national health systems, although all focus on the organisation and delivery of personal medical care services[4]. In contrast, there have been few comparable studies focusing on public health systems[5,6]. From a research perspective, it would be desirable to assess all aspects of national public health institutions and organisations, including central and local governmental and non-governmental organisations, the capacity of the entire public health workforce and the priority given to public health policies. With this information it would be possible to categorise national public health systems and relate these to measures of health status of populations, for example, avoidable mortality. Unfortunately, the data required for such a formal assessment are not available and the methods used in this survey are mostly descriptive.

8.2 Public health in the United Kingdom

The United Kingdom, as the first nation to industrialise, was the first to respond to the major public health problems caused by industrialisation and urbanisation, and for a brief period in the mid-nineteenth century, there was a close relationship between epidemiology and public health. In the twentieth century many of the major developments in epidemiology were initiated in the United Kingdom, including the studies on tobacco and disease by Doll and Hill, medical record linkage studies, mega-trials, clinical epidemiology, and the Cochrane Collaboration. Furthermore, many important intellectual contributions to epidemiology and public health have come from United Kingdom scientists[7]. The academic epidemiology journals published in the United Kingdom have maintained a closer connection with public health than the journals from the United States of America.

Although the United Kingdom public health experience has been a model for other countries, much has been unique to the United Kingdom; many developments differ within the United Kingdom, sometimes on a town-to-town basis[8]. Furthermore, national developments during the 1980s and early 1990s exposed the fragility of public health policies. The Conservative Government, in the 1980s and early 1990s refused to use the word 'inequalities', preferring the milder expression 'variations.' Its policies of deregulation and privatisation widened income inequalities and policies in housing, transport and education increased social exclusion markedly[9]. Many of these policies were continued, or even extended by the Labour government elected in 1997, although its economic policies have led to some redistribution of wealth. Another challenge facing public health has been a breakdown of trust of government[10]. Scandals such as the BSE affair[11] and the acceptance of a large donation from a businessman wishing to retain tobacco advertising in motor racing, have reduced levels of trust. Consequently, when ministers give advice on based on solid evidence, as in the case of immunisation against measles, mumps and rubella, linked by some in the media with autism, they are not believed by a large proportion of the population.

The National Health Service, including its public health elements, has been reorganised repeatedly, and with increasing frequency, over the last three decades[12]. A recently created regional structure survived for only 8 months. These changes have a corrosive effect on public health activities, sapping morale and disrupting relationships with the community.

Returning to the historical roots of public health, the status of public health doctors in the early twentieth century, especially in urban areas, was low, in contrast to their high status in the second half of the nineteenth century. A major feature of the history of public health in the last quarter of the twentieth century has been the struggle by public health physicians to improve their status.

Following the foundation of the National Health Service in 1948, public health in the 1950s and 1960s drifted without a strong identity, but with an increasing concern with the provision of personal preventive services[13]. A split developed between academic social medicine and practical public health in the United Kingdom[13, 14] although some professors of public health were also district public health officers or medical officers of health. In this period academic public health, and especially epidemiology, flourished. In contrast, the practical side of public health declined[15].

The new speciality of Community Medicine was created in the mid-1970s, based on the recommendations of a Royal Commission on Medical Education which suggested the amalgamation of academic social medicine and public health medicine[16]. The new speciality continued to experience the twin tensions of its relationship with the state, on the one hand, and with the rest of the medical profession, on the other. Unfortunately, the public health function was also removed from local authorities, thus precluding a focus on wider public health issues. The role of the medical officer of health was replaced by the 'community medicine physician'; and the requirement for annual reports on the state of public health fell into abeyance[17]. Community medicine became increasingly managerial in focus with an emphasis on the effectiveness and efficiency of personal medical services. The broad mandate of public health was forgotten – perhaps in order to avoid political conflict[18].

The identity of community medicine was closely connected with the structure of the National Health Service and by the early 1980s the position of community medicine was undermined following National Health Service reorganisations. The 1988 Report of the Committee of Inquiry into the Future Development of the Public Health Function advocated returning community medicine to 'public health medicine'[19]. The Report made a detailed set of proposals for the public health function, most of which were adopted by the then Government including the establishment of several new schools and institutes of public health, despite the paucity of staff available to fill academic vacancies[20]. Some were extensions of previous academic departments and others were extensions of service departments with little academic content.

The Report also concluded that the public health role of local health authorities should be made explicit. Regional and district health authorities were given legal responsibility for reviewing the health of the population, setting policy aims and objectives, and evaluating progress. Responsibility was also given to local health authorities to control communicable disease outbreaks. An important aspect of the post-Acheson public health function was the production of annual reports for National Health Service districts and regions[21]. These reports were designed to be a central component of the strategic planning and contracting process with the Health of the Nation document as the guiding plan. There was a tension between the independence of the annual reports and corporate ownership; after all, the annual reports were written by a member of the health authority. The standard of the reports varied greatly from one area to another and their aims were not explicit[22].

According to Acheson, the fundamental role of public health specialists should be to give advice and monitor progress towards specified goals. This would include lobbying on policy issues, coordinating local intersectoral issues, and organising, but not delivering, disease prevention services such as immunisation and screening. Despite the emphasis on prevention and health promotion, the curriculum the Report proposes gives a central place to the analysis of health service needs; the need for research was mentioned only briefly. The increase in the status of public health medicine in the last decade was due more to the indirect impact of health service reforms than to the implementation of the Acheson Report.

A major health service reorganisation in 1989 introduced the internal market to the National Health Service. Health authorities, instead of being given an arbitrary allocation by government to run their services, were allocated a budget based on the population served, adjusted for 'health need' according to a complex formula[23], and expected to buy services from the most appropriate source, the so-called 'purchaser–provider split'. These reforms were welcomed by some public health physicians, although not the Faculty of Public Health Medicine, in contrast to the initial negative reaction of the rest of the medical profession[24].

On balance, the changes seemed to enhance the voice of public health medicine, although a preoccupation with hospital services came at the expense of prevention and health promotion[25]. Many public health physicians believed that the purchaser–provider split was in accord with the Acheson report recommendations[26]. The Conservative Government's Health of the Nation document, published in 1992, set out a strategy for improving health, and included for the first time health goals and targets in several key areas. The criteria used for selecting key areas were that they should be a major cause of death or avoidable ill health; that cost-effective interventions were available; and setting targets and monitoring progress were possible. Although most commentators welcomed the target-setting process, the report was criticised for its failure to grapple with the social origins of ill health, and its lack of attention to health inequalities[27]. A formal evaluation found that it had achieved some successes in shifting resources and incorporating health promotion into contracts but the effects had not been sustained. Its impact had also been weakened by the government's loss of credibility arising from its failure to address the issue of health inequalities[28]. A major limitation of the Conservative Government's strategy was its unwillingness to support local action with appropriate national action, such as legislation to restrict tobacco advertising, or to provide major extra resources for public health programmes. For example, funding for the Health Education Authority for England was radically reduced in 1994.

The election of a Labour government in 1997 heralded a major shift in health policy for the UK. The NHS Plan[29] produced by the new government in 2000 outlined the move away from the purchaser/provider split of the internal market towards a whole systems approach. This model is typified by a greater focus on patient involvement and choice, an emphasis on development of intermediate care and changes to patterns of acute care with greater freedom at a local level. In particular, the reorganisation gives clinicians and primary care organisations the levers to drive improvement in health as well as delivery of health care. Greater awareness of the impact of the wider determinants on health and a government-wide commitment to reducing inequalities were reflected in the creation of a Minister of State for Public Health within the Department of Health, although the post was later downgraded to a junior minister.

The public health agenda of the Labour Government set out in Saving Lives[30] led to a variety of policy initiatives. The Acheson report on inequalities[18] reviewed evidence of effective action to combat health inequalities and emphasised the relatively small contribution of the health service to the reduction of inequalities. The broader social inclusion agenda has also been developed and championed through the work of the Social Exclusion Unit[31]. Increasingly, there is awareness of potential impact on health of government policies from other departments. However, one of the problems in identifying this broad type of activity as central to the work of public health has been the difficulty in gaining public profile and support. For historic reasons the official focus on public health in the United Kingdom continues to sit within the NHS. This positioning is problematic because of the continual over-emphasis in the media and by ministers on acute health services, resulting in a relatively low profile for public health issues. These changes took place against a background of a shift in the nature of public health practice. Full membership of the United Kingdom Faculty of Public Health has been extended to non-medically qualified people, subject to the same post-graduate training, as was recruitment to posts of Director of Public Health in the ever-changing bodies that act as local health authorities. These developments have been accompanied by increased investments in training programmes for medical and non-medical public health professionals.

In summary, the public health workforce in the United Kingdom has benefited from a sustained programme of investment in recent years; it has also been damaged by a permanent process of reorganisation that has largely been driven by attempts to reform the provision of health care. This has led to a situation in which individuals are reluctant to invest efforts in developing long-term programmes because their organisation are unlikely to remain in existence long enough to see them through. The basic sciences of public health are strong, especially epidemiology and biostatistics, but much of the academic public health workforce is concentrated in only a few institutions. In contrast to the earlier decades of the National Health Service, the status of academic public health has diminished as the service role of public health has become dominant. Until recently, little effort was devoted to developing a multidisciplinary and intersectoral approach to health improvement in the United Kingdom. Research funding for universities is dependent increasingly on a formulaic and narrow assessment of the quality and quantity of publications; this exercise makes interdepartmental and multidisciplinary collaboration more difficult. The public health workforce is fragmented and there is little sense of a cooperative movement in which a range of professionals jointly approach the tasks of researching and promoting the health of defined populations.

The outlook for public health in the United Kingdom is, however, more encouraging than in the past[12]. Perhaps the greatest challenge in the United Kingdom is redressing the legacy of under-investment in sectors as diverse as education, housing, and transport, all of which have profound implications for public health. This is particularly apparent in relation to the health of adolescents, who top the league within the European Union in terms of drug use, teenage pregnancy, smoking and hazardous drinking, all signs of a disconnection with society as a whole[32]. This is not, however, a challenge limited to public health; it is recognised increasingly that the low skill levels in the United Kingdom and lack of investment are a major factor in poor economic performance[33]. The rapid pace of change in the organisation and delivery of public health services in the United Kingdom over the last few years does not allow an assessment of whether the new structure will be any more effective in improving the health of the population. The challenges for delivering improved public health include: making health improvement a real priority for primary care; developing new and changing roles for a variety of staff; and making a reality of the opportunities for working with government both at a local level and regional level. There is a need to strengthen the public health capacity so as to develop strong multidisciplinary public health professionals, and this will need to be matched by new investments at all levels of the public health system.

8.3 Public health in Europe

Two agencies, WHO and the European Union, are actively engaged in setting public health policy in Europe. WHO developed a coherent and comprehensive set of 38 health targets[34]. The first major evaluation of progress in implementing the regional targets was completed in 1985 and the second in 1993. In general, progress towards better health was good and moderate progress was made towards the 'lifestyle' and environment targets. The goal of equity, however, remains elusive. The widening gap in health status between the northern/western and the central/eastern parts of Europe, with southern Europe intermediate in most respects, means that many of the health targets for Europe cannot be achieved for the region as a whole[35,36].

In the late 1980s a process of rapid political change began in the countries of Central and Eastern Europe, with an increasing emphasis on market forces as a guiding economic principle[1]. The ramifications of the dissolution of the Soviet Union continue to influence the health of many Europeans. The deterioration of health status in the former Soviet Union is the result of systemic social and economic breakdown consequent on its 'defeat' in the long 'cold war'. The health crisis is unlikely to be resolved until a viable political, economic and social order is established[37].

Most national economies in the region face serious social, economic and political problems and unemployment levels are rising rapidly. By the end of the 1980s, all countries in Central and Eastern Europe for which data were available, except Poland, showed a slow-down in economic growth. Differences in wealth widened, with the rich countries, regions and social groups becoming richer, and the poor relatively poorer.

Striking variations remain in death rates across the continent, and in many countries of Central and Eastern Europe life expectancy at birth declined in the 1980s, especially in men, at a time when it increased by 2.5 years in

Western Europe[38]. The main contribution to the continuing high all cause mortality rates in Central and Eastern Europe since 1970 is from the preventable non-communicable diseases of adults[39]; cardiovascular disease mortality rates, for example, in Central and Eastern Europe are now the highest in the world[34].

A detailed analysis of changes in life expectancy at birth in the 1980s in Czechoslovakia, Hungary and Poland showed that improvements in infant mortality have been counteracted by deteriorating death rates among young and middle-aged people, with the deterioration commencing as young as late childhood in Hungary but in the 30s and 40s in the Czech Republic and Poland. The leading contributors to this deterioration were cancer and cardiovascular diseases. In Hungary, cirrhosis and accidents have also been of great importance, indicating the adverse effect of excessive alcohol consumption[38]. In the early 1990s there was a major improvement in heart disease death rates in Poland possibly due to an increased availability all year round of fruit and vegetables and an increase in the price of dairy products consequent on changes in economic policies[40].

The practice of public health has been weak and poorly coordinated in Central and Eastern Europe and the new Central Asian republics. The first formal school of public health in Poland, established in 1991, reflects a modest resurgence in public health training in Central and Eastern Europe. In many of these countries, public health has taken a prime responsibility for managing the health system[41] and curricula in the new school of public health emphasise health service management[42]. While the latter is a major challenge, given the poor state of the health services in much of Central and Eastern Europe, it continues to distract from the wider goals of public health. The Soros Foundation has established a major workforce development programme that is supporting schools of public health in several central and eastern European countries[43].

Opportunities abound for cooperative international public health efforts to assist the development of public health in Central and Eastern Europe[44]. A priority is the development of a critical mass of trained and experienced public health teachers[45]. Excellent examples of international cooperation in public health training exist, for example, in Hungary where the new programme in public health medicine gives emphasis to non-communicable disease epidemiology, and subjects such as health economics and health promotion have been introduced for the first time[46,47]. It is important that all new ventures are driven by public health needs, not by commercial interests or public health 'entrepreneurs'.

Germany was a pioneer in some aspects of nineteenth-century public health, for example, the work of Virchow. Following the rise of Hitler, however, positive public health developments came to an end and were not reinstituted after the Second World War. Disease prevention is now based largely on health education and there is an aversion to state-supported disease control programmes[42]. Considerable local and regional variation has continued to characterise public health in Germany, and there has been little integration of scientific approaches with public health programmes[48]. Public health training, administration and career structures are also not well developed in Germany and although new postgraduate training initiatives are under way[49], it is unlikely that Germany will provide strong leadership for public health in Europe in the near future.

Paradoxically, France, which was also a pioneer in the early nineteenth-century public hygiene movement, was slow to implement public health measures on a wide scale. Furthermore, the central government has long played a limited role in public health in France[50]. A formal public health training programme has begun in France but it is unlikely, given the weakness of public health in France, that it will provide strong leadership for the rest of Europe. The European Union has a formal interest in public health under Article 129 of the Maastricht Treaty[51]. European Union action in public health has been limited to research, and health information and education concerning, in particular, major non-communicable diseases and drug dependence[52], but its focus is now expanding[53]. Unfortunately, the European Union health policies have been fragmented and influenced strongly by economic policies. The Commission of the European Communities published its Framework for Action in the Field of Public Health in 1993[54], and a proposal for a 5-year public health programme was produced in 1995. The plan immediately ran into strong opposition because of the contradiction between the desire of the Commission to promote health while being involved in huge subsidies to the tobacco and alcohol industries[55,56].

Vested interests within Europe have reduced the impact of the Commission's public health activities. Regional policies in Europe continue to have important adverse effects on the economic performance of poor countries in other parts of the world and thus on their health status. The most notorious example is the EU Common Agricultural Policy (CAP), which is designed to support farmers, with French farmers being the greatest beneficiaries. An average European cow receives approximately $2.20 per day from the CAP in subsidies and other aid; one-half the world's population lives on the same daily amount[57]. The subsidization of tobacco production by the European Union reflects the continued power of tobacco interests and is a major policy anomaly hindering progress on tobacco control; the EU spends approximately Euro 1 billion on tobacco production subsidies and only Euro 10–20 million on agricultural diversification and tobacco control programmes[58].

The European Union policies, to the extent that they are part of a directive, can be enforced, whereas the implementation of WHO policies is voluntary. There is scope for coordinated action by WHO and the European Union on public health strategies, especially in Central and Eastern Europe. The new research programme of the European Union, however, is likely to be too narrow to offer much promise for the development of public health research in Europe; most of the funding will go to biotechnology research[59, 60].

A positive development for public health in Europe is the organisations that have been formed to provide leadership, such as the various European groupings of epidemiologists, the European Public Health Association, the European Public Health Alliance, and the Association of Schools of Public Health in the European Region, which has developed a system of peer review for public health courses[61] and is attempting to coordinate the development of new schools of public health[42]. It is clear that a major influence on health in Central and Eastern Europe for years to come will be the upheavals consequent upon the breakdown of the Soviet Union. The uncritical adoption of the market ideology has reduced the responsibility of most of the governments of the region for population health and at the same time has limited the resources available for public health activities[62].

8.4 Public health in the United States of America

The United States of America epitomises the problems wealthy countries experience when the organisation and practice of public health are neglected[63]. The public health agenda since September 2001 has been driven by the threat of bioterrorism and the research priorities remain focused narrowly on biomedical and genetic research at the expense of a broad public health research agenda[64]. A major dilemma facing public health in the United States continues to be its relationship with the organisation and delivery of medical care services. Until a national and equitable system of medical care is achieved, public health will continue to be neglected and will receive an inadequate share of the vast resources devoted to 'health' in the United States. The tremendous amount spent on medical care, and the reduced national income from taxation because of tax cuts, limit the availability of funds for a whole range of public services, not just for public health services. It is noteworthy that, in the past decade, the average income ($174 million) of the top 400 wealthiest taxpayers increased at 15 times the rate of the income of the bottom 90% of Americans, whose average income rose by only 17% (to $27 000)[65].

8.4.1 Organisation of public health services

The organisation of public health in the United States of America shows large variations among the States[66], reflecting the wide range of governmental (state, local and federal) agencies providing services. Services are also provided at national, state and local levels by environmental, occupational safety, mental health, disability and social service groups. This fragmentation, together with a weak centralised authority driven by a conservative political agenda, leads to great difficulty in the implementation of effective public health programmes. Public health departments have become last resort providers for uninsured patients and for patients rejected by private practitioners. Almost three-quarters of all state and local health departments expenditures are for personal health services[67]. Public health increasingly has been starved of funds and this trend has been exacerbated by the increasing use of federal block grants to states[68,69].

Although the states have primary responsibility for public health in the United States of America, the Federal Government plays a major role in defining health objectives for the nation, providing financial and technical support in achieving these objectives, and in coordinating the efforts of the states[70]. The primary responsibility for public health at the federal level rests with the Department of Health and Human Services. The Public Health Service, one component of the Department, has the central responsibility, although many public health activities are scattered throughout the federal bureaucracy. Within the Public Health Service, the Centers for Disease Control and the Health Resources and Services Administration are the most important public health agencies. Each state has a health agency, although some are components of larger agencies, which also include social welfare and income maintenance services. The vast majority of the funds for public health services come from governmental sources, most from federal agencies.

The state health agency is headed by a state health officer appointed by the Governor in the majority of states. Most state health officers are qualified medically; increasingly, these positions are political appointments. At the local government level, there are approximately 3000 local health departments serving either a single municipality or county or a group of counties. The relationship between the local health departments and local government and state health agencies are variable; some local health departments are district offices of the state health agency, some are autonomous, and some are responsible to both local government and the state health agency. Local health departments are usually responsible for the direct delivery of public health services including non-communicable disease control programmes, and maternal and child health services. A variety of restrictions imposed on local health departments, however, have considerably weakened their role in public health in the 1960s and 1970s. A survey of local health departments found that only 11% of 2263 departments had direct access to a trained epidemiologist or statistician on their staff[71]. The average county and city health department can accomplish only two-thirds of its essential functions[72].

The United States of America has been at the forefront of the process of setting objectives for public health, although antecedents can be found in the Canadian Lalonde Report of 1974[73]. In 1980 several initiatives culminated in a set of quantified goals for 1990, which was followed by a mid-course review in 1985[74]. While broad national goals provided a basis for accountability, no detailed action plans were provided. The over-emphasis on individual responsibility and a downplaying of governmental responsibility for health were other limitations. Some progress has been made towards many of these goals, for example, smoking reduction by adults, and a revised set of objectives were established for the year 2000 and again for 2010[75]. Many of these goals specifically address the need to reduce social and ethnic inequalities in health, although progress has been disappointingly slow in these, and other, areas[74]. Most progress has been made in the delivery of clinical preventive services with less progress occurring in areas that require dealing with substantial countervailing forces[74].

8.4.2 The Institute of Medicine's Report and its impact

A committee was established by the Institute of Medicine (IOM) to review the state of public health in the United States of America in the 1980s because of the perception that the nation had lost sight of its public health goals and had allowed the system of public health activities to fall into disarray[76]. After a 2-year study, the Committee 'viewed with alarm' the state of public health. A range of problems were found: disorganisation, weak and unstable leadership, a lessening of professional public health competence, hostility to public health concepts, outdated statutes, inadequate financial support for public health activities, gaps in data gathering and surveillance and lack of inter sectoral links. The 'core' functions of public health received less than 1% of the health budget[77]. In the Committee's view, these problems reflected a lack of appreciation among the public, policy-makers and the medical profession of the central role of public health in maintaining and improving the health of the public.

The Committee was critical of short-term solutions because they, too, often led to fragmentation, organisational confusion and public disenchantment; in the Committee's word – 'disarray'. Several reasons explain the disarray. Relative success in dealing with many infectious diseases led to the perception that the major public health problems were solved and there was no further need for organised public health involvement. This belief also led to a unidimensional approach to complex public health problems and encouraged the fragmentation of public health programmes among many agencies.

The Report attempted to convey an urgent message to the American public: public health is a vital function, which requires broad public support in order to fulfil society's interest in assuring the conditions in which people can be healthy. The Committee recognised that restoring an effective public health system cannot be achieved by public health professionals alone. The IOM's recommendations would have meant substantial additional resources available for public health, an integration of mental health services into health departments, and an even greater role in the provision of medical services to the poor. Similar conclusions were reached 11 years earlier, after a survey of local public health departments and their directors[78].

The IOM's report received a mixed response. Some questioned the assumption that public health alone can fill the stated mission. Several commentators believed that the Report was unfairly negative towards public health personnel[79], although others concluded that public health practitioners must accept considerable responsibility for the deficiencies in public health. There was even dispute as to whether public health was, in fact, in disarray, given the substantial progress made in improving health status in the United States[80]. The IOM's Report reinforced the central role of states but without addressing adequately the need for federal leadership and planning (Box 8.1)[80]. The bulk of funding for public health comes from federal sources; most public health problems are national in scope and do not respect administrative boundaries. The report did not prioritise recommendations and no evidence was produced to suggest that a structural reorganisation would improve function or outcome.

Practical recommendations to strengthen the public health system in five key areas included the need for improvements in:

- the professional knowledge, skills and abilities of the public health workforce;
- the ability of individual public health officials and their agencies to provide dynamic community leadership;
- the ability of public health workers to access relevant information;
- the ability of public health organisations to engage with the community in planning, priority setting and constituency building; and
- the ability of public health agencies to obtain and utilise fiscal resources[71].

The Institute's report led to considerable further reflection and analyses including a proposal for ten essential public health functions (Box 8.2).

Box 8.1   HIV/AIDS: a public health challenge

The United States' response to the HIV/AIDS epidemic highlights the problems facing public health[80]. Although the HIV problem is huge, the public health response has not been in keeping with that given to other highly virulent, but less devastating, organisms. There was an absence of early national leadership, and inadequate attention was devoted to the epidemic in its early stages; the main driving force of health policy was cost containment[81]. The extreme conservatism of mainstream United States politics in the 1980s limited the ability of the Centers for Disease Control to respond in a timely and appropriate fashion to the emerging epidemic, leading to the charge that the Centers' programmes were afflicted by 'political correctness', rather than being guided by scientific knowledge[82]. The HIV epidemic came at a time when the public health structures within the United States were themselves suffering a 'wasting disease'[83].

Box 8.2   Essential public health functions

- monitor health status to identify community health problems;
- diagnose and investigate health problems and health hazards in the community;
- inform, educate, and empower people about health issues;
- mobilise community partnerships to identify and solve health problems;
- develop policies and plans that support individual and community health efforts;
- enforce laws and regulations that protect health and ensure safety;
- link people to needed personal health services and assure the provision of health care when otherwise unavailable;
- assure a competent public health care workforce;
- evaluate effectiveness, accessibility, and quality of personal and population-based health services; and
- research for new insights and innovative solutions to health problems[84].

These essential public health functions have become a beginning point for a number of public health activities in the US, such as the National Public Health Performance Measures Program, the development of competencies for public health professionals and the development of a research agenda in public health.

A review was completed in 1989 on the implementation of the IOM report's state recommendations, and repeated in 1997, with a companion report on local health departments. Both reported modest improvements in the administrative recommendations issued by the IOM[85, 86]. However, there continued to be erosion of resources provided to health departments in the US, as reflected in the data on revenue to local health departments collected by the National Association of City and County Health Officials[87]. The increasing reliance of health departments on patient care funding reduces their capacity to provide core public health functions. In 2002 two further IOM reports, reaffirmed the general neglect of both the public health workforce and the governmental public health infrastructure and made further recommendations for strengthening the public health infrastructure and workforce[88, 89]. The impact of these reports may be diminished by the continuing focus on the response to bioterrorism and other external threats to national security.

8.4.3 Tobacco control in the USA

The progress made with tobacco control is a reflection of the strength of the national public health workforce. The recent US experience is mixed. As discussed in Chapter 3, tremendous progress was made as a result of litigation, which led to the release of millions of pages of tobacco industry documents and a huge settlement between the tobacco companies and the states in compensation for the costs of treating patients with tobacco-induced diseases[90, 91]. Unfortunately, the promise of using money from the tobacco settlement fund to prevent future smoking has mostly been unfulfilled and several states are using some of these funds to balance budgets[92]. US public health suffered further with the rejection of the Tobacco Control Bill (1998), a healthy public-policy measure that would have curtailed simultaneously both the production and the consumption of tobacco[93]. This bill had much in its favour: it had been negotiated already with the industry; it had been approved by the Senate Commerce Committee with an overwhelming bipartisan majority; it was sponsored by a senior Republican Senator (John McCain); it had strong support from President Clinton; powerful public-health interest groups and professional associations supported it; there is widespread public disdain for smoking, and teenage smoking was a powerful political rallying point; and public opinion polls indicated that 60% of the public supported the measure. However, at the last minute the major tobacco companies, with a huge advertising budget, engineered its defeat by influencing voting patterns in the Congress.

The long-term success of the US public health community will depend, in part, on its response to the defeat on the tobacco issue; the event provides a vivid case study of the politics of public health. Similar confrontations are occurring with other and even more powerful vested interest groups – for example, the gun lobby, the automobile and food industries[93].

8.4.4 Summary

Almost the entire debate on health care reform in the early 1990s centred on the financing and organisation of medical care. Public health was marginalised once again[94]. The major lesson from the United States of America is that public health is unlikely to receive the attention and resources it requires until the delivery of personal medical services is organised more equitably. As long as state public health departments struggle to provide the medical care needs of millions of poor Americans, it is unrealistic to expect these agencies to focus seriously on public health issues. Furthermore, while the Federal Government continues to devolve responsibility for public health to the states, there is unlikely to be a coherent national approach to public health. Public health professionals have failed to overcome the fragmentation of public health initiatives and build public support to counter the strong vested interests, such as the tobacco and food industries[93]. Although there are some promising signs, such as initiatives undertaken by schools of public health and local health departments and the increasing responsibility of managed care programmes for public health action, the outlook for public health in the United States of America is bleak. It is particularly disappointing that a country as wealthy as the United States shows such little constructive leadership in modern global public health. The events of September 11, 2001 and the subsequent experience with anthrax demonstrated the profound impact of an eroded public health infrastructure. These events may lead to major efforts to rebuild that public health infrastructure with a focus on epidemiology and surveillance for both communicable and non-communicable diseases, workforce development, communication and information technology, and laboratory capacity[95]. However, this will occur only if the new resources coming to public health are used to reinvigorate the public health infrastructure in all its complexity – so that it can respond effectively to all public health issues.

8.5 Public health in Japan

From a public health perspective, Japan is of great interest. There have been tremendous improvements in life expectancy in Japan over the last 50 years, and Japan now leads the international life expectancy tables. The rapid growth in wealth and the narrowing of the differences in its distribution, together with the typical diet with its continuing low saturated fat intake and recent decreases in salt intake, have all contributed to this favourable situation[96]. Health care is not likely to be a major factor. The public health system, in particular, mass screening, may also have contributed, but is unlikely to be a major explanation, given the lack of convincing evidence on the effectiveness of screening for most non-communicable diseases.

Despite its long history of isolation and its unique cultural development, Japanese public health has been strongly influenced by Europe. The formal beginning of modern public health in Japan was the 1874 decree named Isei ('medical order'), which was based on developments in Europe, especially Germany, and the United States of America[97]. The Isei consisted of 76 sections and covered a wide range of legislative needs, from public health administration to medical education. Regulations for the prevention of infectious diseases were promulgated in the late 1870s, stimulated by the need to control cholera and smallpox epidemics. From these beginnings, the responsibility for the prevention of infectious diseases rested with the city, town or village. Similarly, in 1890 the responsibility for construction of water supply systems was also decentralised, although the central government provided strong direction.

After the devastation of the Second World War, the new constitution of 1946 stated that 'the state shall try to promote and improve the condition of social welfare and security, and of public health'[96] and the subsequent policies for public health were influenced by this constitutional requirement. The Medical Profession Law of 1948 stipulated that 'the physician shall contribute to improve and promote public health by performing medical care and health guidance, thereby maintaining the healthy livelihood of the nation'[98]. Environmental conditions in Japan deteriorated as industrial growth speeded up in the 1950s, and outbreaks of environmental poisoning led eventually to a new Ministry for the Environment in 1971.

Structurally, the Ministry of Health and Welfare is responsible for health administration, the Ministry of Education for school health, the Ministry of Labour for industrial health, and the Environmental Agency for control of environmental hazards. The Public Health Council, with its expert subgroups, advises the Minister of Health and Welfare. A variety of voluntary agencies play an important role in the delivery of public health services in Japan. Local voluntary organisations have been involved actively in public health campaigns associated with primary health care. Most new public policies and strategies are formulated by central government and implementation is delegated to local government. Preventive services are provided partly by prefectures, and partly by municipal governments. The national government provides between one-third and one-half of the cost of these activities. Public health, as defined by the constitution, also includes medical care, which is largely supplied by hospitals and clinics in the private sector.

A national network of health centres serves as the focus of public health activities including public health campaigns, health education activities, and health checks. The budget for health centres comes from national and local sources and each centre covers about 100 000 people. The range of activities of the health centre is very wide, and includes health education, personal advice on the prevention of disease, as well as maternal and child health guidance. Clinical treatment in the form of medications or operations are not included.

The major response of the Japanese Government to the emergence of non-communicable disease epidemics and the ageing of the population has been legislated requirements for periodic health checks and services for the elderly and an emphasis on health education activities. Mass screening especially for cancer, the leading cause of death, has been the main form of preventive activity in Japan for many decades. Mass screening for gastric cancer, the leading cause of cancer, is one of the programmes supported financially by the 1982 Act for Health of the Elderly; also supported is screening for cervical cancer, breast cancer (including women as young as 35 years), lung cancer and colon cancer. This Act integrated health promotion and medical care for people aged over 40 years and provided financial support for medical cost for people aged over 70 years and to people aged 65–69 with serious handicap. Health promotion programmes are conducted by municipal governments. The financial support for these programmes comes equally from the national, prefectural and municipal governments.

Healthy Japan 21 is a national project launched in April of 2000 to encourage the prevention of disease, mainly through primary prevention and health promotion[99]. The justification for this project is the very rapid expansion of medical expenditure due to the ageing of the population. There are nine areas where goals have been set: nutrition, physical activity, mental health, tobacco, alcohol, dental health, diabetes mellitus, cardiovascular disease and cancer. Each municipal government has to develop its own strategies to achieve the goals with support provided by the national government. The first national project of this kind was developed in 1978 and renewed in 1988. However, these initial projects were of only limited effectiveness because the main focus was the secondary prevention of disease, based on the findings from mass screening programmes.

The fourth phase of the national health promotion programme is another 5-year plan. The priorities are similar to those of the Healthy Japan 21 project. The main targets are cancer, stroke, heart disease and diabetes; other targets are hypertension, hyperlipidemia, and osteoporosis, dementia and periodontal disease which are major causes of reduced quality of life among the elderly. The Japanese government has enacted a law for health promotion, which became effective in May, 2003. This law provides the legal basis to promote the Healthy Japan 21 project and other national health promotion programmes.

The incidence and death rates for gastric cancer are declining, and it is commonly thought that health checks and mass screening have played an important part in this decline, despite the lack of convincing evidence on the value of screening. In 1988 nearly a third of the target population received health checks. An inverse relationship has been reported between the uptake of health checks in adults aged 40 years and over and hospital use by those aged 70 years and over[100]. The survey was based on data from all 509 Japanese cities with a population between 30 000 and 200 000. However, this ecological relationship is far from sufficient to indicate that the periodic health checks have been effective. Death rates from lung cancer are rising rapidly and are not expected to respond to secondary preventive efforts.

Three major challenges face public health in Japan: the ageing population, the rise in the epidemic of tobacco-caused disease, and the westernisation of the diet. Each challenge will require intersectoral collaboration on a scale not yet seen in Japan. The most likely explanation for the striking increase in life expectancy in Japan over the last half century is the increase in wealth, which has been distributed reasonably equitably, and the continuing very healthy diet with low intake of animal fat. The dramatic declines in stroke deaths have been due to specific efforts to prevent high blood pressure, by lowering salt consumption in the entire population, and treatment programmes for hypertensive individuals. While it is impossible to specify the exact contribution of specific public health services to the dramatic improvement in life expectancy, it is clear that these services are not well equipped to deal with the major challenges now facing public health in Japan, including the effects of the recent severe downturn in the economy and the increase in unemployment.

8.6 Public health in Sweden

Sweden is included in this chapter because it is one of the most affluent countries in the world and has a strong reputation as an egalitarian state that pays particular attention to the welfare of its citizens. For example, in 1997 the Swedish Government initiated a broad review of the welfare of its citizens with a strong focus on equity issues[101].

The Swedish health system has been under pressure since the late 1980s due to the poor growth rate of the Swedish economy and demographic changes[102].

As a consequence, the health system has been undergoing major structural transformation; the focus for change has been on medical care services, but public health also has been reorganised[103]. A feature of the Swedish approach to health reform, and in contrast to reform in the United Kingdom and New Zealand, is the slow evolutionary nature of the process and extensive consultation[104, 105].

From a historical perspective, it is noteworthy that a programme for public health in Sweden was initiated more than a 100 years before urbanisation and industrialisation gained momentum in the late nineteenth century[106]. In the second half of the eighteenth century, a variety of strategies were devised to increase the population which was deemed too small. In 1748 a system of national registration, on a parochial basis, was established to monitor population growth and other vital statistics. Nationwide disease registers and the systematic use of national registration numbers ensure that Sweden continues to offer exceptional opportunities for epidemiological research[107].

From an international perspective, health status in Sweden is very high, with low infant and maternal mortality rates and a high life expectancy. Inequalities in health are present as in all other countries, although the gradients are not as great as, for example, in the United Kingdom[108]. During the 1980s, however, smoking differentials by social class increased[109], and social class gradients for all cardiovascular risk factors have diminished among men but increased among women[110]. During the 1990s, however, mortality from cardiovascular disease decreased in all social groups[111].

The county councils were established in the 1860s, mainly to operate hospitals. Their health care tasks have expanded over time and, in the mid-1960s, they took over from central government the responsibility for outpatient and general practitioner services and psychiatric care. The Health and Medical Services Act of 1983 extended still further the areas of responsibility of the county councils. Health care now accounts for 85–90% of the total expenditure of most county councils. The Act requires county councils to plan the development and organisation of the health and medical care needs of the entire county population.

Responsibility for social welfare services and environmental health rests primarily with the municipalities, which number approximately 290 and have populations ranging from about 2500 to 750 000. Until recently private health care has existed only on a limited basis, with about 5% of physicians working full time in private practice.

Health and medical costs have increased very rapidly in recent decades, climbing during the last 15 years by 15–20% annually in current prices. The proportion of the GNP spent on health care reached a peak of 9.1% in 1983–84 but declined to 7.5% by 2000. Health and medical care is financed by proportional income taxes levied by the county councils; between 1960 and 2000 the average county tax increased from about 4.5% to 11% and these taxes now cover 60% of the health and medical care costs with the remainder coming from a variety of national government subsidies and funds.

The national government is responsible for ensuring that the health care system develops efficiently and in keeping with its overall objectives, based on the goals and the constraints of social welfare policy and macroeconomic factors. Central government administration is at two levels: the Ministry of Health and Social Affairs and the relatively independent administrative agencies, chiefly the National Board of Health and Welfare. This Board is involved in planning, monitoring and evaluating health and medical care, supervising the delivery of care and the performance of health care staff, and supervising health information programmes. In 1988 the Government appointed an advisory health policy group, the Public Health Group, to develop preventive health measures from a broad public health perspective. The Group served in an advisory capacity on these matters to the Government and to the Health and Medical Care Advisory Committee, which was established to coordinate matters of health and medical care between the Government and the Federation of County Councils. The Group's duties also included taking independent, executive action to expedite measures in the public sector for improving public health.

In 1991 the Public Health Group published a National Strategy For Health, which proposed a comprehensive strategy for public health with a particular emphasis on counteracting health inequalities through preventive and health promoting measures[112]. The Report endorsed the concept of 'sustainable development for health', in the same way as there is now a consensus on the importance of sustainable economic development. Unfortunately, the implications of this concept were not described. The Report suggested that public health efforts should be based increasingly on measures and programmes at the local level, particularly on those involving active citizen participation. The Public Health Group suggested that the combined government effort to promote health would be made more effective by introducing explicit goals related to public health and equality throughout the public sector. This would require both a review of pre-existing goals and the formulation of new goals and should be implemented in connection with the overhaul of the relevant legislation. An important step was the development of methods for assessing the health impact of decisions and integrating this assessment into government decision, making use, wherever possible, of budgetary directives. This was an important new role for public health professionals in Sweden.

The Public Health Group recommended the formation of a Public Health Fund to subsidise or finance jointly developmental activities within various programme areas. It was suggested that the fund could be financed by a special charge on products hazardous to health. The fund was established, but from general tax revenue. Following another recommendation of the Public Health Group, an Institute of Public Health was established in 1992 to develop, stimulate and support health promotion and disease prevention activities at the national level. The main aims of the National Institute of Public Health are to support local and regional public health efforts and to coordinate national efforts, develop research and disseminate information.

A 1995 Report by the Health Care and Medical Priorities Commission recommended that cost-efficient, population-based, preventive interventions of documented effectiveness be of second priority (behind acute health care, care for immediately life-threatening disorders, and the care of patients with severe suffering and palliative terminal care)[113]. The implications of these priority rankings for resource allocation could be profound and their implementation will, no doubt, be difficult. The Swedish approach to health care priorities is distinctive in that it is led by politicians and represents a consensus[114].

In 2002 the Swedish Parliament accepted for the first time a comprehensive national public health policy, which aims to strengthen health promotion and disease prevention initiatives, contribute to a reduction of health inequalities between groups and make health consequences an important consideration in all decision-making at every level of society[115]. The National Committee for Public Health was commissioned in 1997 to propose national goals for public health as well as strategies for achieving these goals. A number of experts and researchers within various areas collaborated on the development of these goals and 19 different expert-produced reports were published. During the 3 years of its work, the Committee fostered a broad discussion with the public and with politicians and civil servants at State and municipal level, with research workers, and with representatives of different organisations and trades. Furthermore, the Committee invited representatives of different organisations and popular movements to monitor the work actively.

As a basis for its proposals, the Committee used the series of national public health reports and in summarising the health trends, three issues were found to be particularly important:

- the steadily increasing life expectancy;
- the pattern of declining self-estimated good health among young people; and
- the remaining health gap between different social strata.

Contrary to many other national health policies, the Swedish health goals mainly address determinants of health[116]. The goals are directed to the level of society and culture and attempt to put health issues on the political as well as the social agenda. The Swedish public health vision is aiming at good health for all on equal terms. Each individual should be allowed opportunities to achieve the best state of health possible in an environment which promotes health for all while offering special support for those in need. The Committee has formulated six overall strategies, forming the basis for the national goals of public health: strengthening the social capital; growing-up in a satisfactory environment; improving conditions at work; creating a satisfactory physical environment; stimulating health-promoting life habits; and developing a satisfactory infrastructure for health. From these strategies, 18 public health goals were developed and arranged later into 11 target areas[117].

As we have seen, the framework for the practice of public health in Sweden has undergone considerable recent reorganisation. Although the major emphasis has been on personal medical care services, driven, as usual, by cost considerations, the recent overall strategic direction for public health is path breaking by international standards. The major challenge for public health in Sweden is to integrate national public health policies with the local delivery of public health services, which remain the responsibility of local authorities. Many county councils now have public health strategies, and the future of public health in Sweden depends to a large extent on whether the decentralised responsibilities can influence the public's health[118]. On the down side, the public health management capacity at county level is weak, the National Board of Health and Welfare is no longer responsible for the supervision of public health matters but is focused on traditional medical matters, and public health as a distinct medical speciality is threatened.

The evidence from other Scandinavian countries, for example, Finland, on the power of local public health activities, is another cause for optimism. In North Karelia, major gains in the prevention and control of cardiovascular diseases were made as a result of intensive and coordinated local programmes which were taken up nationally. There was a synergy between the national programmes and policies, but the local initiatives paved the way[119]. Local initiatives depend on the political persuasion of local governments and, even in a relatively small country like Sweden, there is a great variation in the emphasis given to public health among the counties. A real possibility as a result of the decentralisation of responsibility for public health, whether it be to states in the United States of America or to counties as in Sweden, is that variations among regions will increase. An ideal approach would combine strong and progressive national guidelines, appropriate legislation and intersectoral support, with local initiatives and responsibilities.

8.7 Public health in New Zealand

The British colonisation of New Zealand, which began in 1840, had a major influence on the evolution of public health, although this was tempered by the different social and political environment in New Zealand[120]. New Zealand has not experienced the problems associated with heavy industrialisation. As elsewhere, public health in nineteenth-century New Zealand was primarily concerned with quarantine and sanitary reform. There was a general reluctance, however, to acknowledge mounting health problems in the colony, and even epidemic outbreaks did not produce a sustained commitment to public health[121]. The Department of Public Health was established in 1901 in response to a plague scare and for a short time prevention was emphasised. In 1909, this Department was amalgamated with the Department of Hospitals and, increasingly, the focus shifted to hospital services, rather than to the health of the whole population.

The social security legislation introduced by New Zealand's first Labour government in 1938 marked the origins of a health care system that was funded primarily by tax revenue and initially provided services free of direct charges. The power of the medical profession prevented the establishment of a national health service. Hospitals and public health services were administered separately with strong central direction until 1989 when 14 area health boards were charged with integrating the public health services (disease prevention and health promotion) and hospital services on a regional basis. Each board had a contractual arrangement with the Minister of Health to provide a comprehensive and integrated range of curative and preventive services with the overall aim of improving the health of the local population. With the publication of the Government's Health Charter and National Health Goals and Targets in 1989, the health service for the first time began to plan coherently with a national focus but with devolved responsibility; priority was given to the reduction in inequalities in health status, especially the higher mortality and morbidity rates experienced by Maori, which have their origin in long-standing socio economic inequalities[122].

In 1990, and driven by concern with the perceived rising cost of health care, the newly elected conservative Government initiated radical changes to the health services[123]. These changes were one outcome of a voluntary, but radical, structural adjustment programme, which had been initiated in 1984 by the

Labour Government – despite its traditional social democratic philosophy[124]. The organisation and delivery of public health services in New Zealand went full circle in a 4-year period beginning in 1991. The major aims of the reforms were to introduce 'the market' into health services and to separate the purchasers of services from the providers.

The main proposal for public health was the separation of its funding and management from that of medical services. The Public Health Commission was established with responsibility for monitoring the state of public health, advising the Minister of Health on matters relating to public health, and for purchasing, or arranging for the purchase, of public health services. The justifications for the changes were the need to develop public health activities and to counter the diversion of resources from public health to medical services. After 2 years of preparation, the Public Health Commission was established formally in legislation in 1993 as a government agency outside the Ministry of Health. Public health services were purchased by the Public Health Commission with the four Regional Health Authorities (which replaced the 14 area health boards) acting as purchasing agencies at the regional level. Public health services were provided by the public health units of Crown Health Enterprises (the revamped hospitals) and other national providers, mostly non-governmental agencies.

The Public Health Commission had an independent board of seven directors, and a statutory obligation to consult with members of the public and professional groups. It embarked upon a process of consultation on a scale never previously attempted in New Zealand in the field of public health. The state of the public health in New Zealand was assessed thoroughly in two annual reports[125]; special reports focused on the health of Maori and Pacific Island people living in New Zealand[126]. Policy advice to the Minister was published in a series of documents. The Public Health Commission had its own budget, less than 3% of the total health budget, of which 93% was spent purchasing services and 7% on information and policy advice. By contrast, in 1980 public funding for public health services was 6.5% of the total health expenditure and 4.2% in 1986[127].

The most important, and in the end critical, feature of the new arrangement was that the Public Health Commission was at arm's length from the Government. This distance encouraged the development of public health advice from a position of semi-independence. The success of this semi-independence depended crucially on the support of the Minister of Health. In its short existence, the Public Health Commission reported to three consecutive Ministers of Health, and only the first was explicitly supportive of the Commission. In December 1994, after less than 2 years of formal existence, the Minister of Health announced plans to disestablish the Public Health Commission. The tasks of the Commission were taken over by the Ministry of Health in July 1995. The main reasons given for the change were the problems of coordination between medical and public health services and between non-regulatory and regulatory public health functions. It appears, however, that an underlying reason for the demise of the Commission was its semi-independent status as a Crown agency at arm's length from the Ministry. Despite the emphasis on 'contestable' advice in the market orientated health sector, the Government appeared uncomfortable receiving such advice from the Public Health Commission.

It is hard to escape the impression that a major reason the Commission was abolished was its tendency to provide the government with advice contrary to the interests of the powerful health-damaging interests in New Zealand, for example, the alcohol and tobacco industries[128]. The New Zealand experiment, with a Public Health Commission separate from the Ministry of Health, must be viewed as a failure[129]. The ultimate evidence of this failure is the premature ending of the Public Health Commission because its semi-independent nature was seen as a threat to the Government. The New Zealand experience suggests that the institutional base for such advice must be securely supported by all major political parties as well as by the public health community. Without strong support, the existence of semi-independent public health agencies will always be precarious.

The future of public health in New Zealand has improved since the election of a Labour Government in 1999. The main new reform is the integration of public health and primary health care services in New Zealand. This will present special challenges to the public health community, and there is a danger that public health activities may become localised and fragmented. There is considerable evidence of engagement with the concerns of the community, but public health is also constrained bureaucratically and sometimes at odds with powerful vested interest groups. Public health practitioners need to work outside established boundaries to respond to health inequalities and to the poor health of Maori. There remain tensions between technical and advocacy models, between enforcement and empowerment strategies, between professional and lay concepts of public health, and between State-sponsored and community-inspired agendas for action. Public health policy has evolved from a history of medical dominance to an accommodation of multiple interest groups, while public health practice has shifted similarly from a rather narrow to a much broader approach, which acknowledges diverse perspectives. There are some signs that a next stage may well be one of more integrative practice and a greater emphasis on investment for health, but much will depend on the cohesion of the public health professions.

8.8 Conclusions

This review of the recent history and current status of public health practice in five wealthy countries indicates that none has fully solved the problem of how best to organise and support public health services adequately; Sweden provides the best example. The current state of public health organisation and services is summarised subjectively for these five countries in Table 8.1. There is little relationship between the public health capacities and policies and the health status indicators. In none of these countries has the public health profession played a

Table 8.1. *The state of public health in five wealthy countries*

	United Kingdom	United States of America	Japan	Sweden	New Zealand
Public health status					
Life expectancy at birth[130]	77.7	77.0	81.0	79.7	77.6
Probability of surviving to age 65 [130]					
Male	81.5	77.4	84.0	84.8	80.9
Female	88.3	85.7	92.1	90.8	87.6
Probability of dying (per 1000)<5[131]					
Male	7	9	5	4	7
Female	6	7	4	3	6
Probability of dying (per 1000) between 15 and 59[131]					
Male	109	144	97	84	106
Female	69	83	47	54	68
Infant mortality rate[130]	6	7	4	3	6
Immunisation coverage DPT3 (%)[132]	94	94	85	99	92
Socio-economic indicators[130]					
Unemployment 2000 (%)	5.5	4.0	4.7	4.7	6.3
Ratio of income of highest 20% of households to lowest 20%	7.1	9.0	3.4	3.6	
Public health capacities					
Education	++	+++	+	+++	+++
Research	++	++	+	++	+
Professional organisations	+	+++	+	+	+
Public health policies					
National plan	Yes	Yes	No	Yes	Yes
Financial support	Low	Low	Low	Low	Low
Priority of prevention	Low	Low	Low	High	Low

Key: + + +strong, ++moderate, +weak.

central role in the recent health service reform debates. Where reorganisation of public health services has taken place, for example, in the United Kingdom and New Zealand, the process has not been driven by a primary concern with population health levels and the outcome has not been a general strengthening of the practice of public health.

The major gains in health status in Japan over the last few decades have not been due primarily to public health programmes. Rather, the driving force seems to have been economic growth and relative equality in income distribution. Specific features of Japanese society probably have also contributed, for example, the healthy diet and the supportive social networks, although even these are now under challenge from the recent period of severe economic slowdown. In the United Kingdom, public health has been dominated medically and close to clinical medicine and health services delivery. In the United States of America, the public health service has been distracted by its major responsibility for the delivery of medical services to the poor, and now by the focus on bioterrorism. Only in Sweden has the public health profession emerged as a strong advocate for a broad definition of public health with a focus on the social and economic determinants of health and disease. There are few positive lessons for poor countries from the current state of public health services in wealthy countries. Fortunately, there are important lessons to be learnt from several poor countries, as we see in the next chapter.

Chapter 8   Key points

- The health status of populations within wealthy countries varies, as do socio-economic indicators.
- There is no obvious relationship between the organisation and delivery of public health services and health status.
- In all five wealthy countries, public health services are of low priority compared with medical care services.
- In none of these countries have public health professionals emerged as key players in the health reform process.
- There are few positive lessons for poor countries from the current state of public health services in wealthy countries.

References

1. McKee, M. & Zatonski, W. Public health in eastern Europe and the former Soviet Union. In: Beaglehole, R. (ed.). *Global Public Health: A New Era*. Oxford: Oxford University Press, 2003.

2. Mackenbach, J.P. & Stronks, K. A strategy for tackling health inequalities in the Netherlands. *Br. Med. J.* 2002; **325**: 1029–32.

3. Powles, J.W. & Gifford, S. Health of nations: lessons from Victoria, Australia. *Br. Med. J.* 1993; **306**: 125–7.

4. Roemer, M.I. *National Health Systems of the World*, vol 1. New York: Oxford University Press, 1991.

5. Mosbech, J. Provision of public health services in Europe. In: Holland, W.W., Detels, R. & Knox, G. (eds.). *Oxford Textbook of Public Health: Influences of Public Health*. Oxford: Oxford University Press, 1991.

6. Beaglehole, R. (ed.). *Global Public Health: A New Era*. Oxford: Oxford University Press, 2003.

7. Rose, G. *The Strategy of Preventive Medicine*. Oxford: Oxford University Press, 1992.

8. Hamlin, C. State medicine in Great Britain. In: Porter, D. (ed.). *The History of Public Health and the Modern State*. Amsterdam: Editions Rodopi B.V., 1994.

9. Toynbee, P. *Hard Work: Life in Low Pay Britain*. London: Bloomsbury, 2003.

10. McKee, M. & Lang, T. Secret government: the Scott report. Links with industry cast doubt on the government's role in public health. *Br. Med. J.* 1996; **312**: 445–6.

11. Editorial. The Phillips report on BSE and vCJD. *Lancet* 2000; **356**: 1535.

12. Griffiths, S. Public health in the United Kingdom. In: Beaglehole, R. (ed.). *Global Public Health: A New Era*. Oxford: Oxford University Press, 2003.

13. Lewis, J. *What Price Community Medicine? The Philosophy, Practice and Politics of Public Health Since 1919*. Sussex: Wheatsheaf Books, 1986.

14. Madeley, R. Public health and paradigms. *J. Pub. Hlth Med.* 1993; **15**: 223–5.

15. Porter, D. How soon is now? Public health and the BMJ. *Br. Med. J.* 1990: **301**: 738-40.

16. *Report of the Royal Commission on Medical Education 1965–68*. London: HMSO Cmd, 3569, 1968.

17. Anon. Public health advocacy: unpalatable truths. *Lancet* 1995; **345**: 597–9.

18. Department of Health. Independent Inquiry into Inequalities in Health, Chair: Sir Donald Acheson. London: HMSO, 1998.

19. Committee of Inquiry into the Future Development of the Public Health Function. *Public Health in England*. London: HMSO, Cmd, 289, 1988.

20. Holland, W.W., Fitzsimons, B. & O'Brien, M. 'Back to the future' – public health research into the next century. *J. Pub. Hlth Med.* 1994; **16**: 4–10.

21. Budden, D. & McKee, M. Change and challenges – public health reporting in the United Kingdom. In: *The German Health Reporting System and Current Approaches in Europe*. Berlin: Robert Koch Institute, 2002: 99-102.

22. Fulop, N. & McKee, M. What impact do annual public health reports have? *Pub. Hlth* 1996; **110**: 307–11.

23. Sheldon, T.A. Formula fever: allocating resources in the NHS. *Br. Med. J.* 1997; **315**: 964.

24. Whitty, P. & Jones, I. Public health heresy: a challenge to the purchasing orthodoxy. *Br. Med. J.* 1992; **304**: 1039–41.

25. Griffiths, R. & McGregor, A. Public health services in the UK. In: Holland, W.W., Detels, R. & Knox, G. (eds.). *Oxford Textbook of Public Health: Influences of Public Health*. Oxford: Oxford University Press, 1991.

26. Milner, P. Unsettling times for public health. *J. Pub. Hlth Med.* 1994; **16**: 1–3.

27. Smith, R. *Health of a Nation: The BMJ View.* London: *British Medical Journal* 1991.
28. Fulop, N., Elston, J., Hensher, M., McKee, M. & Walters, R. Lessons for health strategies in Europe: the evaluation of a national health strategy in England. *Eur. J. Pub. Hlth* 2000; **10**: 11–17.
29. Department of Health. *The NHS Plan.* London: HMSO, 2000.
30. Department of Health. *Saving Lives: Our Healthier Nation.* London: HMSO, 1999.
31. Social Exclusion Unit. *A New Commitment to Neighbourhood Renewal: National Strategy and Action Plan.* London: HMSO, 2001.
32. McKee, M. Sex, drugs and rock and roll: Britain can learn lessons from Europe on the health of adolescents. *Br. Med. J.* 1999; **318**: 1300–1.
33. Turner, A. *Just Capital.* London: Macmillan, 2001.
34. World Health Organization Regional Office for Europe. *Targets for Health For All.* Copenhagen: World Health Organization, 1985.
35. World Health Organization. *The Health of Europe.* Copenhagen: WHO Regional Publications European Series No. 49, 1993.
36. World Health Organization Regional Office for Europe. *The European Health Report 2002.* Copenhagen: WHO Regional Publications, European Series, No. 97, 2002.
37. Field, M.G. The health crisis in the former Soviet Union: report from the 'post-war' zone. *Soc. Sci. Med.* 1995; **41**: 1469–78.
38. Chenet, L., McKee, M., Fulop, N. *et al.* Changing life expectancy in central Europe: is there a single reason? *J.Pub. Hlth Med.* 1996; **18**: 329–36.
39. Boys, R.J., Forster, D.P. & Jozan, P. Mortality from causes amenable and non-amenable to medical care: the experience of eastern Europe. *Br. Med. J.* 1991; **303**: 879–83.
40. Zatonski, W., McMichael, T. & Powles, J. Ecological study of reasons for sharp decline in mortality from ischaemic heart disease in Poland since 1991. *Br. Med. J.* 1998, **316**: 1047–51.
41. Jamrozik, K. A glimpse at public health in Eastern Europe. *Aust. J. Pub. Hlth* 1994; **19**: 102–3.
42. Rissel, C. Impressions of public health in Germany and Europe. *Aust. J. Pub. Hlth* 1994; **19**: 103–4.
43. Soros Foundation at http://www.soros.org/.
44. Gellert, G.A. & Kaznady, S.I. Melting the Iron Curtain: opportunities for public health collaboration through international joint ventures. *Br. Med. J.* 1991; **302**: 633–5.
45. Colomber, C., Lindstrom, B. & O'Dwyer, A. European training in public health. *Eur. J. Pub. Hlth* 1995; **5**: 113–15.
46. McKee, M., Bojan, F. & Normand, C. A new programme for public health training in Hungary. *Eur. J. Pub. Hlth* 1993; **3**: 60–5.
47. McKee, M., White, M., Bojan, F. & Østbye, T. Development of public health training in Hungary – an exercise in international co-operation. *J. Pub. Hlth Med.* 1995; **17**: 438–44.
48. Weindling, P. Public health in Germany. In: Porter, D. (ed.). *The History of Public Health and the Modern State.* Amsterdam: Editions Rodopi B.V., 1994.
49. Kolip, P. & Schott, T. The Postgraduate Public Health Training Programs in Germany. In: Laaser, U., de Leeuw, E. & Stock, C. (eds.). *Scientific Foundations for a Public Health Policy in Europe.* Weinheim: Juventa, 1995.

50. Ramsey, M. Public Health in France. In: Porter, D. (ed.). *The History of Public Health and the Modern State*. Amsterdam: Editions Rodopi B.V., 1994.
51. Ashton, J. Setting the agenda for health in Europe. *Br. Med. J.* 1992; **304**: 1643–4.
52. Allen, P. The Treaty of Maastricht and public health. *Hlth Trends* 1992; **24**: 5–6.
53. Joffe, M. Recent initiatives by the European Union. A new opportunity for promoting health. *Br. Med. J.* 1994; **308**: 610–11.
54. Commission of the European Communities. *Commission Communication on the Framework for Action in the Field of Public Health*. Brussels: Commission of the European Communities (LO3L93/559), 1993.
55. Rogers, A. Obstacle to EU public health initiative. *Lancet* 1995; **345**: 507.
56. Joossens, L. & Raw, M. Are tobacco subsidies a misuse of public funds? *Br. Med. J.* 1996; **312**: 832–5.
57. Green, D. & Griffith, M. *The Rough Guide to the CAP. A CAFOD Briefing*. London: CAFOD, 2002. http://www.cafod.org.uk/policy/roughguidetothecap 200209.shtml.
58. Expenditure FEOGA/EAGGF – communication from DG AGRI – Directorate E (Organisation of markets in specialised crops). In: *European Network for Smoking Prevention, Community Fund of Tobacco Research and Information*, ENSP Briefing Document, January 2002.
59. McCarthy, M.J. Public health in The new European Union research Programme. *J. Epidemiol. Commun. Hlth* 2003; **57**: 236-7.
60. Editorial. The EU's answer to future public health challenges. *Lancet* 2002; **359**: 229.
61. ASPHER. *Quality Improvement and Accreditation of Training Programmes in Public Health*. Lyon: Foundation Merieux-ASPHER, 2001.
62. Robbins, A. A Prague winter for public health. *Am. J. Pub. Hlth* 1995; **110**: 295–7.
63. Garrett, L. *The Betrayal of Trust: The Collapse of Global Public Health*. Oxford: Oxford University Press, 2001.
64. Horton, R. Bioterrorism: the extreme in public health. In: Beaglehole, R. (ed.). *Global Public Health: A New Era*. Oxford: Oxford University Press, 2003.
65. Johnston, D.C. Very richest's share of income grew even bigger, data shows. *New York Times*, 26 June 2003.
66. Fee, E. Public Health and the State: The United States. In: Porter, D. (ed.). *The History of Public Health and the Modern State*. Amsterdam: Editions Rodopi B.V., 1994.
67. Fee, E. The origins and development of public health in the United States. In: Holland, W.W., Detels, R. & Knox, G. (eds.). *Oxford Textbook of Public Health: Influences of Public Health*. Oxford: Oxford University Press, 1991.
68. Omenn, G.S. & Nathan, R.P. What's behind those block grants in health? *New Engl. J. Med.* 1982; **17**: 1057–60.
69. Reichman, L.B. How to ensure the continual resurgence of tuberculosis. *Lancet* 1996; **347**: 175.
70. Hinman, A.R. & Bradford, W.R. Public health services in the United States. In: Holland, W.W., Detels, R. & Knox, G. (eds.). *Oxford Textbook of Public Health: Influences of Public Health*. Oxford: Oxford University Press, 1991.
71. Roper, W.L., Baker, E.L. Dyal, W.W. & Nicola, R.M. Strengthening the public health system. *Pub. Hlth Rep.* 1992; **107**: 609–15.

72. McGinnis, J.M. Health in America – the sum of its parts. *J. Am. Med. Assoc.* 2002; **287**: 2711–12.
73. Lalonde, M. *A New Perspective on the Health of Canadians.* Ottawa: National Health and Welfare, 1974.
74. McGinnis, J.M. Setting objectives for public health in the 1990s: experience and prospects. *Ann. Rev. Pub. Hlth* 1990; **11**: 231–49.
75. US Department of Health and Human Services. *Healthy People 2010.* Washington, DC: US Department of Health and Human Services, 2000.
76. Committee for the Study of the Future of Public Health. *The Future of Public Health.* Washington: National Academy Press, 1988.
77. Trevinor, F.M. & Jacobs, J.P. Public health and health care reform: the American Public Health Association's perspective. *J. Pub. Hlth Pol.* 1994; **15**: 397–406.
78. Miller, C.A., Brookes, E.F., DeFriese, G.H., Gilbert, B., Jain, S.C. & Kavaler, F. A. survey of local public health departments and their directors. *Am. J. Pub. Hlth* 1977; **67**: 931–9.
79. Brumback, C.L. The IOM Report, the future of public health. *J. Pub. Hlth Pol.* 1990; **11**: 106–9.
80. Annas, G.J. Back to the future: the IOM Report reconsidered. *Am. J. Pub. Hlth* 1991; **81**: 835–7.
81. Fox, D.M. AIDS and the American health policy: the history and prospects of a crisis of authority, *Millbank Mem. Fund Q.* 1986; **64**: 733.
82. Frances D.P. Toward a comprehensive HIV prevention program for the CDC and the nation. *J. Am. Med. Assoc.* 1992; **268**: 1444–7.
83. Kuller, L.H. & Kingsley, L.A. The epidemic of AIDS: a failure of public health policy. *Milbank Mem. Fund Q.* 1986; **64**: 56–78.
84. Harrell, J. & Baker, E. *The Essential Services of Public Health.* Washington, DC: American Public Health Association, 1997.
85. Scutchfield, F.D., Beversdorf, C.A., Hiltabiddle, S.E. *et al.* A survey of state health department compliance with the recommendations of the Institute of Medicine report: The Future of Public Health. *J. Pub. Hlth Pol.* 1997; **18**: 13–29.
86. Scutchfield, F.D., Hiltabiddle, S.E., Rawding, N. *et al.* Compliance with the recommendations of the Institute of Medicine report: The Future of Public Health: a survey of local health departments. *J. Pub. Hlth Pol.* 1997; **18**: 155-66.
87. National Association of County and City Health Officials. 2001. MAPP Project, available at http://nacchoweb.naccho.org/MAPP_Home.asp.
88. Institute of Medicine. *Who Will Keep the Public Healthy? Educating Public Health Professionals* for the 21st Century. Washington, D.C.: The National Academic Press; 2002.
89. Institute of Medicine. *The Future of the Public's Health in the 21st Century.* Washington, D.C.: The National Academic Press; 2003.
90. Hurt, R.D. & Robertson, C.R. Prying open the door to the tobacco industry's secrets about nicotine. The Minnesota Tobacco Trial. *J. Am. Med. Assoc.* 1998; **280**: 1173–81.
91. Mitka, M. Smoke and mirrors. *J. Am. Med. Assoc.* 2001; **285**: 1008.
92. Campaign for Tobacco-Free Kids. Special Report. State Tobacco Settlement. http://tobaccofreekids.org/reports/settlements/.

93. McKinlay, J.B. & Marceau, L.D. Upstream healthy public policy: lessons from the battle of tobacco. *Int. J. Hlth Serv.* 2000; **30**: 49–69.
94. Navarro, V. The future of public health in health care reform. *Am. J. Pub. Hlth* 1994; **84**: 729–30.
95. Susser, E. & Susser, M. The aftermath of September 11: what's an epidemiologist to do?. *Int. J. Epidemiol.* 2002; **31**: 719–21.
96. Marmot, M.G. & Davey-Smith, G. Why are the Japanese living longer? *Br. Med. J.* 1989; **299**: 1547–51.
97. Tatara, K. The origins and development of public health in Japan. In: Holland, W.W., Detels, R. & Knox, G. (eds.). *Oxford Textbook of Public Health. Influences of Public Health.* Oxford: Oxford University Press, 1991.
98. Koizumi, A. Development of public health in Japan. *Asian Med. J.* 1982; **25**: 14–20.
99. Healthy Japan 21. http://www.mhlw.go.jp/english/org/policy/p10-11.html.
100. Tatara, K., Shinsho, F., Suzuki, M., Takatorige, T., Nakanisch, N. & Kuroda, K. Relation between use of health checkups by middle aged adults and demand for inpatient care by elderly adults in Japan. *Br. Med. J.* 1991; **302**: 615–18.
101. Lundberg, O. & Palme, J. A balance sheet for welfare: Sweden in the 1990s. *Scand. J. Pub. Hlth* 2002; **30**: 241–3.
102. Lundberg, O., Diderichsen, F. & Yngwe, M.A. Changing health inequalities in a changing society? Sweden in the mid-1980s and mid-1990s. *Scand. J. Pub. Hlth* 2001, Suppl **55**: 31–9.
103. Wall, S., Persson, G. & Weinehall, L. Public health in Sweden: facts, vision and lessons. In: Beaglehole, R. (ed.). *Global Public Health: A New Era.* Oxford: Oxford University Press, 2003.
104. Ham, C. Reforming the Swedish health services. *Br. Med. J.* 1994; **308**: 219–20.
105. Glennerster, H. & Matsaganis, M. The English and Swedish health care reforms. *Int. J. Hlth Serv.* 1994; **24**: 231–51.
106. Johannisson, K. The people's health: public health policies in Sweden. In: Porter, D. (ed.). *The History of Public Health and the Modern State.* Amsterdam: Editions Rodopi B.V., 1994.
107. Adami, H.-O. A paradise for epidemiologists? *Lancet* 1996; **347**: 588–9.
108. Leon, D., Vågerö, D. & Otterblad Olausson P. Social class differences in infant mortality in Sweden. A comparison with England and Wales. *Br. Med. J.* 1992; **305**: 687–91.
109. Rosen, M., Hanning, M. & Wall, S. Changing smoking habits in Sweden: towards better health but not for all. *Int. J. Epidemiol.* 1990; **19**: 316–22.
110. Branström, I. A cardiovascular community intervention project in Northern Sweden, PhD thesis. University of Umeå, Sweden, 1994.
111. National Committee for Public Health. Health in Sweden – The National Public Health Report 2001. *Scand. J. Pub. Hlth* 2001, Suppl. **58**.
112. The Public Health Group. *A National Strategy for Health: Summary Report Series No. 13.* Stockholm: Public Health Group, 1991.
113. The Ministry of Health and Social Affairs. *Priorities in Health Care. Ethics, Economy, Implementation.* Stockholm: Swedish Parliamentary Priorities Commission, 1995.
114. McKee, M. & Figueras, J. Setting priorities: can Britain learn from Sweden? *Br. Med. J.* 1996; **312**: 691–4.

115. Health on Equal Terms – national goals for public health. *Scand. J. Pub. Hlth 2001*, Suppl **57**: 1–68.

116. Pearson, T.A. Scandinavia's lessons to the world of public health. *Scand. J. Pub. Hlth* 2002: **28**: 161–3.

117. Ministry of Health and Social Affairs. *Public Health Objectives*. Fact Sheet No 2. Stockholm: Ministry of Health, January 2003.

118. Ovretveit, J. Purchasing for health gain: the problems and prospects for purchasing for health gain in the 'managed markets' of the NHS and other European health systems. *Eur. J. Pub. Hlth* 1993; **3**: 77–84.

119. Puska, P., Tuomilehto, J., Nissinen, A. & Vartiainen, E. *The North Karelia Project. 20 Year Results and Experiences*. Helsinki: National Public Health Institute (KTL), 1995.

120. Davis, P. & Lin, V. Public health in Australia and New Zealand. In: Beaglehole, R. (ed.). *Global Public Health: A New Era*. Oxford: Oxford University Press, 2003.

121. Bryder, L. A New World? Two hundred years of public health in Australia and New Zealand. In: Porter, D. (ed.). *The History of Public Health and the Modern State*. Amsterdam: Editions Rodopi B.V., 1994.

122. Beaglehole, R. & Davis, P. Setting national health goals and targets in the context of a fiscal crisis: the politics of social choice in New Zealand. *Int. J. Hlth Serv.* 1992; **22**: 417–28.

123. Salmond, G., Mooney, G. & Laugesen, M. Introduction to health care reform in New Zealand. *Hlth Policy* 1994; **24**: 1–3.

124. Kelsey, J. *The New Zealand Experiment: A World Model for Structural Adjustment?* Auckland: Auckland University Press, 1995.

125. Public Health Commission. *Our Health, Our Future: The State of Public Health in New Zealand*. Wellington: Public Health Commission, 1993 and 1994.

126. Public Health Commission. *The Health of Pacific Islands People in New Zealand*. Wellington: Public Health Commission, 1994.

127. Muthumal, D. & McKendry, C.G. *Health Expenditure Trends in New Zealand, 1980–92*. Wellington: Ministry of Health, 1993.

128. Barnett, P. & Malcolm, L. To integrate or de-integrate? Fitting public health into New Zealand's reforming health system. *Eur. J. Pub. Hlth* 1998; **8**: 79–86.

129. Armstrong, W. & Bandaranayake, D. *Public Health in New Zealand: Recent Changes and Future Prospects*. Monograph No 1. Department of Public Health, Wellington School of Medicine, 1995.

130. United Nations Development Programme. Human Development Report. *Deepening Democracy in a Fragmented World*. Geneva: World Health Organization, 2002.

131. World Health Organization. *World Health Report. Reducing Risks, Promoting Healthy Life*. Geneva: World Health Organization, 2002.

132. www.who.int/vaccines-surveillance.

9

Public health organisation and practice in poor countries

9.1 Introduction

Poor countries demonstrate tremendous diversity from a public health perspective. Some, such as China and Cuba, have shown remarkable improvements in health status over a few decades. Others, especially in sub-Saharan Africa, lag far behind the rest of the world. Many of the poorer countries have suffered recent economic setbacks which have had negative impacts on health. In this chapter, the organisation and delivery of public health activities are described and analysed in China, Cuba and the state of Kerala in India. These countries are success stories in that they each made major health gains and offered hope for other countries striving to find health at low cost[1,2]. However, all these countries have suffered major set backs over the last decade. This chapter ends with a discussion of the role of international agencies in promoting public health in Africa, the region most in need of effective public health programmes.

9.2 China: public health a political priority – but faltering progress

The evolution of public health in China has, from a global perspective, more importance than developments in most other countries. With an estimated population in 2000 of 1.3 billion, China accounts for over 20% of the world's population and almost one-third of the population living in poor countries.

The history of public health in China over the last half century is a cause for cautious optimism, although more recent changes raise many questions and concerns[3]. Since 1949, when the People's Republic of China was established, social and economic changes have led to dramatic improvements in the health status of the Chinese people. Life expectancy more than doubled

227

from 32 years in 1950 to 71 years in 1998[3]. China's success in improving the health of its people far exceeds what could be expected at its stage of economic development, raising interesting questions about the relationships between development and health. Much of China's success has been attributed to the national health system and to improvements in the provision of safe water and sanitation, nutrition, education (especially of women), and to family planning services[2].

Chinese medicine is probably the world's oldest body of continuous medical knowledge, with a history of over 4000 years of observation and theory[4]. Many Chinese discoveries predated Western discoveries. For example, by the beginning of the sixteenth century the Chinese had discovered the value of variolation for the prevention of the more serious, naturally acquired, form of smallpox. From China the technique was brought to Turkey and then to England at the beginning of the eighteenth century.

The outbreak of pneumonic plague in Manchuria in 1911 advanced the cause of western medicine in China; the Peking Union Medical College was established in 1916 with support from the Rockefeller Foundation. At this time, there were no national or municipal health services in China. A programme in public health was developed at the Peking Union Medical College and between 1924 and 1942 trained (in English) 313 graduates. The most impressive aspect of this public health work was a rural health programme in Tingxian. This scheme, although having little impact on the health of the villages because of the widespread poverty, was ahead of its time in training village health workers.

The health challenges facing the new People's Republic of China in 1949 were staggering. Preventive medicine, despite its honourable tradition, was nonexistent in most of China, and modern therapeutic medicine was unavailable in rural areas where 85% of China's population lived. Four basic guidelines for the organisation of health care were specified at the first National Health Congress in 1950:

- Medicine should serve the workers, peasants and soldiers;
- Preventive medicine should take precedence over therapeutic medicine;
- Chinese traditional medicine should be integrated with western medicine; and
- Health work should be combined with mass movements.

The last principle was put into action with dramatic effect[5]. One of the best known of many campaigns was aimed at eliminating the 'four pests', originally defined, although not in all areas, as flies, mosquitoes, rats and grain-eating sparrows. When the elimination of sparrows appeared to be unsound ecologically, other pests were substituted[4]. Campaigns against specific diseases were also mounted, for example, against schistosomiasis.

The basic concept of the mass health campaigns was the involvement of people in dealing with important health problems, a foreshadowing of the Ottawa Charter concept of empowerment within the constraints of Chinese society. The first campaign was launched in 1951, and over the next 30 years there were an average of four or five campaigns a year. These campaigns were conducted under the leadership of the 'National Patriotic Health Campaigns Committee' and required an effective political, administrative and economic network, and unpaid volunteer labour. Although the mass campaigns were dramatic, the rapid expansion of health services infrastructure also contributed to the control of epidemic and endemic infections[6]. The key organisations were the anti-epidemic stations, which became the best staffed and organised component of the public health service. These units had responsibility for all aspects of disease monitoring and control.

China made considerable progress in the 1950s and 1960s in solving the problems of infectious disease epidemics and in the provision of safe water and sanitation. Progress was not linear. A major famine in 1958–61, due to policies that de-emphasised the rural sector and encouraged urban growth, and adverse climatic factors that resulted in a dramatic decline in grain output, was responsible for up to 30 million premature deaths[7]. This was the largest famine in human history and went almost unrecognised outside China; major international relief aid was not attempted or even requested. A similar, but less destructive, period of disruption took place during the Cultural Revolution of the late 1960s.

In the first decades of the People's Republic of China, there was an ongoing tension between the Communist Party leadership and the professionals within the Ministry of Public Health (MPH). This tension resulted in a fragmentation of responsibility for health care, which was most apparent during the Great Leap Forward (1957–58). Health services, however, remained almost entirely in the public sector and curative and preventive care were closely integrated. Of overriding importance in the rapid improvements in health status in China was the attention given to increasing literacy and the provision of adequate housing and nutrition, all based, at least in principle, on the notion of collective responsibility.

China has now experienced four decades of communist leadership inspired by Mao Zedong, and almost three decades of economic and structural reform since his death in 1976. The latest period of reform has improved living standards for many Chinese, although death rates differ markedly between urban and rural areas[8], with a substantial burden of sickness and premature death being especially apparent in poor rural areas. The recent reforms, however, have dismantled much of the health and medical system inspired by the early Chinese leadership, including the cooperative medical system in rural areas and the 'barefoot doctor' system[9–11]. In most rural areas, health care has shifted to a fee-for-service system, although urban residents are generally covered by a state insurance system because of work-related benefits[12]. The modernisation reforms of the 1980s encouraged all institutions to generate revenues, including public health institutions, which resulted in an increase in the share of service charges from 27% in 1984 to 53% in 1994. This reduced the demand for, and utilisation of, preventive services. The immunisation coverage rate dropped from 75% in 1979 to 39% between 1984 and 1986[13]. Preventive services suffered as the privatisation process pushed 'barefoot doctors' to focus on curative services; maternal and child services were especially at risk.

Ageing of the population represents a major challenge for China, with 10% of the population in 2002 over 65 years of age. The family planning policy of one-child families has major long-term ramifications for the future care and support of the elderly, especially in rural areas. China's experience shows that population growth can be controlled rapidly, although this required coercive measures in the 1970s and early 1980s. In 1979 the one child per family policy was introduced because the birth rate was again increasing. Public compliance with the policy has been strong, but it remains to be seen if the stated goal of stabilising the population at about 1.3 billion is attainable; the population growth rate in major cities is now below replacement level. Another major health challenge facing China is the emerging non-communicable disease epidemics, especially the tobacco-induced epidemics. It has been projected that there will be over two million smoking-related deaths each year by the year 2025[14]. An important environmental issue is the heavy pollution of many Chinese cities, from both industrial and household sources.

The control of sexually transmitted diseases (STDs) was one of the triumphs of the first public health revolution. STDs began to re-emerge in the early 1980s, with the 'opening up' of China, although there was no longer a formal reporting system. The first case of HIV was identified in 1985 and was considered an imported case. The development of HIV/AIDS in China is characterised by three stages: from the mid-1980s to 1988, there were sporadic, imported cases amongst foreign travellers in coastal provinces; from 1989 to 1993, following the identification of 146-HIV-positive drug users in Yunnan, there was geographically limited spread; and from 1994 there has been sharp rise among drug users and in sexually transmitted HIV, and beyond Yunnan to Sichuan (1995), Xinjiang (1996), and Guangxi (1997). AIDS related to blood transfusion and blood products emerged in the late 1990s as a result of impoverished villagers and migrant workers earning money from blood donation. It has been estimated that there were about 600 000 HIV-positive individuals in China at the end of 2000. If no effective interventions take place in China, UNAIDS estimates that there may be as many as 6 million testing HIV-positive by the year 2005 and more than 10 million by the year 2010[15].

Chinese health policy has been remarkably consistent in providing substantial resources for health. Total health expenditure has increased from 3.5% of GDP in 1990 to 5.33% of GDP in 2000[16]. The proportion of government expenditure has, however, declined while individual out-of-pocket expenditure has increased, reflecting a shift in emphasis to curative care. The share of public health services in total government budget has decreased from 12.4% in 1980 to 10.6% in 1995[13] and this may reflect government emphasis on development of hospitals at county and above levels during this period. None the less, appropriate training and multisectoral and integrated policies have been emphasised despite the challenges from broader economic reforms. Much preventive medicine in China is organised vertically, with central responsibility for specific disease control programmes. Separate programmes are all administered by the epidemic prevention stations of the provincial and county health bureaux and this encourages integration across the programmes, particularly in rural areas. Control of the non-communicable disease epidemics will require strong government leadership, comprehensive policies and programmes and changes in the training of health personnel. Inevitably, the success of the preventive efforts has increased the demand for curative care. The preventive approach is not as prominent with non-communicable diseases as it was with communicable diseases, although smoking control programmes are being initiated belatedly; the establishment of a new Centre for Non-communicable Diseases, within the National Centre for Disease Control, suggests that non-communicable diseases prevention programs will now move vertically downwards to all levels. Furthermore, new policy initiatives to develop community health services across China are likely to reinstate and re-emphasise the importance of primary care and the integration of public health and primary care approaches.

It is too early to assess the impact of the continuing social and economic reforms on public health in China, although the available evidence is not encouraging[13]. The approach adopted by the Chinese to the new public health problems, especially the non-communicable diseases and the emergence of HIV/AIDS, will be of great interest. The priority given to health in the early post-revolutionary era and the willingness to allocate resources to effective programmes, along with economic gains, had a huge impact on the health of Chinese. This occurred principally by reducing infectious diseases mortality and controlling population growth. The recent experience with the epidemic of severe acute respiratory syndrome (SARS), which originated in south China in late 2002, exposes the neglect of the public health infrastructure[17]. After more than a decade of focusing on economic growth rather than on the social infrastructure, the provincial health care systems are far less capable of coping with new epidemics of infectious diseases than before. The rapid economic development over the past 20 years, the accelerated pace of industrialisation and urbanisation, and the widening of the income gap between population groups, will determine the current and future health needs of the Chinese population. A sustainable and successful approach to these challenges will require the incorporation of the underlying social, cultural and economic factors into public health interventions and strong government and public health leadership.

9.3 Cuba: public health at all cost

Cuba is home to about 11 million people and possesses some of the most favourable health indicators in the Americas. Cuba's overall achievements in health, education and general social and economic development since the overthrow of the old regime in 1959 have been remarkable. These successes are all the more impressive in the face of the enduring opposition of the United States of America which has, amongst other tactics, maintained a trade blockade, including an embargo on food and medicine. This embargo has been described as 'a war against public health with high human costs'[18]. The Cuban experience is another indication that population health status can be improved early on in the process of 'development'.

Some of Cuba's success can be attributed to the support of the former Soviet Union. More important, however, has been the priority given to health by the Cuban government. Public health according to President Castro 'became a challenge and a battleground between imperialism (United States of America) and ourselves, . . . and this multiplied our efforts. That is why we have developed this field and are striving to become a medical power with the best possible health indices'[19].

Cuba's achievements are now under severe threat. The tightening United States trade embargo, the collapse of the main trading partners in Central and Eastern Europe, and natural disasters, have created a situation of increasing scarcity[20]. This situation threatens not only the health system, and the health of all Cubans, but perhaps even the government itself. Cuba is now in a period of uncertainty, which will inevitably have adverse health effects. These threats highlight Cuba's public health achievements over the last four decades.

The trade embargo of the United States of America was first imposed in 1960 and since then has been implemented to varying degrees[21]. The United States 'Cuban Democracy Act of 1992' reimposed third-country sanctions that had been rescinded in 1975, thus prohibiting United States subsidiaries in other countries from trading with Cuba. Of the various factors causing difficulty for Cuba in the 1990s, the embargo is the only deliberate factor and is the only one that could, in the interests of the health of Cubans, be easily reversed. Unfortunately, the prospects for such a reversal are slim, at least in the short term.

The extent of Cuba's achievement in health are reflected in the health statistics, which are now considered reliable[19]. In 1960, life expectancy at birth was 64 years and the infant mortality rate (IMR) was 65 per 1000 live births. In 2001, life expectancy at birth had increased to 77 years, the infant mortality rate was 7.2 per 1000 live births and the probability of dying under the age of 5 years was down to 11 for males and 8 for females per 1000[22]. By comparison, life expectancy at birth in the United States of America was also 77 years in 2001 and the probability of dying under the age of 5 years was 9 for males and 7 for females per 1000[23]. So at least in terms of life expectancy, Cuba has reached its goal of parity with the United States and Cuba now ranks among the 25 countries in the world with the lowest infant mortality[24]. It remains to be seen how long this equality will be maintained in the face of the social and economic problems now facing Cuba. The health advances have been achieved despite the poverty of Cuba. Cuba's GNP per capita, adjusted by purchasing power parity, was estimated to be 1692 international dollars in 1998 (USA's was 29 240). In terms of income inequality, the median value of the ratio of the richest to the poorest population quintile (the 20/20 income ratio) during the 1990's decade was 5.0 for Cuba and 10.7 for USA[23]. Even under the most difficult economic constraints, the Cuban government has made health a top priority, both because of its concern for Cubans and for symbolic reasons.

Despite Cuba's success in the health field, it is unlikely that other poor countries will wish, or have the resources, to emulate Cuba's health systems. Cuba developed a health system in which primary health care was based on the central role of physicians. Furthermore, there has been a strong emphasis on expensive technology. This approach could be developed only under a political system in which decision making was highly centralised and planned and in which health commanded a high level of resources. A central directive from President Castro established a School of Medicine in each province and led to the production of a 'physician surplus' that is over 58 doctors per 10 000 population, the highest in the world. Part of this surplus is directed to international cooperation (2600 Cuban doctors are presently working in international medical missions) and part is channelled through extending family, community, labour doctors and other medical schemes[25,26].

Primary health care in Cuba was based initially on polyclinic teams of physicians and nurses and other health workers, which provided services for a defined population of between 25 000 and 30 000 people. The teams worked to guidelines established by the Ministry of Public Health, and the collection and standardisation of high quality statistical data on the population has been encouraged. The teams were to focus on prevention, but in practice there was too little time for preventive work[19]. In an effort to solve this and other problems with primary health care, the Cuban Government established the Family Doctor Programme as the central component of the medical system, beginning with a pilot project in 1984. This programme aimed to integrate primary health care with the community by putting a doctor and nurse team on every city block and in every rural community. A central task of the team is to monitor the health of the entire population, not just the sick, with each team responsible for between 120 and 150 families or about 600–700 people[19]; in most poor countries this ratio would be much greater.

By 1991, the Family Doctor Programmes scheme covered over 60% of the population. The primary health care system now comprises 31 000 doctors and nurses organised in a network that encompasses 442 polyclinics, 64 rural hospitals, and some 22 000 family doctor clinics. For every 15 to 20 family doctor and nurse teams (the so-called basic health care teams) there is a basic provider group (of which there are 969 nation-wide), formed by specialists in internal medicine, paediatrics, gynaecology and obstetrics, and psychology, in addition to technical experts in public health and epidemiology, statistics and social work. As at the end of 2000, 99.1% of the Cuban population was covered by the health care system[22,23].

The major causes of death and disease in Cuba are now the non-communicable diseases, especially heart disease and cancer. A focus of the Family Doctor Programme is, therefore, on non-communicable disease risk factors, especially smoking, obesity, nutrition and physical inactivity. The top priority of the Family Doctor Programme has been the use of health education and popular participation in the implementation of health programmes. Health education takes place through lectures and the media, as well as at the individual level. To combat physical inactivity, the government promoted individual and group exercises and sports. One of the few benefits of the economic crisis of the 1990s was the increase in regular physical activity as a result of fuel shortages.

High levels of smoking present particular problems for the Cuban government because tobacco is an important export crop. Cuba is the second largest producer of tobacco in Latin America, after Brazil, and tobacco is second to sugar as a source of foreign exchange. In 1970, half the adult population (15 years and over) smoked regularly (two-thirds of men and one-third of women). In 1980, the pattern was unchanged despite the encouragement of non-smoking since 1960. The most recent campaign began in 1986 and was assisted by a reduction in the availability of tobacco products in the early 1990s as part of the economic austerity programme. By 1995, 37% of the adult population was reported to be smoking regularly (48% of men and 26% of women)[27]. As in other countries, smoking is more prevalent among people with the least education, although the gradients are less than in many rich countries[28].

Mass participation in public health programmes in Cuba has been used to great effect. For example, the campaign against haemorrhagic dengue fever in the early 1980s relied for its success on mass participation to eradicate the mosquito vector. Few other countries, apart from China, have demonstrated such an ability to mobilise the population to combat epidemic disease.

The public health approach to non-communicable disease prevention adopted by the Cuban Government raises interesting questions[29]. In particular, there are many similarities between the emphasis on health education of individuals in Cuba and in most other countries. The anti-smoking campaign, for example, focuses on education and information, but not apparently on other important policy instruments such as taxation, although cigarettes have not been advertised in Cuba since 1960. Since 1971, tobacco has been marketed in two ways: on the rationed market, where the prices are kept low, and on the open market where prices are high. It is forbidden to sell cigarettes to people under the age of 16 years[28]. Recently, legislative reforms have been introduced to restrict smoking in public places. The Cuban approach to disease prevention, involving health education and mass participation, is more equitable than in other countries because of the relatively equal distribution of goods and services in Cuba. Power in Cuba still resides firmly with the Government, although much responsibility for health is devolved to the citizens.

The difficulties faced by the Cuban Government in providing adequate food and services for the people will lead to questioning of the Government's legitimacy. In some ways, it is a surprise that the Government has survived for so long after the collapse of its trading partners in Central and Eastern Europe. No doubt its long success in meeting the health needs of the people is part of the explanation for the Government's ability to maintain control. In the meantime, the humanitarian crisis has been averted because the Government has maintained a high level of budgetary support for the health care system[24]. The official US position is that the fundamental problem in Cuba is the 'Government's allegiance to economic and political doctrines that have failed elsewhere'[30].

One manifestation of the difficulties faced by Cuba was the epidemic of optic and peripheral neuropathy in 1992–1993, which affected approximately 50 000 people, about 0.5% of the population[31]. The *proximal* cause of the Cuban epidemic neuropathy is believed to be a toxic–metabolic one: micronutrient deficiency associated with an increased or excessive metabolic demand for thiamine and other B-group vitamins. The hardening of the US economic and commercial embargo, the impact of the Soviet dissolution on the Cuban economy and on its food supply were, on the other hand, *distal* causes or macrodeterminants of that epidemic situation[32–34]. Most patients were adults – mostly farmers – between the ages of 15 and 65 years, suggesting that children and old people were protected by their larger rations of milk and eggs[35]. In typical Cuban fashion, a massive mobilisation of resources was undertaken to deal with the epidemic, including experts from the United States of America. Beginning in May 1993, the entire population received multi-vitamin tablets daily to overcome the possible nutritional deficiency and the epidemic rapidly subsided[31]. Even though the adverse health consequences of the US embargo on the Cuban population go beyond the epidemic neuropathy, the US policy remains resistant to public health concerns[33].

It is unlikely that the unique health system built up over the last three and a half decades will survive if the Government should fall. If the Cuban health and social system crumbles, the health of Cubans will deteriorate and health inequalities increase, perhaps on the same scale as occurred in Central and Eastern Europe following the collapse of the Soviet Union.

9.4 Kerala State: public health at low cost – but faltering progress

Kerala, a state in the south west of India, is discussed because of the contrast it provides with the rest of the Indian subcontinent. The health of Keralites is considerably better than might be expected, based on the enduring poverty of the state. The public health situation of Kerala is all the more remarkable when it is put into the context of India as a whole.

Modern public health in India is influenced strongly by the colonial experience. The system is geared to the priorities of the Government and is remote from the bulk of the population and inappropriate to many of their needs[36]. The provision of public health services in British India grew out of, and continued to be shaped by, anxieties aroused by the Indian mutiny of 1857. The strong driving force was the unhealthy state of the British troops[37,38]. The public health infrastructure evolved as one response to these concerns, but the emphasis was always on the needs of the military. Although the British believed they had done much to improve the health of Indians, there was a huge gap between the rhetoric and the reality[36]. This pattern was repeated by other colonising nations[39].

Despite British rule, India continued to be ravaged by major epidemics, which led to negative population growth; between 1896 and 1914 bubonic plague killed over eight million people; malaria and tuberculosis killed more than twice as many over a similar period and the influenza epidemic of 1918–19 was even more devastating. The plague epidemic evoked fear and panic not caused by other epidemics[40], especially as control measures had little impact on the epidemic. By its inaction in the face of these epidemics, the colonial government missed the opportunity of adopting a broad public health approach based on sanitary measures, which was used successfully in many other countries[38]. By contrast, the plague outbreak of 1994 was more remarkable for the fear it generated, rather than for the deaths caused[41,42], although the root cause was the same[43].

The reasons for the slow progress with public health in India were many[37]. British rule had itself created many health problems. For example, the military expeditions of the early nineteenth century contributed to the spread of cholera, and agricultural developments disrupted traditional systems of drainage, exposing large tracts of the country to malaria. Furthermore, there was little consensus among colonial officials concerning medical policy in India. Medical experts contributed to the disagreements; the longstanding dispute over the control of malaria (mosquito eradication and general sanitation vs. quinine prophylaxis) prevented vigorous action[38,44].

Improvements in public health in British India depended on resources and cooperation between colonial officials and Indians. Neither the government nor key sections of the local population demonstrated the necessary long-term commitment to the provision of effective sanitary measures[40]. Public health in India under British rule must be judged a failure, with only Europeans and a small sector of the Indian urban population receiving benefits. Unfortunately, this legacy persists[36]. A slowing of the infant mortality rate in India has been observed in recent years; the IMR in India as a whole was 68 per 1000 live births in 2001, equivalent to that reached by Kerala 40 years ago (Table 9.1).

Kerala State was formed in 1956 by integrating the princely states of Travancore and Cochin with the Malabar district of the former Madras Presidency. The former two states traditionally had considered the provision of health care facilities a primary duty of the Maharajah. The northern part of Kerala, previously part of Madras, lagged behind the rest of the state in health status. Infant mortality, for example, in the north of Kerala was about twice as high as the rest of

Table 9.1. *Literacy rates, infant mortality rates, and life expectancy at birth, Kerala and India, 1961–2001*[45,46]

	Kerala					India				
	1961	1971	1981	1991	2001	1961	1971	1981	1991	2001
Literacy rates (%)										
Men	65	77	85	94	91	34	40	—	53	76
Women	39	54	66	87	80	13	18	25	32	54
Infant mortality rates										
Per 1000 live births	66	61	37	17[a]	14	114	138	119	83	68
Life expectancy at birth										
Males	46.2	60.5	60.6	66.9	69.9	41.9	46.4	54.1	60.6	59.7
Females	50.0	61.1	62.1	72.8	75.5	40.6	44.7	54.7	61.7	60.9

[a] 1992.

Kerala in 1956[47]. Of great interest is the extension to the whole of Kerala of the policies, which had been successful in Travancore and Cochin and which produced similar outcomes within 35 years[47].

In 2000, Kerala's population was 32 million, under 4% of India's total[48]. For many years Kerala has differed markedly from the rest of India in having an overall more favourable health profile[49]. Table 9.1 shows the comparative data for infant mortality rates, life expectancy at birth, and literacy rates for men and women[50,51].

Until the 1920s, infant mortality rates were similar to the rest of India[47,52]. Since then, the infant mortality rates have been consistently lower in Kerala and have declined much more rapidly. Similarly, life expectancy at birth has been higher and has increased more than in India as a whole since 1961. However, Kerala is endemic for diseases associated with poor environmental conditions[53]. Literacy rates, especially in women, are now much higher in Kerala than in India as a whole, and the sex difference in literacy in Kerala is very small. A matriarchal caste in Kerala historically was interested particularly in the education of women and by the end of the nineteenth century every village in Kerala reportedly had a school. Other social and economic indicators do not, however, show Kerala to be at any advantage in comparison with other states. For example, the per capita income for Kerala for the year 1981–82 ranked 11th among the Indian states, and the percentage below the poverty line in 1977–78 was estimated to be 47 for Kerala and 48 for India as a whole; in 1987–88, 32% were estimated to be below the poverty line[47]. In 1997–98, the per capita domestic product was US$208 (Rs 2490) in Kerala and US$237 (Rs 2840) in India as a whole[54]. The modest increases in per capita income which occurred in Kerala, largely through remittances from migrant workers in the Middle-Eastern Gulf countries, were complemented by social policies[47].

The nutritional intakes of Keralites also appear to be very similar to the rest of India[52]. Safe water supply coverage in Kerala is less than for the rest of India. Per capita government expenditure on health care in Kerala, however, has been one of the highest among all Indian states. The achievement of Kerala in human development would not have occurred without the commitment of financial resources by the State Government; as in China, international aid agencies played only a minor role.

The gains in infant mortality have been attributed to the expansion of immunisation programmes and possibly to an expansion of health facilities in the northern region[55]. The explanation for the overall better health experiences in Kerala is more complex. The role of health care has been influenced strongly by the level of education and health consciousness, especially of women; schooling encourages pupils to identify with the whole modern system, including health centres and recommended treatments[2].

The emphasis on rural, primary and female education has historically been greater in Kerala and this continued post-Independence. The high degree of literacy in Kerala is due to both government policy, which especially influenced the timing at which particular groups of people became literate in Kerala, and cultural attitudes towards women, and women's attitudes about themselves, which encouraged the acquisition of literacy[56]. Education is not merely a proxy for wealth. Education seems to have its impact on health by changing expectations and raising awareness, as much as by a direct impact on the behaviour of mothers[57]. With greater education and independence, mothers make more decisions more rapidly. Educated mothers are more likely to ensure a healthier distribution of food on a year-round basis and utilise appropriate health[58]. Even so, a child of an uneducated mother living in a highly educated society has a much better chance of survival than a child of an educated woman living in a largely uneducated society[58], indicating the critical influence of social context on the absolute level of risk.

Unfortunately, it is not easy to reproduce in other countries the complex social, cultural and political circumstances that have generated a high degree of political awareness and the educational structure of Kerala. Education is no magic bullet; an effective and accessible health system is also required. Kerala provides several important lessons for other poor countries. Within a surprisingly short time, the quality of life for the broad majority of Keralites has improved, demonstrating that high levels of health and social development can be achieved in the absence of high rates of economic growth. Kerala's success occurred within the context of a country that has been notably unsuccessful in its attempts to achieve a similar improvement in quality of life for its citizens using conventional western approaches, such as medical care services and family planning programmes. Kerala's success is a result of a particular set of mutually supporting and reinforcing factors, not just education or 'political will', with equity considerations being of fundamental importance[2].

A recent development in Kerala is the creation of the Achutha Menon Centre for Health Science Studies, which has offered a modern MPH course since 1998 but still with only a small number of students, relative to the need in India. This centre is the public health wing of the Sree Chitra Tirunal Institute for Medical Sciences and Technology. This Institute was established by an act of parliament in 1977 and is now an 'institution of national importance' under the National Government Department of Science and Technology and has the status of a university.

The Kerala experience indicates that vigorous public action can transform the level of social development and can cause major improvements in social and health indicators, even at relatively low levels of per capita income and within a single generation. These achievements are now under threat from the reduced remittances from overseas Keralites, especially in the Gulf States, and by the continuing poor economic situation in the State.

9.5 Africa: poor health at high cost and with major setbacks

Africa is a huge continent comprising over 50 nations with a total population of approximately 600 million, including 500 million in sub-Saharan Africa (SSA). The history of Africa's self-development, before foreign rule began, is impressive[59]. Africa now faces a remarkable range of complex problems whose origins are many and varied. Responsibility for much of the present crisis in Africa lies within the nation states, which in turn were a creation of the colonial powers and the 'tribes' they empowered, as Africa began to emerge from colonial rule in the 1950s[59].

The slave trade devastated Africa, especially West Africa, for almost two centuries. This trade was one of the precursors of deteriorating health standards and social breakdown in Africa, although it undoubtedly contributed to the rising standard of living in Europe[60]. Further destruction of African society took place after the colonial partition in the 1880s[61]. The continuing transfer of wealth to the rich countries of the north, environmental degradation, natural disasters, harsh governments and dictatorships and civil strife, have compounded Africa's problems over the last half century. Disease epidemics, of which HIV/AIDS is the most recent, have added to the African misery.

From a public health perspective, all is not despair. Despite its social, economic and political problems, the health of most Africans has improved; however, in comparison with all other countries, African countries are towards the bottom of the health tables. For example, in 1999, seven of the 48 SSA countries had a lower life expectancy than in 1970, while eight countries have seen an increase in infant mortality rate between 1981 and 1999. Life expectancy in 17 of 48 countries declined between 1981 and 1999, probably through a combination of: average per capita incomes of less than US$1 per day, the impact of the HIV epidemic, declines in health service provision and conflict[62].

Adult mortality rates in sub-Saharan Africa are difficult to ascertain in the absence of accurate mortality statistics. Where data are available, the situation is bleak. For example, in a rural district in Tanzania in the period 1992–95, mortality was over 40 times higher in 20–24-year-old women than in the same aged women in England and Wales[63]. During the 1960s and 1970s considerable progress was made in promoting education and health care; child mortality rates more than halved between 1960 and 1990, an achievement that took more than a century in Europe. However, from the late 1970s most countries have experienced severe economic crises, precipitated by rises in oil prices, increasing debt and interest rates, a reduction in prices for exports from poor countries, and a fall in tax revenues. Poor countries have had to borrow on the international market to continue to govern; debt servicing requirements increased dramatically, and by the early 1980s many countries in Africa were unable to meet these repayments. Structural adjustment programmes were designed by the World Bank and the International Monetary Fund to overcome these difficulties in return for debt rescheduling,[64, 65] although the real need is for debt alleviation.

Structural adjustment programmes are now in place in many poor countries, not just in Africa. Most debt relief and overseas aid are dependent now on recipient countries agreeing to these programmes[65]. The imposition of these programmes by agencies such as the World Bank and the International Monetary Fund is one indication of the recent ascendancy of these agencies over health affairs in Africa; the World Health Organization has too often been relegated to a subsidiary role[66].

Structural adjustment programmes include a wide range of measures: trade liberalisation, currency devaluation, increased interest rates, introduction of user charges for medical care, and most importantly for health, a decrease in spending on social welfare programmes. The ultimate aim is to stimulate economic growth. The evidence on the positive impact of these programmes on long-term economic growth is limited, although a few countries, especially in South America, have responded positively – at least in the short term. These programmes have resulted in significant macroeconomic policy changes and public sector restructuring and reduced social provisioning, with negative effects on education, health and social services for the poor. A recent review of available studies on structural adjustment and health for a WHO Commission states: 'The majority of studies in Africa, whether theoretical or empirical, are negative towards structural adjustment and its effects on health outcomes'[67]. Child mortality rates have risen in several African countries, malnutrition has increased, and several endemic diseases have become more prominent[62]. It is difficult to blame structural adjustment for all these problems but popular discontent, the so-called 'IMF food riots', has been directed at the international agencies; non-governmental aid agencies have been strongly critical of structural adjustment[66].

The colonial powers extracted great wealth from their colonies. Money has continued to move from poor countries in the South to rich countries in the North. In 1992, for example, there was a net flow of US$19 billion from the 40 poorest countries in the world to the richest. These poor countries, 30 of them in sub-Saharan Africa, received $16 billion in aid, but paid $35 billion in debt repayments and interest. They defaulted on $12 billion, which was added to their debt, which reached $450 billion[66]. Other aspects of the modern phase of globalisation have also had detrimental effects on Africa. For example, the development of agreements under the World Trade Organization (WTO), notably Trade-related Intellectual Property Rights (TRIPS) and its interpretation by powerful corporate interests and governments, have threatened to circumscribe countries' health policy options. The best known case relates to the recent legal battle around the attempt by South Africa to secure pharmaceuticals, especially for HIV/AIDS, at a reduced cost[62].

While spending on health and other social services has been reduced, military spending has increased and armies continue to flourish in Africa, in the midst of human misery. Efforts to balance government budgets were directed not unfortunately to reducing military spending; social services were an easier target. Much of the blame for this spending rests with rich countries, which have not done enough to phase out military assistance or arms sales. The United States of America and the former Soviet Union accounted for over 60% of the export trade in military equipment between 1996 and 2001, with the total value of this trade being about $120 billion[68].

The steps required to ease the immediate economic problems in Africa are straightforward. Of most importance is the removal of the crushing debt. The World Bank and International Monetary Fund (IMF) debt cannot be cancelled for constitutional reasons, only its repayment delayed. The most recent move to reduce debt is the Heavily Indebted Poor Countries (HIPC) initiative, launched by the World Bank and the IMF in 1996 to provide comprehensive debt relief to the world's poorest, most heavily indebted, countries. For 28 low human development countries included in this initiative, debt servicing fell from 5% of GDP in 1990 to 3.6% in 2000[68]. Unfortunately, prospects for debt relief are not great despite the widespread publicity brought to this issue by the Jubilee 2000 campaign. No concrete progress on this issue was made at the 2001 United Nations World Summit for Sustainable Development, which considered proposals for the reduction of global poverty, now encompassing more than one billion people[69]. Wealthy nations reiterated their belief that free trade and deregulation will lead to economic growth which, in turn, will reduce global poverty; poor counties resented being told what to do.

The second step is to ensure that economic restructuring puts the needs of poor people first, especially their needs for health and education. The World Bank is apparently changing its policy and giving more emphasis to health and social issues, although the impact of these changes has yet to be felt[65]. Public support for these measures is vital. Health professionals have a key role to play, given the impact of structural adjustment on health. Of equal importance to short-term economic reform is the need to rebuild African societies – a challenge which is made even more difficult by HIV/AIDS which is threatening the very survival of several SSA countries. In the long term, the politics of mass participation offer the most hope for overcoming the ongoing strife that affects Africa[59]. The prospects for much of Africa remain bleak. However, in 1993 the apartheid regime in South Africa came to a surprisingly peaceful end, although the public health challenges remain formidable[70]. In addition, new global health initiatives such as The Global Fund to Fight AIDS, Tuberculosis and Malaria[71] present an opportunity for African countries to mount a response to their health crises. However, unless these resources contribute to the development of infrastructure, human capacity and management processes, the response is likely to have only a short-term impact on Africa's most pressing health problems.

9.6 Conclusions

The experience of Kerala and China and a few other countries such as Sri Lanka and Costa Rica, which achieved high levels of population health at relatively low cost, indicates that unusually low mortality can be achieved if several conditions are met[2]. Sufficient female autonomy is a prerequisite and this, in turn, is influenced strongly by the dominant culture. However, as we have seen, good continuing progress is not guaranteed and the changing socio-economic and political context can affect past gains adversely. Many of the countries that have performed, from a health perspective, below that expected on the basis of their national wealth are Muslim, which, in general, does not support female autonomy. Religion is not, however, an absolute barrier to progress because some eastern Muslim countries, such as Malaysia, have achieved a better health status than would be expected on the basis of per capita income. Adequate levels of nutrition are another prerequisite, as is the widespread dissemination of the research-based knowledge, which underpins modern public health. Sufficient resources must also be devoted to the public health infrastructure and to efficient and accessible health services and education, especially for females, in order to ensure the uptake of this knowledge. Preventive health services must be available, for example, childhood immunisation and pre- and postnatal services.

Political consensus on the priority of high levels of education and health is a central requirement. This does not require a broad consensus on all political issues, only that successive governments are not able to overturn the advances of their predecessors. The central role of policy analysis in reforming the health sector in poor countries requires more attention[72]. Above all, it is clear from the poor countries that have made rapid gains in health status, that progress will not occur simply as a by-product of economic growth. Government leadership at national and regional levels is essential and must take precedence over the operation of market forces. Unfortunately, in most countries of the world today, this lesson has not been acted upon yet.

Chapter 9   Key points

- Most poor countries have poor health statistics.
- A few poor countries have achieved remarkably good health statistics at relatively low cost; these gains are now under threat.
- The experience from these countries suggest the following conditions are required:
  - political consensus on the high priority of education and health services;
  - female autonomy;
  - adequate nutrition; and
  - efficient and accessible health services, including preventive services.

References

1. Halstead, S.B., Walsh, J.A. & Warren, K.S. (eds.). *Good Health at Low Cost*. New York: Rockefeller Foundation, 1985.
2. Caldwell, J.C. Routes to low mortality in poor countries. *Pop. Dev. Rev.* 1986; **12**: 171–220.
3. Lee, L., Lin, V., Wang, R. & Zhao, H. Public health in China: history and contemporary challenges. In: Beaglehole, R. (ed.). *Global Public Health: A New Era*. Oxford: Oxford University Press, 2003.
4. Sidel, R. & Sidel, V.W. *The Health Of China: Current Conflicts In Medical And Human Services For One Billion People*. Boston: Beacon Press, 1982.
5. Xu, W. Flourishing health work in China. *Soc. Sci. Med.* 1995; **41**: 1043–5.

6. Taylor, C.E., Parker, R.L. & Dong-Lu, Z. Public health policies and strategies in China. In: Holland, W.W., Detels, R. & Knox, G. (eds.). *Oxford Textbook of Public Health*. Oxford: Oxford University Press, 1991.

7. Ashton, B., Hill, K., Piazza, A. & Zeita, R. Famine in China, 1958–61. *Pop. Dev. Rev.* 1984; **10**: 613–45.

8. Lawson, J.S. & Lin, V. Health status differentials in the People's Republic of China. *Am. J. Pub. Hlth* 1994; **84**: 737–41.

9. Shi, L. Health care in China: a rural–urban comparison after the socioeconomic reforms. *Bull. WHO* 1993; **71**: 723–36.

10. Chen, X., Hu, T. & Lin, Z. The rise and decline of the cooperative medical system in rural China. *Int. J. Hlth Serv.* 1993; **23**: 731–42.

11. Hsiao, W.C.L. The Chinese health care system: lessons for other nations. *Soc. Sci. Med.* 1995; **41**: 1047–55.

12. Zheng, X. & Hillier, S. The reforms of the Chinese health care system: county level changes: the Jiangxi Study. *Soc. Sci. Med.* 1995; **41**: 1057–64.

13. Liu, X. & Mills, A. Financing reforms of public health services in China: lessons for other nations. *Soc. Sci. Med.* 2002; **54**: 1691–8.

14. World Health Organization. *Tobacco Alert*. Geneva: WHO, April 1995:3.

15. UNAIDS. *China Update*. Geneva: UNAIDS, 2000.

16. Ministry of Health. *Chinese Health Statistical Digest*, 2001. Beijing: Ministry of Health, 2001.

17. Ashraf, H. China finally throws full weight behind efforts to contain SARS. *Lancet* 2003: **361**: 1439.

18. Eisenberg, L. The sleep of reason produces monsters – human costs of economic sanctions. *New Engl. J. Med.* 1997; **336**: 1248–50.

19. Feinsilver, J.M. *Healing the Masses: Cuban Health Politics At Home And Abroad.* Berkeley: University of California Press, 1993.

20. Ochoa, F.R. & Pardo, C.M.L. Economy, politics, and health status in Cuba. *Int. J. Hlth Serv.* 1997, **27**: 791–807.

21. Kuntz, D. The politics of suffering: the impact of the US embargo on the health of the Cuban people: report of a fact-finding trip to Cuba, 6–11 June 1993. *Int. J. Hlth Serv.* 1994; **24**: 161–79.

22. Organización Panamericana de la Salud. *Situación de Salud en Cuba: Indicadores Básicos 2000*. La Habana: Ministerio de Salud Pública. 2001.

23. Pan American Health Organization (PAHO). *Health in the Americas*, edition 2002; Volume II.; Washington, D.C., 2002.

24. Chelala, C. Cuba shows health gains despite embargo. *Br. Med. J.* 1998; **316**: 493.

25. Soteras, L., Fernández, B., Serrano, M., Antúnez, P. & Castro, O. (1993): Planificación de los recursos humanos para la salud. *Educ. Méd. Salud* 1993; **27**: 160–77.

26. Granma April, 23, 2002. http://www.granma.cu/espanol/abril02-4/17prueba5-e.html.

27. Mackay, J. & Eriksen, M. *The Tobacco Atlas*. Geneva: World Health Organization, 2002.

28. A Report of the Pan American Health Organization. *Tobacco or Health: Status in the Americas*. Washington, D.C., Pan American Health Organization/Pan American Sanitary Bureau: Regional Office of the World Health Organisation, 1992.

29. Tesh, S. Health education in Cuba: a preface. *Int. J. Hlth Serv.* 1986; **16**: 87–104.
30. Albright, M.K. Economic sanctions and public health: a view from the Department of State. *Ann. Int. Med.* 2000; **132**: 155–7.
31. Centers for Disease Control. Epidemic neuropathy – Cuba, 1991–1994. *J. Am. Med. Assoc.* 1994; **271**: 1154–5.
32. Rojas, F. Neuropatía Epidémica en Cuba 1992–1994. Editorial Ciencias Médicas; La Habana, 1995.
33. Roman, G.C. On politics and health: an epidemic of neurologic disease in Cuba. *Ann. Int. Med.* 1995; **122**: 530–3.
34. Roman, G.C. Epidemic neuropathy in Cuba: a public health problem related to the Cuban Democracy Act of the United States. *Neuroepidemiology* 1998; **17**: 111–15.
35. Barry, M. Effect of US embargo and economic decline on health in Cuba. *Ann. Int. Med.* 2000; **132**: 151–4.
36. Arnold, D. Crisis and contradiction in India's public health. In: Porter, D. (ed.). *The History of Public Health and the Modern State.* Amsterdam: Editions Rodopi B.V., 1994.
37. Harrison, H. *Public Health in British India: Anglo-Indian Preventive Medicine 1859–1914.* Cambridge: Cambridge University Press, 1994.
38. Ramasubban, R. Imperial health in British India, 1857–1900. In: MacLeod, R. & Lewis, M. (eds.). *Disease, Medicine and Empire.* London: Routledge, 1988.
39. MacLeod, R. Introduction. In: MacLeod, R. & Lewis, M. (eds.). *Disease, Medicine and Empire.* London: Routledge, 1988.
40. Chandavarkar, R. Plague panic and epidemic politics in India, 1896–1914. In: Ranger, T. & Slack, P. (eds.). *Epidemics and Ideas: Essays on the Historical Perception and Pestilence.* Cambridge: Cambridge University Press, 1992.
41. Madan, T.N. The plague in India, 1994. *Soc. Sci. Med.* 1995; **40**: 1167–8.
42. John, T.J. Final thoughts on India's 1994 plague outbreaks. *Lancet* 1995; **346**: 765.
43. Cook, G.C. Plague: past and future implications for India. *Pub. Hlth* 1995; **109**: 7–11.
44. Worboys, M. Manson, Ross and colonial medical policy: tropical medicine in London and Liverpool, 1899–1914. In: MacLeod, R. & Lewis, M. (eds.). *Disease, Medicine and Empire.* Routledge: London and New York, 1988.
45. TATA Institute of Fundamental Research. The Third International Workshop on Medical Certification of Causes of Death for India. *Proceedings of the International Meeting on Verbal Autopsy and on the Epidemiological Aspects of the Sample Registration System.* New Delhi, 2001.
46. *State of India's Population.* New Delhi: Population Foundation of India. 1998.
47. Krishnan, T.N. *The Route to Social Development in Kerala. Social Intermediation and Public Action: a retrospective study, 1960–1993.* New York: UNICEF, 1996.
48. Jayant Kumar Banthia. Registrar General and Census Commissioner of India. Census of India 2001. Series 1. Provisional Population Totals. Paper-1 of 2001 supplement District Totals. Published by the Controller, Dept. of Publications, Civil Lines, Delhi – 110 054.
49. Jeffrey, R. *The Politics of Health in India.* Berkeley: University of California Press, 1988.
50. UNICEF. *The State of the World's Children.* Oxford University Press, 1995.

51. Gulati, L. Population ageing and women in Kerala State, India. *Asia-Pac. Pop. J.* 1993; **8**: 53–63.

52. Nag, M. The impact of social and economic development on mortality: comparative study of Kerala and West Bengal. In: Halstead, S.B., Walsh, J.A. & Warren, K.S. (eds.). *Good Health at Low Cost*. New York: Rockefeller Foundation, 1985.

53. John, T.J. & White, F. Public health in South Asia. In: Beaglehole, R. (ed.) *Global Public Health: A New Era*. Oxford: Oxford University Press, 2003.

54. Planning Commission Government of India. *National Human Development Report 2001*. Planning Commission March 2002. Table 2.1 Per capita State Domestic products. Page 146.

55. Krishnan, T.N. Health statistics in Kerala State, India. In: Halstead, S.B., Walsh, J.A. & Warren, K.S. (eds.). *Good Health at Low Cost*. New York: Rockefeller Foundation, 1985.

56. Jeffrey, R. Governments and culture: how women made Kerala literate. *Pacific Affairs* 1987; **60**: 447–72.

57. Caldwell, J.C., Caldwell, P., Gajanayake, I., Orubuloye, I.O., Pieris, I. & Reddy, P.H. Cultural, social and behavioural determinants of health and their mechanisms: a report on related research programs. In: Caldwell, J., Findley, S., Caldwell, P. *et al. What We Know About Health Transitions*, vol 2. Canberra: Australian National University, 1990.

58. Caldwell, J.C., Reddy, P.H. & Caldwell, P. The social component of mortality decline: an investigation in South India employing alternative methodologies. *Pop. Stud.* 1983; **37**: 185–205.

59. Davidson, B. *The Black Man's Burden: Africa and the Curse of the Nation-State*. London: James Currey Limited, 1992.

60. Turshen, M. *The Political Ecology of Disease in Tanzania*. New Brunswick: Rutgers University Press, 1984.

61. Kanji, N., Kanji, N. & Manji, F. From development to sustained crisis: structural adjustment, equity and health. *Soc. Sci. Med.* 1991; **33**: 985–93.

62. Sanders, D., Dovlo, D., Meeus, W. & Lehmann, U. Public health Africa. In: Beaglehole, R. (ed.). *Global Public Health: A New Era*. Oxford: Oxford University Press, 2003.

63. Kitange, H.M., Machibya, H., Black, J. *et al.* Outlook for survivors of childhood in sub-Saharan Africa: adult mortality in Tanzania. *Br. Med. J.* 1996; **312**: 216–20.

64. Godlee, F. Third world debt: what's the point of immunising children if we are then going to starve them? *Br. Med. J.* 1993; **307**: 1369–70.

65. Logie, D.E. & Woodroffe, J. Structural adjustment: the wrong prescription for Africa? *Br. Med. J.* 1993; **307**: 41–4.

66. Godlee, F. The World Health Organization in Africa. *Br. Med. J.* 1994; **309**: 553–4.

67. Breman, A. & Shelton, C. Structural adjustment and health: a literature review of the debate, its role players and the presented empirical evidence. WHO Commission on Macroeconomics and Health Working Paper WG 6:6. Geneva: WHO, 2001.

68. United Nations Development Programme. *Human Development Report 2002: Deepening Democracy in a Fragmented World*. New York: UNDP, 2002.

69. Vidal, J. Ten years on – slow progress on sustainable development. *Lancet* 2002; **360**: 737.
70. Geiger, H.J. Letter from South Africa. *Pub. Hlth Rep.* 1995; **110**: 114–16.
71. Brugha, R. & Walt, G. A global health fund: a leap of faith? *Br. Med. J.* 2001; **323**: 152–4.
72. Walt, G. & Gilson, L. Reforming the health sector in developing countries: the central role of policy analysis. *Hlth Pol. Planning* 1994; **9**: 353–70.

10

Public health at the crossroads

10.1 Introduction

Public health is at a crossroads, and not for the first time. In 1926 Winslow described public health in the United States of America as standing 'at the crossroads' because of challenges posed by the emerging epidemics of non-communicable diseases[1]. The dramatic adverse effects on health of the industrialisation of the northern states in the USA had been controlled by the application of the sciences of sanitary engineering and bacteriology in the last quarter of the nineteenth century. Life expectancy in New York increased by almost 17 years from 36 years in the 40-year period up to 1920, largely as a consequence of reductions in communicable disease mortality rates. Winslow concluded that the main challenge facing public health was 'the application of medical knowledge to the individual patient at a time when that knowledge can really exert a maximum effect'. Winslow advocated the secondary prevention approach to chronic diseases based on their early detection and management when effective treatment might still be possible. He was also an early advocate for a national community-based health service – still a long way off in the USA.

An important question now is whether public health practitioners took the best path 80 years ago. Even more important questions are whether we are on the right path now and are the public health infrastructure and workforce strong enough to take advantage of current opportunities for collective action to advance the health of entire populations[2]. In hindsight, Winslow and colleagues did not set us off in the right direction; for one thing, the knowledge base for effective therapeutic interventions for chronic disease was almost non-existent, as was the evidence concerning the environmental determinants of the chronic disease epidemics. Winslow had misplaced confidence in the power of early detection and treatment and not enough confidence to explore alternative and more fundamental strategies for the prevention of epidemics of chronic diseases.

From a historical perspective, there are strong parallels between the state of public health today and the situation at the end of the nineteenth century. Mid-nineteenth century epidemiology and public health practice were relatively successful in controlling the epidemics of infectious diseases. Unfortunately, towards the end of the century epidemiology and public health lost their way and became dominated by bacteriology and by the identification of high risk populations. A similar cycle is now recurring. Following the successes in controlling the major non-communicable disease epidemics in many countries in the second half of this century, epidemiology and public health are in danger of succumbing to a new paradigm. Molecular and genetic approaches to the control of disease and the new focus in several wealthy countries on threats of bioterrorism are influencing the research, policy and practice agendas. In both historical periods, a fundamental failing of the public health profession has been the inability of public health specialists to articulate and act upon a broad vision of public health and to confront the underlying causes of premature death and disability.

At the beginning of the twenty-first century, the public health movement is under threat in both wealthy and poor countries[3]. Fortunately, this also represents an opportunity for reinvigoration. This chapter summarises the challenges facing public health practitioners and the steps that need to be taken to move public health towards the centre stage of health and social policy and become a force for global democracy.

10.2 Public health: definitions and scope

Public health has always been pulled in two different directions: towards a broad focus on the underlying social and economic causes of health and disease and towards a narrow medical focus. These two pathways are summarised in Table 10.1.

Public health movements in most countries are heading down the narrow disease-focused route under the influence of the prevailing social and economic ideology and the pressures from international aid donors. Only a serious and concerted effort will divert public health to a broader perspective. Public health professionals will need to ensure that the alternative routes and their implications are widely debated and discussed. A failure to take this initiative will lead inevitably to further movement down the narrow public health pathway.

To be most effective, public health practitioners require a firm sense of identity, based on a broad and inclusive definition of public health. The plethora

Table 10.1. *Two directions for public health*

Characteristics	Broad	Narrow
Definition of health	Based on WHO constitution	Absence of disease
Underlying theory	Socio-Structural	'Lifestyle'
Motivating concerns	Inequalities in health; alleviating poverty to improve health; sustainable development	Individual risks of disease
Major public health activities	Linkage of public health sciences with policy and programmes	Cost-containment; disease prevention, especially in high risk groups
Place of epidemiology	Balanced by other methods; participatory research	Emphasis on technique and clinical and molecular epidemiology
Advantages	Potential long-term global benefits	Short-term benefits
Disadvantages	Risk of failure because of breadth of concerns	Failure to address fundamental threats to global health

of definitions suggests the need for a short and succinct definition of public health that is broad in scope and of wide appeal; such a definition will make it easier for public health practitioners to gain greater understanding by the public of the importance of their work. We support the following definition: 'collective action for sustained population-wide health improvement'[2] which emphasises the hallmarks of public health practice: the focus on actions and interventions, which require collective (or collaborative or organised) actions; sustainability, that is, the need to embed policies within supportive systems; and the goals of public health: population-wide health improvement, which implies a concern to reduce health inequalities. The importance of this definition is that it is broad enough to include oversight of the activities of the medical care system and recognises the importance of responding to the underlying social, economic and cultural determinants of health and disease.

The integration of medical care under the public health umbrella would facilitate the process of setting broad health goals and targets and encourage resources to flow to prevention. At the same time, public health specialists would contribute to the organisational aspects of universally accessible and effective medical care and to the further development of evidence-based medicine.

There is tremendous potential for merging the two disciplines, public health and medical care, because both sets of activities are usually under the direction of the same government department. Furthermore, many public health programmes can be delivered only through the medical care system, and new resources for prevention could flow from a closer integration with medical care programmes. The national health goals and targets movements of the late 1980s had this overall objective[4]. Such a policy redirection requires strong political leadership and is more likely to achieve the desired ends if it has been motivated by a real desire to support public health and to strive for equality of opportunity for health rather than for the need to legitimise cost containment.

An important task for public health practitioners is to balance effort devoted to controlling individual risk factors and to deal with the underlying social and economic causes of health. It is relatively easy to research a 'new' risk factor or to implement a high risk disease control strategy[5]. It is much harder to develop an innovative research programme exploring the impact of income inequality on health or to present evidence-based policy advice on the need – from a health perspective – for income redistribution. The latter requires input from many different social policy and public health scientists.

A refocusing 'upstream' involves a move away from a predominant concern with individual risks towards the social structures and processes that generate health and disease[6]. This is not to deny that there is still much to be gained from dealing with specific causes of premature death and disease using effective public health measures. For example, in many countries cigarette smoking is the most readily preventable cause of disease. The public health significance of smoking, however, is closely related to global and national economic, social and political issues. The complex reasons for the continuing high rates of smoking by disadvantaged groups, including women, highlight the strong links between social forces and high risk behaviour[7].

Strategies that concentrate solely on the high risk approach to the prevention of disease, for example, screening, have associated costs that may divert resources from more fundamental public health activities. A resolution of the dilemma posed by the disease prevention – medical care imbalance is yet to be achieved. Public health professionals, by recognising explicitly their chosen path of action, can assist in reaching the necessary balance.

Apart from a firm sense of direction, public health also requires a strong and clearly articulated theoretical foundation based on a clear appreciation of the history of public health, in order to avoid being at the mercy of the prevailing ideology[8]. Progress in public health will be easier when there is a return to a more sympathetic attitude towards collective endeavour.

Unfortunately, the term 'public health' is a source of confusion. 'Public' can refer either to the action of individual members of the community or to the social groups of which individuals are part. The meaning adopted is critical for the practice of public health; different interpretations lead to the dominance of either individual or collective strategies. Regrettably, the individualistic interpretation and practice are currently dominant, especially in the USA, although public health is still underpinned in most countries by collective strategies such as garbage collection and clean water supplies.

Similarly, the meaning of 'health' is of central importance to the orientation of public health activities. If 'health' is equated with the absence of disease, as it is in much of epidemiology, disease prevention will receive more emphasis. If, on the other hand, 'health' is interpreted in a broader sense, involving the equitable distribution of the foundations for health, health promotion will be emphasised[9]. A definition of public health based on a strong commitment to collective endeavour and a broad view of health will lead to public health activities quite distinct from a definition that emphasises the individualistic approach to health.

10.3 Recent public health movements

10.3.1 New public health

The term 'new public health', first used in 1916, is unfortunate because every generation can appropriate the term 'new'. Its original use referred to a narrow view of public health based on bacteriology[10]. Identification and treatment of individual carriers of tuberculosis was seen as the solution to this epidemic, rather than an improvement of living conditions of the whole population.

The most recent use of the term 'new public health' emerged from a recognition that major health problems cannot be solved by medical care[11]. This was articulated most clearly by the Lalonde Report from the Canadian Government, published in 1974 under the name of the then Minister of National Health and Welfare[12]. This report led to the first wave of modern health promotion. The report proposed the 'health field concept', which included four elements: human biology, environment, lifestyle and health care organisation. This 'new perspective' aimed to direct more resources into a positive approach to health with greater emphasis on health promotion. Unfortunately, for a variety of reasons, not least the economic crisis of the late 1970s, most health promotion energy was diverted towards the 'lifestyle' health field, with health education as the favoured strategy.

The United States Surgeon General followed in 1979 with a report that led to an ambitious set of quantified health goals and targets which have now been reformulated for 2010 (see Chapter 8); most of the goals focused on disease prevention and emphasised individual lifestyle strategies[13]. Many other countries adopted a similar approach to health goals and targets, with health education being the prime strategy and cost containment the underlying motivation. Sweden has developed the most ambitious approach to health goals with a focus on the underlying determinants of health (see Chapter 8).

At a global level, the response of WHO was Health For All by the Year 2000, a proposal which recognised that the main determinants of health are outside the health care sector; primary health care was seen as the key to achieving this goal at the Alma Ata conference in 1978[14]. Primary health care, as originally formulated, stressed the importance of equity in access to community-based services, and encouraged a comprehensive approach to improving health including actions outside the health sector. It did not take long, however, for this comprehensive approach to be replaced by selective and targeted strategies for disease control such as childhood immunisation. Such vertical programmes rely heavily on specific and focused activities[15]. Although vertical programmes have contributed to population health improvement, for example, the polio eradication campaigns[16], they are hard to sustain in the absence of a strong public health infrastructure and represent an important departure from the original Health For All concept[17].

10.3.2 The Ottawa Charter: new dimensions to health promotion

The Lalonde Report and related documents were criticised because of the perceived emphasis on victim blaming and the neglect of the social and economic determinants of health. In contrast, the Health for All proposal was rejected as being too ambitious. Out of these criticisms came the second wave of modern health promotion under the banner of the Ottawa Charter for Health Promotion, largely developed by the World Health Organization (Box 10.1)[18, 19].

The Ottawa Charter was influenced strongly by the more difficult economic environment of the 1980s. The Healthy Cities project, launched in 1986 as both a vision and a movement, has been one of the major instruments for the implementation of the Ottawa Charter[20]. Healthy Cities grew as a series of local community experiments, usually led by health promotion practitioners. Although some of these projects have achieved success and have been sustained, many more have struggled and, by focusing on individual cities, the wider social and economic and political factors have often been ignored[20]. In the final analysis, unless they are translated into policies, projects are only of limited value in demonstrating possible approaches to health promotion. The reintegration of the Ottawa Charter and lifestyle approaches has begun with a people-centred approach to health promotion, which focuses on personal and community development and on the need to complement top-down approaches with the empowerment of local communities[21,22]. More generally, this approach seeks to build ecologically and economically self-reliant local economies interlinked as part of a global system.

Box 10.1   The Ottawa Charter and health promotion

The Ottawa Charter breaks health promotion into five action areas:

- Building health public policy;
- Creating supportive environments;
- Strengthening community action;
- Developing personal skills; and
- Re-orienting health services.

The Ottawa Charter is primarily a philosophical document and it has not been easy to translate into practical use. The Ottawa Charter approach to health promotion down-plays the lifestyle (health education) approach to health and emphasises the importance of social structures and policy as key health determinants. Health is placed firmly in the socio-political domain, well outside the individual and biological realms. This major shift in focus has not been easy to apply in practice and the conceptual vagueness leads to difficulties in evaluation.

10.3.3 Ecological public health

The term 'ecological public health' emerged from a perception of the need to integrate health and the environment[23,24]. The survival of humanity depends on the development of an ecological balance between humans and the biosphere. Globally, this balance requires a rate of resource and energy use at a level of about one-fifth of that of modern high technology societies, raising fundamental questions about the type of societies required for a sustainable future[25]. As with the term 'new public health', there is little need for the term 'ecological public health' as public health is, by definition, ecological. 'Public health' is an evolving term; the addition of new labels is sometimes confusing and often unnecessary. Ideally, public health should be dynamic and flexible, incorporating the most appropriate elements of earlier public health movements: disease prevention, health promotion, health education, health policy, environmental concern and community empowerment.

10.3.4 Population health

The population health movement had its origin in the work of the Canadian Institute for Advanced Research and its publications of the early 1990s[26,27]. This work has recently been re-evaluated[28]. The original model reflected the view that the social environment was critical for health and that the health care system contributes only a little to overall population health status. Japan was said, for example, to have high health status because little of the national wealth was spent on the armed forces. However, the definition of population health has always been ambiguous; it has been defined as the 'health outcomes of a group of individuals, including the distribution of such outcomes with the group'[29]. The impact of this movement outside of Canada, and even within Canada, seems to have been minimal[30,28]. This movement has been criticised for ignoring the socio-political determinants of health and for providing little encouragement for human agency in improving health[31].

10.4 A critical connection: public health and epidemiology

At its formal beginnings in the middle of the nineteenth century, epidemiology was linked intimately with the public health movement. Indeed, improvement in the public's health was the justification for the foundation of the London Epidemiological Society in 1850. As we have seen, however, epidemiology has become divorced from public health practice and policy.

For epidemiology to become reintegrated with public health practice, changes will be required in both the education and training of epidemiologists, and in the practice of public health. It will not be easy for epidemiology to regain its whole population purpose and closer connection with healthy public policy; 'a social policy approach to healthy lifestyles' rather than the current 'lifestyle approach to social policy' is required[32].

There is now sufficient evidence to support the population approach to prevention. Risk factors are distributed normally and the majority of new events occur in people in the middle range of the distribution; the small proportion of the population at high risk of disease, at least as identified by single risk factors, produces only a minority of the new cases of disease. A major challenge, however, with the population-wide strategy is the prevention paradox:

'a preventive measure that brings large benefits to the community affords little to each participating individual[33]. The high risk strategy is attractive because it yields a large benefit to sick or high risk individuals, although it affords little benefit to the community as a whole and does nothing to prevent ongoing development of epidemics. A difficult task for epidemiologists is to focus attention on strategies for whole populations and this requires evidence-based advocacy[34].

There is potential for making strategies directed at individuals more effective with the increasing recognition that clinical decisions should be based on measures of absolute risk rather than of relative risk, that is, the actual risk of disease an individual faces should be an important consideration in the patient's decision about therapeutic options. With the development of clinical guidelines based on sound epidemiological data, epidemiology is changing clinical practice. For example modern guidelines for the treatment of mild hypertension encourage the treatment of older people, especially those with other risk factors, rather than middle-aged people[35,36].

Epidemiology, along with the other disciplines of public health, is indispensable to the process of health policy formation, but epidemiologists require a clearer understanding of the policy-making process. A closer integration of public health sciences with policy-making will ensure that health policy is influenced by evidence[37], just as clinical medicine is moving towards an evidence-based approach. If new policies are accompanied by a statement of the supporting evidence and by a full assessment of the political risks and benefits, engagement with the policy-making process may become easier for public health scientists.

10.5 A growing foundation: public health education and training

Although postgraduate public health education has a long history in the United States of America and in the United Kingdom, dating back to early last century, in most of the world public health education is a relatively new development, and funding for public health training is limited. The separation of public health from medical schools had a deleterious impact on both schools of public health and on medical schools[38]. The former became divorced from medicine and the latter could safely neglect public health. On both accounts, the health of the public suffered.

Public health education is developing in many countries and new schools and institutes of public health have been established[39]. In Australia the resurgence began in the mid-1980s stimulated by the election of a Labour government and a review of public health education[40]. In Germany and Eastern Europe and Central Asia developments occurred in the 1990s[40–42]; prior to these developments, Germany had no experience with modern postgraduate training in public health.

There are now approximately 60 schools of public health in Europe and most are stand-alone research and training institutions or are departments of public health within a medical school[43–45]. Innovative broad-based institutional initiatives, which are closely related to public health practice, are rare[46]. There are now 30 schools of public health in the United States of America (and approximately 130 medical schools), seven of which have been established in the last decade[47]. Many are developing strong links with local departments of public health and with community organisations. The enormous growth in research grants, however, has overshadowed commitment to teaching and community practice. There is a serious lack of appropriate public health training opportunities in most of the developing world. For example, India has only one or two modern public health training institutions, and the entire South East Asian region has approximately 12 schools of public health for a population of well over 1.5 billion people[48]. There is also a need to shift from traditional approaches to public health training to an applied approach which addresses the reality of global public health practice in resource-constrained settings[49].

Where strong schools of public health exist, closer ties with medical schools and local departments of public health are desirable. This integration is important especially in poor countries, which cannot afford either an elite medical profession modelled on European or North American lines, or a weak public health profession. The hope that the public health approach would permeate medical schools has, so far, proved illusory. Changing the dominant philosophy of medical schools is difficult, especially if they remain isolated from their communities; few medical schools have responsibility for the health and health care needs of their local communities. On the other hand, if medical schools embrace public health and establish close links with their communities, public health will flourish. Of central importance is that public health sees itself as a speciality in its own right – not as a sub-speciality of medicine – and develops close and collaborative links with medical care.

The development of public health training peer review and accreditation systems to ensure public accountability for the training activities is a priority in all countries. Such systems can be developed collegially and constructively using peer review mechanisms as a first stage in the accreditation process[43,50].

In the short term, the institutional base for public health training matters little; the nature of the training and the orientation are paramount. However, for developing countries local training has many advantages. A key goal is the strengthening of the partnership between the two processes of education and practice[51]. The appropriate institutional base will be determined by local and national history and current practicalities. Whatever the base, strong institutional support and leadership of public health education and training is essential to bridge the gulf between academic and practical public health and to ensure that students are socialised in the values of public health. Similarly, strong links between public health practice and the delivery of medical care will support the implementation of preventive programmes; this interaction is essential in all societies and especially in poor countries.

10.6 The promise of public health research

Public health research has been one important contributor to the increase in life expectancy over the last century, along with the growth in education opportunities which facilitate the uptake of this knowledge. Formal public health programmes play a role but health gains can occur in their absence[52]. There is still much more to be learnt, however, and an even more urgent task is the translation of existing knowledge into policies and effective programmes[53]. Public health research is a multidisciplinary activity. It involves the application of the whole range of biological, social and behavioural sciences to the health problems of human populations. All too often, however, it is limited to epidemiological and health systems research. The real research challenge is the exploration of the interaction between social, economic and environmental factors and disease.

Public health research is under-funded and researchers are in short supply[54]. Globally, about US$70 billion is spent on health research overall, with an estimated 10% spent on researching the 90% of the world's health problems, thus neglecting the health needs of poor countries[55]. In Australia less than 2% of total health expenditure was spent on health research and development in 1990–91 and less than a quarter of this went on public health research[56]. In New Zealand the proportion of health-related research expenditure directed to public health is similar; the relative under spending on public health research was one justification for transforming the Medical Research Council into the Health Research Council of New Zealand. This transformation had a beneficial but short-lived impact on public health research funding. Innovative methods of funding public health research are required in order to build effective multidisciplinary research groups rapidly.

At the international level, the World Bank and the World Health Organization identified research topics with the potential to contribute rapidly to health improvements. The major public health research challenges identified include:

- the continuing epidemics of preventable childhood infectious diseases, which are aggravated by poverty and under nutrition;
- the economic, social and environmental changes, which lead to emerging and re-emerging infectious diseases;
- the growing epidemics of non-communicable diseases and injuries; and
- the assessment of the effectiveness and efficiency of public health programmes.

This exercise, built upon the 1993 World Bank Report *Investing in Health*[57], and shaped the long-term priorities of the main international health research agencies. Regrettably, the emphasis has been on research on disease-specific interventions and 'best buy' packages at the expense of broad social and public health research addressing the underlying causes of premature death and disease[58].

Much public health and epidemiological research has become repetitive and divorced from both practice and problem-solving[59]. Closer integration of public health agencies and academic institutions will improve the quality and relevance of public health research. Public health researchers will increase their relevance to the needs of policy-makers if they pay more attention to the policy environment and to the process of policy-making[60]. Some of the irrelevance of public health research would be reduced if researchers adhered to the motto of an independent research organisation, the New England Research Institutes, which reads 'no research without therapeutic or policy benefit'[61].

The value of using the appropriate research method for the appropriate question is now recognised[62,63]. As epidemiology moves from a focus on individual risk factors and towards the more difficult task of exploring community influences and social and economic structures, it will need to work much more closely with other public health sciences. The great strength of qualitative research is that it has the potential to illuminate the nature of quantitative relationships. Similarly, interaction with medical and biological scientists is essential for good public health research[64].

10.7 Public health advocacy: an important skill

A key aspect of public health practice is advocacy[65]. All countries require a strong advocacy group for public health, yet few have an established and vigorous public health association that takes advocacy seriously. The American

Public Health Association, the Canadian Public Health Association and the Australian Public Health Association are examples of agencies that have good visibility and an impact on health policy. A new Public Health Advocacy Institute was established in the United States of America in 2000 to make public health considerations and analytical methods an integral part of legal discussions and debates[66].

Public health scientists, in comparison with their medical colleagues, have a low public profile; public health is rarely a public relations success. Too often, public health practitioners are portrayed as moralists preaching against pleasurable behaviours such as drinking and smoking. In addition, public health practitioners, unskilled in media advocacy, are reticent to take credit for their contributions to health improvements. Extravagant claims and promises from laboratory scientists and clinicians are often left unchallenged, and journalists occasionally let their enthusiasm overshadow balanced reporting[67].

Public health practitioners must work constructively with the media, which always have an important influence on policy debates[68,69]. The strategic use of mass media to advance a social or policy initiative is a powerful public health tool and can be used to strengthen community action. Media advocacy functions by setting agendas, framing debates, and stressing the need for policy solutions to personal problems. Tobacco control activists have been particularly successful as media advocates[70].

Advocacy is especially difficult for public health practitioners employed by government agencies. Practitioners employed by more independent agencies such as universities have a special responsibility to speak publicly on the underlying causes of population health levels and on the most appropriate public health strategies. One solution is for professional associations to play a much stronger collective advocacy role[71].

10.8 Participation: the key to a strong public health movement

Public participation is the key to a strong and vigorous public health movement. True participation implies effective two-way consultation and joint ownership of public health programmes[22,72]. Much of this community-based work is unrecognised, at least in economic terms, as it is unpaid and undertaken largely by women. Public health practitioners need to appreciate the existence of popular beliefs about disease causation and occurrence. For example, members of the public put a greater emphasis on the role of 'stress' and often invoke fatalism to explain death and disease[7,73]. A top-down approach to health promotion is unlikely to be effective, as it ignores the active way in which people construct explanations of health and disease[74].

The Alma Ata declaration recognised that 'people have the right to participate individually and collectively in the planning and implementation of their health care'[14]. A continuing major challenge is to encourage effective participation in countries in which involvement in public affairs is rare. The poor remain poor because they are marginalised from the political and economic decision-making process[75]. Poor people take no part in the allocation of health resources or in the more general allocation of public resources. Economic and social decisions are inevitably, but unfairly, more influenced by powerful and entrenched vested interest. There is a strong case for a Global Development Organization to advocate for global action on human development and to coordinate development programmes[76].

Global progress in public health is related closely to the development of mass participatory democracy, beginning at the community level and extending throughout society[75]. The basis of social cohesiveness and democracy are cooperative civic networks[77]. The experience of the few countries, which achieved high population levels of health at relatively low cost, emphasises the need for a strong social consensus on the importance of health and educational services. This, in turn, often reflects a vigorous democracy, especially at the local level[78]. Unfortunately, the prospects for democratic participation in much of the world is bleak. Public health practitioners must continue to stress the need for this participation and to advocate with the communities they serve[79]. Further, the 'success stories' of the last few decades have all suffered major setbacks over the last decade (see Chapter 9).

Public health practitioners must also take a leadership role in keeping the public health vision alive – and implementing it – rather than awaiting the spontaneous development of mass movements for public health. In many countries environmental issues are the impetus for building a public health constituency. Public health researchers and practitioners can foster the development of a community voice by forming close links with community groups. This is easier when the research stems directly from community concerns. There is often a fine line between community participation and community manipulation. Inevitably, public health programmes challenge established power bases; enduring successes will occur only when there is a strong alignment between community concerns and public health policies and programmes. Public health practitioners have an obligation to articulate strong health arguments for equitable and sustainable development.

10.9 Public health, human rights and ecological constraints

Although the modern origins of the idea of human rights go back at least as far as the eighteenth century, health as a human right is a relatively recent concept[80]. The United Nations in 1948 adopted the Universal Declaration of Human Rights, which includes a statement that 'everyone has the right to a standard of living adequate for the health and well being of himself and his family'. This right was expanded further by the United Nations in 1966 in an International Covenant on Economic, Social and Cultural Rights (Article 12), which included the obligation for states ratifying the covenant to take steps to:

- reduce stillborn and infant mortality rates;
- promote the healthy development of the child;
- improve all aspects of environmental and industrial hygiene; and
- prevent, treat, and control epidemic, endemic, occupational and other diseases.

These general statements, although important and legally binding in international law, do not make it easy to determine the specific obligations involved[81]. Signatories are obliged to work towards achieving these rights, by adopting legislative measures, but progress is limited because action is conditional on the availability of resources (Article 2). The human rights approach to public health was advocated strongly as the basis of the response to HIV/AIDS[82]. It is now more widely interpreted by the UN Committee on Economic, Social and Cultural Rights to include the underlying determinants of health[83,84].

The formation of the World Health Organization provided the first international agency to lead the movement for health as a human right. WHO's constitution proclaims 'the enjoyment of the highest attainable standard of health is one of the fundamental rights of every human being' and WHO's objective is 'the attainment by all peoples of the highest possible level of health'. The legal implications of the WHO definition of health are that nations have duties both to promote health, social and related services as well as to prevent or remove barriers to the realisation and maintenance of health[85].

International and national statements on health as a human right mean little when there is no enforceable mechanism for making them effective. Even where legal mechanisms are available, they are not often used. These statements, however, have tremendous symbolic value. Unfortunately, fewer than 40 countries have an agency responsible for human rights and very few of these agencies have any responsibility for health. Furthermore, most international statements have a strong 'western' flavour and assume the equality of men and women; many religious and cultural groups do not acknowledge this equality. While equity in opportunities for health is an important public health goal, it is obvious that this view is not held widely in most countries. Public health professionals are able to point out the consequences of ignoring equity in health as a fundamental human goal.

10.9.1 Principles of public health ethics

The four basic principles of medical care ethics also apply to the practice of public health: respect for autonomy, non-maleficence, beneficence and justice, as described in Chapter 6. From a public health perspective, all four principles are important, but public health practice is fundamentally different from medical practice[86]. In general, people seek advice and help from doctors and other health care professionals; few ask for public health advice. In the interests of beneficence, the principle of 'doing the most good', public health practitioners make judgements about healthy lifestyles and thus run the risk of paternalism. Public health practitioners will achieve more by focusing on the provision of health-enabling conditions and opportunities as well as supporting the case for access to affordable treatments.

Issues of rights are involved in all aspects of public health programmes from analysis to implementation and monitoring[87]. Each stage can involve a conflict of rights, for example, rights to privacy vs. access to data for epidemiological purposes. The moral basis for public health interventions is not always explicit and ranges from a desire to inform people by health education, to the promotion of the 'common good' through policy advocacy[88]. There is always tension in public health between autonomy of the individual and the desire to protect and promote the health of the whole population. All public health programmes must attempt to balance individual and collective rights[89].

Public health and human rights are linked in three general ways[90]. Firstly, public health policies can have both a positive and a negative impact on human rights, especially when state power is used to limit the 'rights of a few for the good of many', as is often the case in the control of communicable disease; however, there need not be a conflict between human rights and public health. For example, the control of the HIV/AIDS pandemic requires increased attention to the promotion of the human rights of people most at risk of infection. AIDS is inextricable from individual and collective behaviour, strongly influenced by broad social forces, and directly linked with social discrimination. Dramatic progress in reducing the risk of HIV transmission will be difficult until discrimination on the basis of sexual preference and gender is prohibited legally and anti-discrimination measures and educational programmes are promoted widely and enforced.

The second link is the health impact of violations of human rights. Unfortunately, there is all too much evidence to support this linkage, ranging from medically sanctioned and culturally accepted torture[91], genital mutilation of girls, or the systematic rape and elimination of refugees or political opponents[92, 93].

The third, and most fundamental consideration, is that health and human rights are linked inextricably in the struggle to advance human well-being within the context of the closed biosphere[59]. To die because of the absence of the fundamentals of health, whether it be medical care or adequate nutrition, is a violation of human rights. The striking and enduring inequalities in health within, and especially between, countries is both a public health and a human rights issue. The reduction of inequalities represents a great opportunity for improving the health of all populations, but this goal will require both public health and socio-economic policy interventions. Public health practitioners have a responsibility to continue to draw attention to the importance of the linkage between human rights and public health and to develop methods of assessing the impact on human rights of health policies and programmes and health reforms[94].

10.10 The globalisation of public health

10.10.1 The daunting global context

A major challenge facing public health is to sustain and extend the health gains that have been made over the last half century and to ensure that the setbacks are reversed. Several interrelated global developments have a profound influence on public health:

- the unequal relationship between wealthy and poor countries;
- the prevailing ideology which stresses the role of the 'free market' and 'individualism'; and
- the threats to the environment.

The globalisation of the economy, with attendant changes in world trade and the spread of free market policies and service-based economies, has a profound impact on health, both positive and negative[95]. Unfortunately, the security of the globalised economy is far from guaranteed, as evidenced by the recent generalised economic down-turn which shows no sign of abating. The marked inequality in wealth between countries is rooted firmly in the exploitative relationship between rich and poor countries, with poor countries viewed largely as a market for the products of wealthy countries and as a source of cheap – and often skilled – labour. Indeed, the rich countries have achieved their wealth by exploiting the poverty of the poor[96]. The extent of global poverty, poor nutrition, the debt crisis and the deterioration of the environment all demand attention[97], as does population growth, which interacts with poverty and over-consumption to aggravate the environmental pressures.

In the face of these problems, current development aid for poor countries is both grossly inadequate and often ineffective, especially when it is tied to free trade agreements, economic growth and to western notions of individual liberty. Wealthy countries have pledged repeatedly to give at least 0.7% of GNP to official development assistance programmes, yet only a few countries, Norway, Sweden, Denmark and the Netherlands, have achieved this modest goal[98]. These countries vary enormously in the degree to which their policies support development. On a 10-point scale, the overall score ranges from 5.6 in the Netherlands with Japan and the USA being the only countries to score under 3 as shown in Fig. 10.1[99].

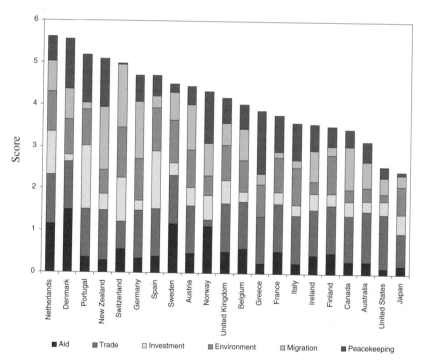

Fig. 10.1. Ranking the rich: summary of overall scores for members of the Development Assistance Committee (except Luxembourg). *Source:* Center for Global Development

The health impact of the World Trade Organization (WTO) initiated in 1994, and now with 124 members, has been mixed. On the one hand, the growth in trade has increased global wealth dramatically, although this has not been distributed equitably. On the other hand, several of the WTO Multilateral Trade Agreements severely limit public health policy options at a national level, for example, by restricting access to affordable pharmaceuticals[100, 101]. Further constraints result from the conditions imposed by the World Bank and the International Monetary Fund, for example, the reductions in government spending on health and social services. The World Bank is now, in financial terms, the most important agency in world health[102]. International governmental agencies (such as the World Health Organization) and non-governmental organisations are relatively powerless, at least in financial terms.

Since 1945 at least five United Nations organisations have become involved heavily in international health activities: WHO, World Bank, UN Children's Fund (UNICEF), UN Population Fund (UNFPA), and UN Development Programme (UNDP). Although WHO is still the lead technical agency, this view is not always shared by other agencies and there is serious lack of coordination and cooperation among agencies[103].

The World Bank puts much faith in the involvement of the private sector in the provision of health care in poor countries. The route to good health, as envisaged by the World Bank, is through economic development and medical science, and to a lesser extent, through increased education. In this sense, the World Bank has strongly influenced international health development. Although the World Bank's 1993 report *Investing in Health* recognised that poverty and ill health are causally related, it did not advocate for the redistribution of wealth as a means of improving health[104]. The WHO Health For All emphasis on a broad social and economic approach has not been endorsed strongly by the World Bank, and indeed even the commitment of WHO to this approach has been questioned[76]: a fundamental issue remains the need for debt relief for poor countries. Recent World Development Reports have shifted away from the World Bank's long-term *laissez-faire* doctrine. The Bank now acknowledges that massive inequalities are a barrier to rising prosperity and growth, and recognises the need for stronger government leadership, strong trade unions and greater equality in poor countries, although the messages are not always consistent[105].

The World Bank continues to support the use of specific cost-effective interventions. This approach is reminiscent of 'magic bullet' medicine, which attempted to identify pharmaceutical agents for each disease. The strongest contender for the 'public health magic bullet' is the education of women. While the World Bank deserves credit for stressing the importance of education, the social and cultural barriers that limit the opportunities for girls and young women also need to be addressed.

10.10.2 WHO: struggling to respond to multiple global health challenges

Health problems have never respected national boundaries and most health issues need coordinated international action. There is a desperate need for strong global leadership for health. WHO, for several decades after its founding in 1948, provided this leadership. During its first three decades, WHO focused successfully on providing scientific and technical advice and on setting international standards. It reached its highest standing with the smallpox eradication campaign, successfully completed in 1977 and formally certified in 1979. Partial victory at minimal cost has also been achieved in WHO's campaign to eradicate guinea worm disease[106] and considerable success has been achieved towards the eradication of polio[16], although the target date has been postponed in several countries, notably in India and Nigeria, where eradication will be especially difficult because of the weak health infrastructures and the lack of strong and continued government support.

In the early 1980s, WHO provided a second round of leadership by firmly advocating a broad vision of health under the banner of Health For All by the Year 2000; this advocacy led the Organization into politically sensitive areas. A weakness of efforts to implement the Health For All philosophy was the assumption that equity in health can be achieved by health services and by narrowly defined disease prevention and health promotion activities. Although the Health for All vision and rhetoric were broad initially and encompassed social and economic change, selective primary care rapidly became the prime strategy followed by a rapid retreat from the comprehensive Health for All strategies. Abundant evidence demonstrates that this approach will not achieve equity[27, 80].

Unfortunately, the unattainability of the Health For All goal may have weakened the Organization indirectly. The rhetoric has not been matched by the achievements, in part because of insufficient resources[107]. The status of WHO declined in the early 1990s. Lack of effective leadership, confused vision, poor accountability and an unwieldy bureaucratic structure, all contributed to the Organization's inability to translate policy into action[107]. The power of member states to promote vested interests and to lobby for political appointments has led to fragmented and ineffective programmes and to a poorly defined set of priorities. WHO's country operations have been limited because of the need to work through national health ministries; WHO has had relatively little money to spend at the country level and much of its impact is indirect and takes years to be apparent.

Undoubtedly, many areas of high achievement continue in WHO, especially in the particular programmes supported by extra budgetary funds from the wealthiest member states[108]. These funds provide a way for donors to support programmes. Unfortunately, this has led to competition for both funding and implementation at the country level which, in turn, has undermined the process of developing integrated primary health care systems in many poor countries[109].

In 1998, Gro Harlem Brundtland, a former Prime Minister of Norway, was appointed Director General, with wide support from within the Organization. Under her leadership WHO began a period of major strategic and structural reform. Rapid change during the past 5 years and a focus on a few priorities under central leadership reinvigorated WHO and restored its international credibility[110, 111]. Many new programmes and partnerships were established and the Organization has elevated health successfully on the international development agenda. Several of these initiatives have been remarkably successful, for example, the Tobacco Free Initiative's work on the Framework Convention on Tobacco Control, which was approved by the World Health Assembly (WHA) in May 2003. Other activities have been less successful, for example, Roll Back Malaria (RBM) which has been criticised for poor and confused leadership[112]. The World Health Report of 2002[34] used controversial methods to rank national health systems and stimulated a torrent of criticism of the Organization but did little to assist countries improve the performance of their health systems[113].

The Organization has also been criticised for its willingness to enter into public–private partnerships[114, 115]. The issue of partnerships is critical to WHO. On the one hand, WHO is unable to fulfil its mandate acting alone and with its limited resources; on the other hand, there is a danger in the loss of control which comes from entering into partnership with a wide range of agencies, often with competing agendas. Furthermore, the contributions of private organisations to WHO represent a tiny fraction of the external funds received, yet they consume a disproportionate amount of administrative energy. The many external successes achieved under Dr Brundtland were accompanied by poor internal management, which blunted the morale of the Organization and were difficult to address.

In late 2002, Dr Brundtland unexpectedly announced her retirement after just one term. She was replaced by Dr JW Lee, a South Korean with over 20 years of experience working for WHO in July 2003. Three of his goals are to focus on the Millennium Development Goals (MDGs), to devolve more resources to the regions, and to strengthen county level work. Although the WHO leadership undoubtedly is important in positioning the Organization internationally, it is an intergovernmental agency and must report to its governing body, the World Health Assembly, and is thus subject to pressure from major donor countries. This pressure may be responsible for some of the apparent compromises in positions taken by WHO, for example, with regard to the effect of TRIPS on limiting access to affordable pharmaceuticals[110]. Of course, pressure on WHO from vested interests has a long history; it has been best documented with regard to the tobacco industry[116]. More recently, WHO has come under blatant pressure from elements of the food industry in the USA, which objects to its recommendations for reducing the consumption of sugar[117].

WHO must continue to articulate a realistic and shared vision of public health, which includes a comprehensive primary health care system and an integrated intersectoral approach to health.

10.10.3 Recent global health initiatives: the promise of public–private partnerships

Over the last few years several important global health initiatives have begun to shape the response to major public health challenges; the most important examples are listed in Table 10.2. Many of the new activities have been established as public–private partnerships, for example, The Global Alliance for Vaccines and Immunization (GAVI), and Roll Back Malaria (RBM) initiated by WHO, and most recently, the Global Fund to Fight AIDS, Tuberculosis and Malaria (GFATM)[114]. Considerable new resources have come to these initiatives from philanthropic foundations, notably from the Bill and Melinda Gates Foundation – which had granted almost US$ 3 billion in health funding by the end of 2002.

GAVI was launched as a public–private partnership in 2000 with an initial donation from the Gates Foundation of US$ 750 million for 5 years. After a decade of falling immunisation coverage levels, GAVI aims to raise coverage and introduce new and underused vaccines. GAVI provides eligible countries with new vaccines, safe equipment and financial support to strengthen immunisation services. A review of the early phases of the GAVI work in sub-Saharan African countries found several serious problems ranging from weaknesses in the cold chain necessary for effective immunisation services to lack of planning for long-term financial sustainability if the GAVI funding stops after 5 years as planned currently[118].

RBM refers to a movement against malaria. It was launched in 1998 as one of the major initiatives of Dr Brundtland, Director General of WHO, with the aim

Table 10.2. *Selected recent global health initiatives*

Initiative launch date	Main partners	Main aim	Comments
GAVI, 2000 www.vaccine alliance.org	WHO, UNICEF Gates	Improve access to sustainable immunisation services	Overly ambitious, sustainability questioned
RBM, 1998 www.rbm.who.int/	WHO, UNICEF, WB, UNDP, DFID, USAID	Raise support for malaria control; progress towards MDG targets	Continuing lack of progress
TFI, 1998 www.who.int/tobacco/en/	WHO	Promote global tobacco control	FCTC approved by WHO, May 2003
GFATM www.global fundatm.org	UN, G8, WB, WHO, UNAIDS	Raise funds for three priority diseases	Running out of funds
CMH, 2001 www.who.int/whosis/cmh	WHO	Increased investment in health to reduce poverty	Follow-up continuing at country level

of seeking greater support for malaria control, after many unsuccessful campaigns. The specific aim now is to make progress towards the relevant MDG which is to 'have halted and begun to reverse the spread of HIV/AIDS, the scourge of malaria and other major diseases that afflict humanity' by 2015. An external review of RBM carried out in 2002 noted the many achievements, especially in advocacy for the control of malaria. However, the reviewers were concerned that a lack of progress on malaria control threatens to undermine the credibility of the partnership and may even undercut future global initiatives[112].

✴ The Tobacco Free Initiative (TFI) was one of Dr Brundtland's flagship initiatives and has concentrated on developing the Framework Convention on Tobacco Control, the first public health treaty initiated by WHO. The Convention was approved by the World Health Assembly in May 2003, despite major and continuing objections by the USA which wanted a 'reservation' clause included to enable countries to sign the Convention but with national exceptions permitted[119]; many tobacco control groups felt that the draft presented to the WHA was already too much of a compromise. The next steps in implementing the Convention are for it to be ratified by 40 countries, when it will then come into force in international law. The challenge for WHO and its partners is to build on the Convention and to develop strong protocols on specific issues and then assist countries implement their obligations.

The GFATM was established in 2002 by the UN Secretary General as an independent Fund to raise and disburse funds for the control of three priority diseases with the target of raising US$ 10 billion a year. Over US$ 2 billion have been pledged to the Fund over 5 years but so far less than 1 billion has been delivered to the Fund and several major donors are still short of committing what might be considered a fair share. The Fund has completed two rounds of disbursements, not without controversy[120], but does not have sufficient funds to meet the expected requirements of successful bids from the third round of applications[121, 122]; and despite being a public–private partnership it has received only a token amount from the private sector. By mid-2003, about US$ 600 million had been committed to programmes in about 50 countries, although a much smaller amount actually has been spent[122]. There has been concern from some ministers of finance in recipient countries that the grants from the fund will distort national macroeconomic policies[123], although this concern has been overcome[124]. The USA is committing $15 billion for AIDS in Africa but only a small proportion of this will be for the Fund; most will go to bilateral programmes for 14 countries in Africa and the Caribbean.

The WHO Commission on Macroeconomics and Health refocused the attention of the development community on the importance of health for economic growth and estimated the sums needed to advance the health of the poor[125]. Although the amount suggested – $ 27 billion a year by 2007 – sounds large, it is relatively little compared with the approximately $100 billion spent on the war in Iraq in 2003 or the tax cuts approved in the USA in 2003; currently about $6 billion per year is provided for international aid in health. The Commission estimated the likely economic return of investments in health and, although they seem impressive, the evidence base for these estimates is weak[126]. The Commission suggested that countries should establish their own macroeconomic commissions on health to advance the process and several countries have done so. The major criticism of the Commission is that it is encouraging a vertical approach to disease control with much less emphasis on the need to build health infrastructures; there is also great concern that its call for major new resources for health development is not likely to be met[127].

Perhaps the most important initiative is the establishment by the United Nations member states in 2000 of the Millennium Development Goals (MDGs). The baseline for the goals has been set at 1990 and the goals are to be achieved by 2015. The overall ambition of the MDGs is poverty alleviation and this has great relevance for health improvement. Three of the eight specific goals refer to health – infant mortality, maternal mortality, and HIV/AIDS, malaria and other diseases; in addition, 9 of the 16 targets are health related, as are 18 of the 48 indicators to be used to measure progress (Table 10.3).

Table 10.3. *Millennium Development Goals and targets related to health*

Goals	Health targets	Health indicators
Child mortality	Reduce under-5 mortality by two-thirds	• Under-5 mortality rate (probability of dying between birth and age 5) • Infant mortality rate
Maternal health	Reduce maternal mortality by three-quarters	• Maternal mortality ratio • Percentage of births attended by skilled health personnel
HIV/AIDS, malaria and other diseases	Halt and reverse spread of HIV/AIDS	• HIV prevalence among pregnant women aged 15 to 24 • Condom use rate of the contraceptive prevalence rate • Number of children orphaned by HIV/AIDS
	Halt and reverse incidence of malaria and other diseases	• Prevalence and death rates associated with malaria • Proportion of malaria risk areas using effective malaria prevention and treatment measures • Prevalence and death rates associated with tuberculosis • Proportion of tuberculosis cases detected and cured under directly observed and treated short courses • Proportion of population in malaria risk areas using effective malaria prevention and treatment measures • Percentage of 1-year-old children immunised for measles
Environmental sustainability	Access to safe drinking water	• Percentage of population using solid fuels • Percentage of population with sustainable access to an improved water source, urban, rural
	Improved sanitation	• Percentage of population with access to improved sanitation
Global partnership	Access to drugs	• Percentage of population with access to affordable essential drugs on a sustainable basis
Poverty and hunger	Halve hunger	• Prevalence of underweight children under 5 years
Universal primary education		
Gender equality		

All the other goals are also important for health, for example, the goal on education is critical for health improvement. The MDGs now occupy a central place in global development strategies and, because of the prominence given to health targets, the central place of health in the development agenda has been confirmed. Although the MDGs reaffirm the importance of health to development, there is a risk of narrowing the health agenda and reinforcing the vertical approach to disease control; after all, there is much more to health improvement than the specific problems targeted by the MDGs, especially in middle and higher income countries, and health systems must focus on a broader range of problems than those covered by the MDGs even in the poorest countries.

An interim assessment of progress towards the goals in Africa suggests a discouraging situation; despite some progress, in the absence of dramatic changes in rates of improvement, the MDGs will not be reached for most indicators in most countries[128]. Given the understandable desire to demonstrate progress towards the goals by 2015, there is also a danger that the benefits of this progress may be concentrated in the more privileged sections of the countries concerned, thus further disadvantaging the poorest populations.

Some details on these global health initiatives and summary comments are shown in Table 10.2, together with the relevant websites. Each of these initiatives has much to contribute to health improvement, and each has limitations; it is not easy to make a balanced judgement on the total package, indeed, it might be premature. However, it is obvious that fragmentation and lack of coordination is a real risk because of the large number of new activities. It remains to be seen whether the public private partnerships can add value over previous approaches to global health problems, which were dominated by the public sector through WHO[115].

10.11 Prospects for public health: cautious optimism still justified

There is good reason to be cautiously optimistic about the future prospects for public health. Major improvements have taken place in global standards of health in the last half century. However, there have also been major setbacks. Health conditions have improved more in the past 50 years than in the whole of previous human history. Life expectancy has increased in most countries and most of the improvement in population health status in poor countries has been a result of government leadership and social and public health interventions.

On a less positive note, the twenty-first century started with a confusing global disorder[96]. The 'new world order' since the early 1990s has not, in general been supportive of public health practice. The global economy is integrated increasingly under the banner of 'free trade' and 'market forces'. The crisis over the safety of British beef and the potential threat to public health from the link between bovine spongiform encephalopathy and Creutzfeldt–Jakob disease is a specific example of the unintended adverse effects of neo-liberal economic theory. At least some of the responsibility for the crisis can be traced to the government policy of deregulation, which allowed cattle to be fed meat rendered from sheep infected with scrapie[129, 130]. At a more general level, the reduction in spending by governments on health and other social services has weakened the public health infrastructure seriously. Although overall levels of health are improving, there are still marked variations in health between and within regions, and social class variations in health are increasing in many countries. The situation in sub-Saharan Africa and in Central and Eastern European countries is particularly bleak with HIV/AIDS responsible for much of the fall in life expectancy in Africa[131].

Global challenges to health, apart from market forces, are mounting. The dominance of the ideology of individualism causes serious difficulties for the collective actions, which are the core of effective public health policy and programmes. American exceptionalism, that is withdrawal by the USA from many multilateral arrangements, is a particularly worrying trend[132]. The general response to global environmental change has been minimal so far. Our vulnerability to disease could be exposed readily by subtle environmental changes or by a breakdown in basic public health services. New diseases, such as AIDS and, to a lesser extent, SARS, expose the sharp divisions within society and the lack of attention to the public health infrastructure . The control of 'old' diseases such as tuberculosis is limited by drug resistance, limited funding, inadequate strategies and lack of attention to the underlying social conditions[133]. SARS will have an important adverse effect on economic growth, especially in Asia, at a time when the global economy is depressed and this will have additional longer-term adverse effects on the health of the poor[134].

The global burden of non-communicable diseases inevitably will increase as populations age and the major risk factors become entrenched in all but the poorest populations. Population growth remains excessive in many parts of the world and reinforces poverty. The threat posed by the ongoing spread of nuclear weapons is controlled precariously and the dissemination of small-scale weapons of destruction is out of control[135, 136]. Civil wars continue unabated, aggravated by ethnic and religious rivalries, especially in Africa but also in Central and Eastern Europe and the Middle East. In short, the struggle to improve the health of the public will be never ending as new threats and problems emerge.

In the absence of a strong and cohesive international movement, public health is ill-equipped to face these challenges. Public health education and research are poorly organised and inadequately funded at both national and international levels; undergraduate and non-tertiary public health education are poorly developed. The public health work force is fragmented and often demoralised. Internationally, public health under the influence of the World Bank and the major donor countries is defined primarily as selected technical interventions against a limited range of priority diseases.

Public health competes with other values, such as liberty and material prosperity. Fortunately, health is compatible with other important and inclusive social goals, especially conserving the environment and sustainable development. The realisation that a high degree of wealth is not essential for a healthy population leads to the challenges of ensuring 'health at (relatively) low cost' and a more equitable distribution of the available wealth. A priority for public health practitioners is to keep health as a social goal high on the political agenda, at the same time avoiding prescribing 'healthy lifestyles'. People will then be in a better position to make choices, especially around issues of consumption, fully informed of the health consequences for them as individuals and for society as a whole.

Opportunities exist for the public health movement to exert a more central role in human affairs. The economic pendulum will swing back towards a more collectivist approach as the ill-effects of the free market are recognised, especially by the huge marginalised segments of the world's population. Public health practitioners, however, cannot await a more favourable political environment passively.

In many countries postgraduate education in public health is undergoing a renaissance, and new leadership will emerge from the ranks of these students. A more considered approach to building and supporting this leadership is required. Public health service agencies welcome newly trained graduates increasingly in public health. Participatory public health research is increasing, especially around local environmental issues and among indigenous people. The major new public health research issues concerning the impact of global environmental change are under active investigation by multidisciplinary teams. The need for integration of research methods is recognised widely and linkages are being developed between public health education and research institutions and policy agencies.

A heavy responsibility rests on current public health practitioners. If, at this critical stage in the evolution of public health, we continue on the narrow, individualistic path of least resistance, we will become marginalised as, at best, a poor relation of clinical medicine. If, on the other hand, we choose a broad and inclusive vision of public health and translate this into practice, there is a real prospect for a true 'golden age of public health'. Above all, there is the need for a collective, international responsibility that addresses the requirements of future generations through coordinated multi-sectoral action at local, community, national, regional and international levels. If public health practitioners are successful in framing these debates and in communicating their importance, public support for public health activities will increase and, collectively, we will be able to reduce the threats to the health of all populations.

10.12 Conclusions

For global public health movements to claim a central position in public policy, several actions must be taken. An international debate is required to reach a consensus on the broad scope of public health, its theoretical underpinning and on its ethical and moral basis. Epidemiology and the other public health sciences must reclaim their close linkages with public health policy and practice. Public health professionals must recognise that evidence-based advocacy is a legitimate public health activity, which must be taught and practised by all public health professionals. A strong public health movement will require community participation in setting the public health research agenda. Above all, given the interdependence of global political and socio-economic movements, strong global public health leadership is required.

Chapter 10   Key points

- The global context for public health is daunting.
- Strong international leadership is required because of the global nature of the threats to public health.
- Public health is at the crossroads: the choice is between a narrow focus on individual health issues or a broad focus on the major health determinants and problems.
- If public health practitioners adopt a broad focus and implement appropriate strategies, there are good prospects for a true 'golden age of public health'.

References

1. Winslow, C.E.A. Public health at the crossroads. *Am. J. Pub. Hlth* 1926; **16**: 1075–85.
2. Beaglehole, R., Bonita, R., Horton, R. *et al.* Public health for the new era: collective action for health improvement. *Lancet*, in press.
3. Garrett, L. *The Betrayal of Public Health: The Collapse of Global Public Health*. Oxford: Oxford University Press, 2001.
4. Beaglehole, R. & Davis, P. Setting national health goals and targets in the context of a fiscal crisis: the politics of social choice in New Zealand. *Int. J. Hlth Serv.* 1992; **22**: 417–28.
5. Beaglehole, R. & Magnus, P. The search for new risk factors for coronary heart disease; occupational therapy for epidemiologists? *Int. J. Epidemiol.* 2002; **31**: 1117–21 and 1134–5.
6. Anon. Population health looking upstream. *Lancet* 1994; **343**: 429–30.
7. Lawlor, D., Frankel, S., Shaw, M. *et al.* Smoking and ill health: does lay epidemiology explain the failure of smoking cessation programs among deprived populations? *Am. J. Pub. Hlth* 2003; **93**: 266–70.
8. Nijhuis, H.G.J. & Van Der Maesen, L.J.G. The philosophical foundations of public health: an invitation to debate. *J. Epidemiol. Commun. Hlth* 1994; **48**: 1–3.
9. Seedhouse, D. The way around health economics' dead end. *Hlth Care Anal.* 1995; **3**: 205–20.
10. Hill, H.W. *The New Public Health*. New York: Macmillan, 1916.
11. Ashton, J. & Seymour, H. *The New Public Health*. Milton Keynes: Open University Press, 1988.
12. Lalonde, M. *A New Perspective on the Health of Canadians*. Ottawa: National Health and Welfare, 1974.
13. McGinnis, J.M. Setting objectives for public health in the 1990s: experience and prospects. *Ann. Rev. Pub. Hlth* 1990; **11**: 231–49.
14. World Health Organization. *Alma-Ata. Primary Health Care (Health For All Series No.1)*. Geneva: World Health Organization, 1978.
15. Walsh, J.A. & Warren, K.S. Selective primary health care: an interim strategy for disease control in developing countries. *New Engl. J. Med.* 1979; **301**: 967–74.
16. Aylward, R.B., Acharya, A., England, S. *et al.* Global health goals: lessons from the worldwide effort to eradicate polio. *Lancet* 2003; **362**: 909–14.
17. Rifkin, S.B. & Walt, G. Why health improves: defining the issues concerning 'comprehensive primary health care' and 'selective primary health care'. *Soc. Sci. Med.* 1986; **6**: 559–66.
18. Kickbush, I. The contribution of the World Health Organization to a new public health. *Am. J Pub. Hlth* 2003; **93**: 383–8.
19. Ottawa Charter for Health Promotion. *Hlth Prom.* 1992; **1**: i–v.
20. Baum, F.E. Healthy cities and change: social movement or bureaucratic tool? *Hlth Prom. Int.* 1993; **8**: 31–40.
21. Raeburn, J. & Rootman, I. *People-Centred Health Promotion*. London: John Wiley, 1997.
22. Raeburn, J. & Macfarlane, S. Putting the public into public health: towards a more people-centred approach. In Beaglehole, R. (ed.). *Global Public Health: A New Era*. Oxford: Oxford University Press, 2003.

23. World Commission on Environment and Development. *Our Common Future.* Oxford: Oxford University Press, 1987.
24. World Health Organization Commission on Health and the Environment. *Our Planet, Our Health.* Geneva: WHO, 1992.
25. Boyden, S. & Shirlow, M. Ecological sustainability and the quality of life. In: Brown, V. (ed.). *2020: A Sustainable Healthy Future. Towards an Ecology of Health.* Melbourne: La Trobe University, 1989.
26. Evans, R.G. & Stoddart, G.L. Producing health, consuming health care. *Soc. Sci. Med.* 1990; **31**: 1347–63.
27. Evans, R.G., Barer, M. & Mamor, T.R. (eds.). *Why Are Some People Healthy and Others Not? The Determinants of Health in Populations.* New York: Aldine de Gruyter, 1994.
28. Evans, R.G. & Stoddart, G.L. Consuming research, producing policy? *Am. J. Pub. Hlth* 2003; **93**: 371–9.
29. Kindig, D. & Stoddart, G. What is population health? *Am. J. Pub. Hlth* 2003; **93**: 380–3.
30. Friedman, D. & Starfield, B. Models of population health: their value for US public health practice, policy and research. *Am. J. Pub. Hlth* 2003; **93**: 366–70.
31. Coburn, D., Denny, K., Mykhalovskly, E. *et al.* Population health in Canada: a brief critique. *Am. J. Pub. Hlth* 2002; **93**: 392–6.
32. McKinlay, J.B. Paradigmatic obstacles to improvements in women's health. Paper presented at the Symposium on Women's Health, Puerto Rico, USA. December 1994.
33. Rose, G. *The Strategy of Preventive Medicine.* Oxford: Oxford University Press, 1992.
34. World Health Organization. *World Health Report 2002: Reducing Risks, Promoting Healthy Life.* Geneva: WHO, 2002.
35. Jackson, R. Guidelines on preventing cardiovascular disease in clinical practice. *Br. Med. J.* 2000; **320**: 659–61.
36. Jackson, R., Barham, P., Bills, J. *et al.* The management of raised blood pressure in New Zealand. *Br. Med. J.* 1993; **307**: 107–10.
37. Brownson, R.C., Baker, E.A., Leet, T.L. & Gillespie, K.N. *Evidence-based Public Health.* New York: Oxford University Press, 2003.
38. White, K.L. *Healing the Schism. Epidemiology, Medicine, and the Public's Health.* New York: Springer, 1991.
39. Ashton, J. Institutes of public health and medical schools: grasping defeat from the jaws of victory? *J. Epidemiol. Commun. Hlth* 1992; **46**: 165–8.
40. Jamrozik, K. A glimpse at public health in Eastern Europe. *Aust. J. Pub. Hlth* 1994; **19**: 102–3.
41. McKee, M., White, M., Bojan, F. & Ostbye, T. Development of public health training in Hungary – an exercise in international co-operation. *J. Pub. Hlth Med.* 1995; **17**: 438–44.
42. Kolip, P. & Schott, T. The postgraduate public health training programs in Germany. In: Laaser, U., de Leeuw, E. & Stock, C. (eds.). *Scientific Foundations for a Public Health Policy in Europe.* Weinheim: Juventa, 1996.
43. Association of Schools of Public Health in the European Region (ASPHER). *Quality Improvement and Accreditation of Training Programmes in Public Health.* Lyon: Foundation Merieux-ASPHER, 2001.

44. Association of Schools of Public Health in the European Region (ASPHER) http//www.ensp.fr/aspher.
45. De Leeuw, E. European schools of public health in state of flux. *Lancet* 1995; **345**: 1158–60.
46. Navarro, V. European schools of public health. *Lancet* 1995; **345**: 1511.
47. Association of Schools of Public Health. http://www.asph.org/.
48. Jain, S.C. Education and training – capacity building. *J. Hlth Pop. Dev. Countries* 2000; **3**: 39–42.
49. Bertrand, W.E. *Public Health Schools Without Walls: New Directions for Public Health Resourcing.* New York; The Rockefeller Foundation, Draft, March 1999.
50. Public Health Accreditation project. *The Final Report of the Accreditation Working Party.* Canberra: Commonwealth Department of Human Services and Health, 1995.
51. Rotem, A., Walters, J. & Dewdney, J. The public health workforce education and training study. *Aust. J. Pub. Hlth* 1995; **19**: 437–8.
52. Powles, J. & Comim, F. Public health knowledge and infrastructure. In: Smith, R., Beaglehole, R., Woodward, D. & Drager, N. (eds.). *Global Public Goods for Health.* Oxford: Oxford University Press, 2003.
53. Beaglehole, R. Global cardiovascular disease prevention: time to get serious. *Lancet* 2001; **358**: 661–3.
54. Holland, W.W., Fitzsimons, B. & O'Brien, M. 'Back to the future' – public health research into the next century. *J. Pub. Hlth Med.* 1994; **16**: 4–10.
55. Global Forum for Health Research. *The 10/90 Report on Health Research 2001–2002.* Geneva: Global Forum for Health Research, 2002.
56. Nichol, W., McNeice, K. & Goss, J. (eds.). *Expenditure on Health Research and Development in Australia. Welfare Division Working Paper No. 7.* Canberra: Australian Institute Health & Welfare, 1994.
57. World Development Report. *Investing in Health, World Development Indicators.* New York: Oxford University Press, 1993.
58. World Health Organization Ad Hoc Committee on Health Research Relating to Future Intervention Options. *Investing in Health Research and Development.* Geneva: World Health Organization, 1995.
59. McMichael, A.J. Prisoners of the proximate: loosening the constraints on epidemiology in an age of change. *Am. J. Epidemiol.* 1999; **149**: 887–97.
60. Walt, G. How far does research influence policy? *Eur. J. Pub. Hlth* 1994; **4**: 233–5.
61. Network: The newsletter of the New England Research Institutes. Summer/Fall 1995.
62. Black, N. Why we need qualitative research. *J. Epidemiol. Comm. Hlth* 1994; **48**: 425–6.
63. Baum, F. Researching public health: behind the qualitative–quantitative methodological debate. *Soc. Sci. Med.* 1995; **40**: 459–68.
64. Holland, W.W. The hazards of epidemiology. *Am. J. Pub. Hlth.* 1995; **85**: 616–7.
65. Weed, D.L. Science, ethics guidelines, and advocacy in epidemiology. *Ann. Epidemiol.* 1994; **4**: 166–71.
66. The Public Health Advocacy Institute. http://www.phaionline.org.
67. Anon. SIDS theory: from hype to reality. *Lancet* 1995; **346**: 1503.
68. Wallack, L. Media advocacy: a strategy for empowering people and communities. *J. Pub. Hlth Pol.* 1994; **15**: 420–35.

69. Chapman, S. & Lupton, D. *The Fight For Public Health: Principles and Practice of Media Advocacy.* London: Br. Med. J. Publishing Group, 1994.
70. Chapman, S. A David and Goliath Story: tobacco advertising in Australia. *Br. Med. J.* 1980; **281**: 1187–90.
71. Editorial. The when and how of advocacy. *Lancet* 1997; **349**: 891.
72. Macfarlane, S., Racelis, M. & Muli-Musiime, F. Public health in developing countries. *Lancet* 2000; **356**: 841–6.
73. Davison, C., Frankel, S. & Smith G.D. The limits of lifestyle: re-assessing fatalism in the popular culture of illness prevention. *Soc. Sci. Med.* 1992; **34**: 675–85.
74. Bury, M. Health promotion and lay epidemiology: a sociological view. *Hlth Care Anal.* 1994; **2**: 23–30.
75. United Nations Development Programme. *Human Development Report 2002. Deepening Democracy in a Fragmented World.* New York: UNDP, 2002.
76. Horton, R. The case for a Global Development Organisation. *Lancet* 2002; **360**: 582–3.
77. Putnam, R.D., Leonardi, R. & Nanetti, R.Y. *Making Democracy Work.* Princeton: Princeton University Press, 1993.
78. Caldwell, J.C. Routes to low mortality in poor countries. *Pop. Dev. Rev.* 1986; **12**: 171–220.
79. Labonte, R. A holosphere of healthy and sustainable communities. *Aust. J. Pub. Hlth* 1993; **17**: 4–12.
80. Susser, M. Health as a human right: an epidemiologist's perspective on the public health. *Am. J. Pub. Hlth* 1993; **83**: 418–26.
81. Leary, V. The right to health in international human rights law. *Hum. Rights* 1994; **1**: 24–57.
82. Mann, J.M. Human rights and the new public health. *Hlth Hum. Rights* 1995; **1**: 229–33.
83. Hunt, P. The right to health: from the margins to the mainstream. *Lancet* 2002; **360**: 1878.
84. Gruskin, S. & Loffe, B. Public health and human rights. *Lancet* 2002; **360**: 1880.
85. Cook, R.J. *Women's Health and Human Rights. The Promotion and Protection of Women's Health through International Human Rights Law.* Geneva: World Health Organization, 1994.
86. Wikler, D. & Cash, R. Ethical issues in global public health. In Beaglehole, R. (ed.). *Global Public Health: A New Era.* Oxford: Oxford University Press, 2003.
87. Kass, N.E. An ethics framework for public health. *Am. J. Pub. Hlth* 2001; **91**: 1776–82.
88. Cole, P. The moral bases for public health interventions. *Epidemiology* 1994; **6**: 78–83.
89. Gostin, L.O. Public health law reform. *Am. J. Pub. Hlth* 2001; **91** 1365–8.
90. Mann, J., Gostin, L., Gruskin, S., Brennan, T., Lazzarini, Z. & Fineberg, H.V. Health and human rights. *Hlth Hum. Rights* 1994; **1**: 6–23.
91. Silove, D. Overcoming obstacles in confronting torture. *Lancet* 2003; **361**: 1555.
92. Krug, E.G., Mercy, J.A., Dahlberg, L.L. *et al.* The world report on violence. *Lancet* 2002, **360**: 1083–8.
93. World Health Organization. *World Violence Report.* Geneva: WHO, 2002.

94. Gostin, L. & Mann, J. Towards the development of a human rights impact assessment for the formulation and evaluation of health policies. *Hlth Hum. Rights* 1994; **1**: 58–81.

95. Stiglitz, J. *Globalization and its Discontents.* London: Allen Lane, 2002.

96. Hobsbawm, E. *Age of Extremes: The Short Twentieth Century, 1914–1991.* London: Michael Joseph, 1994.

97. Singer, P. *One World: The Ethics of Globalization.* New Haven: Yale University Press, 2002.

98. UNICEF. *The State of the World's Children.* New York: Oxford University Press, 1995.

99. Center for Global Development. *Ranking the Rich: The First Annual Center for Global Development and Foreign Policy Commitment to Development Index.* www.cgdev.org/rankingtherich.

100. Report of the Commission on Intellectual Property Rights. *Integrating Intellectual Property Rights and Development Policy.* London: Commission on Intellectual Property Rights, 2002.

101. Editorial. Patently robbing the poor to serve the rich. *Lancet* 2002; **360**: 885.

102. Editorial. The World Bank, listening and learning. *Lancet* 1996; **347**: 411.

103. Lee, K., Collinson, S., Walt, G. & Gilson L. Who should be doing what in international health: a confusion of mandates in the United Nations? *Br. Med. J.* 1996; **312**: 302–7.

104. O'Keefe, E. The World Bank: health policy, poverty and equity. *Crit. Pub. Hlth* 1995; **6**: 28–35.

105. Elliott, L. World Bank to ease *laissez-faire* policy. *The Guardian Weekly*, April 9, 1992:12.

106. Caincross, S. Victory over guineaworm disease: partial or pyrrhic? *Lancet* 1995; **346**: 1440.

107. Peabody, J.W. An organisational analysis of the World Health Organization: narrowing the gap between promise and performance. *Soc. Sci. Med.* 1995; **40**: 731–42.

108. Vaughan, J.P., Mogedal, S., Kruse, S.E., Lee, K., Walt, G. & de Wilde, K. *Co-operation For Health Development. Extra-budgetary Funds in the World Health Organization.* Australian Agency for International Development, Royal Ministy of Foreign Affairs, Norway, ODA, United Kingdom, 1995.

109. Godlee, F. WHO's special programmes: undermining from above. *Br. Med. J.* 1995; **310**: 178–82.

110. Horton, R. *Second Opinion; Doctors, Diseases and Decisions in Modern Medicine.* London: Granta Books, 2003.

111. Horton, R. WHO: the casualties and compromises of renewal. *Lancet* 2002; **359**: 1605–11.

112. Daniels, D., Dunlop, D., Feachem, C. *et al.* Achieving impact: roll back malaria in the next phase. Final report of the external evaluation of roll back malaria. 29 August 2002. http://mosquito.who.int.

113. Musgrove, P. Judging health systems: reflection on WHO's methods. *Lancet* 2003; **361**: 1817–20.

114. Walt, G. & Buse, K. Partnerships and fragmentation in international health: threat or opportunity? *Trop. Med. Int. Hlth* 2000; **5**: 467–71.

115. Buse, K. & Walt, G. Global public–private partnerships. Part II. What are the issues for global governance? *Bull. WHO* 2000; **78**: 699–709.
116. Zeltner, T., Kessler, D.A., Martiny, A. & Randera A. *Tobacco Industry Strategies to Undermine Tobacco Control Activities at the WHO. Report of a Committee of Experts on Tobacco Industry Documents*. Geneva: WHO, 2000.
117. Ashraf, H. WHO's diet report prompts food industry backlash. *Lancet* 2003; **361**: 1442.
118. Brugha, R., Starling, M. & Walt, G. GAVI, the first steps: lessons for the Global Fund. *Lancet* 2002; **359**: 935–8.
119. Editorial. Agents of mass destruction found in USA. *Lancet* 2003; **361**: 1575.
120. Siringi, S. Tanzania loses Global Fund money because of internal wrangling. *Lancet* 2002; **360**: 1848.
121. Kapp, C. Global Fund faces uncertain future as cash runs low. *Lancet* 2002; **360**: 1225.
122. Feachem, R. Opening Speech. The Global Fund's 5th Board Meeting, 5 June 2003 http://www. Globalfund.org/fifthboardmeeting/openingspeechferachem.html.
123. Wendo, C. Uganda stands firm on health spending freeze. *Lancet* 2002; **360**: 1847–8.
124. Wendo, C. Uganda agrees to increase health spending using Global Fund's grant. *Lancet* 2003; **361**: 319.
125. World Health Organization. *Macroeconomics and Health: Investing in Health for Economic Development. Report of the Commission on Macroeconomics and Health*. Geneva: World Health Organization, 2001.
126. Morrow, R.H. Macroeconomics and health. *Br. Med. J.* 2002; **325**: 53–4.
127. Waitzkin, H. Report of the WHO Commission on Macroeconomics and Health: a summary and critique. *Lancet* 2003; **361**: 523–6.
128. Sahn, D.E. & Stifel, D.C. Progress toward the Millennium Development Goals in Africa. *Wld Developm.* 2003; **31**: 23–52.
129. Gray, J. Nature bites back at human hubris. *Guardian Weekly*, April 7, 1996.
130. Smith, P.G. The epidemics of bovine spongiform encephalopathy and variant Creutzfeldt–Jakob disease: current status and future prospects. *Bull. WHO* 2003; **81**: 123–30.
131. Beaglehole, R. (ed). *Global Public Health: A New Era*. Oxford: Oxford University Press, 2003.
132. McKee, M. & Cocker, R. The dangerous rise of American exceptionalism. *Lancet* 2003; **361**: 1579–80.
133. Lerner, B.H. New York City's tuberculosis control efforts: the historical limitations of the 'War on Consumption'. *Am. J. Pub. Hlth* 1993; **83**: 758–66.
134. Editorial. Will SARS hurt the world's poor? *Lancet* 2003; **361**: 1485.
135. Lown, B. Time to leave behind genocidal weapons. *Br. Med. J.* 1995; **310**: 993–4.
136. Coupland, R.M. The effect of weapons on health. *Lancet* 1996; **347**: 450–1.

Index